Atlas of
Medical
Mycology

Atlas of
Medical
Mycology

Reena Ray Ghosh MBBS, MD (Microbiology)
Associate Professor and In-charge of Mycology
Department of Microbiology
RG Kar Medical College and Hospital
Kolkata, West Bengal

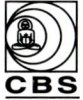

CBS

CBS Publishers & Distributors Pvt Ltd

New Delhi • Bengaluru • Chennai • Kochi • Kolkata • Mumbai
Bhopal • Bhubaneswar • Hyderabad • Jharkhand • Nagpur
• Patna • Pune • Uttarakhand • Dhaka (Bangladesh)

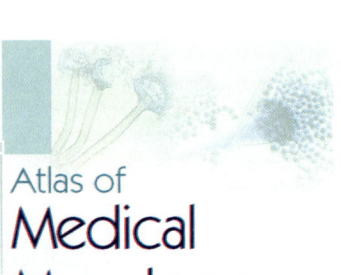

Atlas of
Medical
Mycology

ISBN: 978-93-87964-27-3

Copyright © Author and Publisher

First Edition: 2019

Published by Satish Kumar Jain and produced by Varun Jain for

CBS Publishers & Distributors Pvt Ltd
4819/XI Prahlad Street, 24 Ansari Road, Daryaganj, New Delhi 110 002, India.
Ph: 23289259, 23266861, 23266867   Fax: 011-23243014   Website: www.cbspd.com
e-mail: delhi@cbspd.com; cbspubs@airtelmail.in.
Corporate Office: 204 FIE, Industrial Area, Patparganj, Delhi 110 092
Ph: 4934 4934   Fax: 4934 4935   e-mail: publishing@cbspd.com; publicity@cbspd.com

Branches

- **Bengaluru:** Seema House 2975, 17th Cross, K.R. Road,
  Banasankari 2nd Stage, Bengaluru 560 070, Karnataka, India
  Ph: +91-80-26771678/79   Fax: +91-80-26771680   e-mail: bangalore@cbspd.com
- **Chennai:** 7, Subbaraya Street, Shenoy Nagar, Chennai 600 030, Tamil Nadu, India
  Ph: +91-44-26260666, 26208620   Fax: +91-44-42032115   e-mail: chennai@cbspd.com
- **Kochi:** 42/1325, 1326, Power House Road, Opp KSEB Power House, Ernakulam 682 018, Kochi, Kerala
  Ph: +91-484-4059061-65   Fax: +91-484-4059065   e-mail: kochi@cbspd.com
- **Kolkata:** No. 6/B, Ground Floor, Rameswar Shaw Road, Kolkata-700014 (West Bengal), India
  Ph: +91-33-2289-1126, 2289-1127, 2289-1128   e-mail: kolkata@cbspd.com
- **Mumbai:** 83-C, Dr E Moses Road, Worli, Mumbai-400018, Maharashtra, India
  Ph: +91-22-24902340/41   Fax: +91-22-24902342   e-mail: mumbai@cbspd.com

Representatives

• Bhopal	0-8319310552	• Bhubaneswar	0-9911037372	• Hyderabad	0-9885175004
• Jharkhand	0-9811541605	• Nagpur	0-9021734563	• Patna	0-9334159340
• Pune	0-9623451994	• Uttarakhand	0-9716462459		
• Dhaka (Bangladesh)	01912-003485				

Printed at: HT Media Ltd., Greater Noida, UP, India

Foreword

It is a great pleasure in writing the Foreword to this book *Atlas of Medical Mycology*. The importance of mycology has assumed a great significance throughout the world. Moreover, as there are geographic variations, this atlas will be of tremendous help in this country. Dr Reena Ray Ghosh has been successful in making the subject lucid and interesting to the students, especially for the postgraduate students.

I have seen Dr Reena's uncompromising honesty and sincerity towards her work, something which is very rare in today's scientific field. She was a precious asset to me and my department during my tenure as Head, Department of Microbiology. I am really proud of her.

Her first attempt at documenting the findings of her laboratory in the form of a book has been deeply rewarding. I hope she continues to receive support and modern infrastructure facilities to further her work and to establish molecular studies.

Lastly I hope her book *Atlas of Medical Mycology* becomes the publisher's pride.

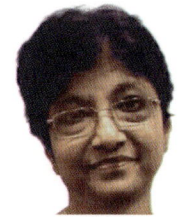

Sujata Bhattacharya

Prof Sujata Bhattacharya
Ex-Head, Department of Microbiology
RG Kar Medical College and Hospital
Kolkata

Foreword

This is a great pleasure to write the Foreword to the book *Atlas of Medical Mycology* by Dr Reena Ray Ghosh dealing with medically important fungi. The mycotic infections are increasing in incidence throughout the world as a result of modern medical practice and increase in the population of those at risk due to use of immunosuppressive therapies, broadspectrum antibiotics and central venous access devices. Technology has led to the improved survival of person with malignancies, transplanted organs, HIV infection, following trauma and at the extreme of ages.

In the modern era there are a number of novel diagnostic techniques for accurate identification of different mycotic pathogens. Despite these advances the approach to the diagnosis of fungal infections still relies on the traditional methods on the subjective microscopic and macroscopic examination of morphological and cultural characteristics as well as histopathological examination. As such, these evaluations rely on the expertise of a trained mycologist.

The author, Dr Reena Ray Ghosh, Associate Professor, Department of Microbiology, RG Kar Medical College and Hospital, Kolkata, is an experienced and enthusiastic medical teacher dealing with different types of mycotic infection particularly the diagnosis for more than a decade. This atlas will ideally be suited for medical and non-medical students, both for the undergraduate and postgraduate courses and also for the clinical microbiologist for diagnosis.

The unique feature of this book is that it has many photographs and photo micrographs of all the common fungi of the clinical specimens commonly available in a tertiary care hospital. This will help the reader to understand and memorise the fungi commonly found in medical practice. At the end of the chapters there are key points with multiple choice questions for self-instruction learning. These are also helpful to the students for understanding the subject.

I am sure this book will win the heart of both undergraduate and postgraduate students as well as practising microbiologists.

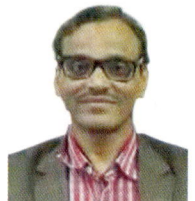

Prof PK Kundu
Principal
Malda Medical College
Malda, West Bengal

Foreword

I am thrilled to finally see the book *Atlas of Medical Mycology* and it makes me immensely proud as it has been written by an expert colleague of mine, Dr Reena Ray Ghosh, Associate Professor, Department of Microbiology, RG Kar Medical College, Kolkata.

The author has got teaching experiences for more than twenty years and she bears her testimony and experiences in this book. The book contains six chapters, each having great importances and merits of its own. Although many books are available in the market but *Atlas of Medical Mycology* is an unique book on this subject and hence, in this perspective, it is a great challenge of its own.

Illustration on various diseases with colour photographs and the brief history will be extremely helpful for diagnosis of different types of cases.

I am sure that this book will be an essential guide not only for the undergraduate and postgraduate students, but also become the quandaries of research workers in this field.

The author has shown her foresightedness and I sincerely appreciate her noble efforts to write such a complete, informative, updated, illustrative and practicable book on mycology.

"Some books are to be tasted, others to be swallowed, and some few to be chewed and digested."

—Bacon

I think the book will be in the category of "Few to be chewed and digested".

I wish that this book will conquer the hearts of the students, research workers and will take an important and eminent space in the field of microbiology.

Prof Suddhodhan Batabyal
Principal
RG Kar Medical College
Kolkata

Foreword

It is my honour to write the Foreword to the book *Atlas of Medical Mycology*. Recently the importance of mycology has gained a significant position throughout the world. This atlas by Dr Reena Ray Ghosh provides a comprised yet broad idea to various medicinally important fungi. She with her hard work has been successful in making the subject interesting to the students especially for the postgraduate students.

I am really proud of Dr Reena for taking the initiative in writing a book on mycology. She is undoubtedly the most hardworking person I have ever seen. I admire her knowledge in mycology. I have seen her honesty and utmost sincerity towards her work and I must say she is an asset to my department.

With this book she has taken a step to show how each subject can be interesting if it is produced in an interesting manner. I salute her for taking such a great step. I hope she continues to receive support to produce such great works in future.

I wish her all the success and hope her book *Atlas of Medical Mycology* becomes the publisher's pride.

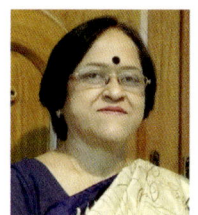

Mitali Chatterjee

Prof Mitali Chatterjee
Head, Department of Microbiology
RG Kar Medical College and Hospital
Kolkata

Preface

There are many encyclopedic books available in many subspecialties of medical microbiology, including mycology. These large texts serve as invaluable pillars for setting a foundation for trainees, as well as being comprehensive guides for practitioners and teachers. But ever so often, descriptions by language, no matter how vivid, expressive or lucid, remain words on paper. Many such times describe in great detail but do not include any visual corroboration. I have noticed that this leads to an indelible deficiency on the part of trainees trying to understand the subject as well as tutors trying to teach. With *Atlas of Medical Mycology*, I have tried to fill this knowledge gap. As Louis Pasteur once put it:

"Dans les champs de l' observation le hasard ne favoriseque les espritspréparés."

In the fields of observation chance favours only the prepared mind.

With pertinent and comprehensible laboratory and clinical photographs, I hope the atlas fulfils this intention. Since complete absence of explanatory text, would again lead to lack of clarity on the approach and appreciation of each image, I was compelled to add small descriptions that serve as "bridge-text" joining information read from extensive manuscripts and this atlas.

I hope postgraduate trainees, teachers and practitioners find this book useful. Any suggestions for further improvement and refinement from the students are welcome.

Reena Ray Ghosh

Acknowledgements

It gives me immense pleasure to personally express my gratitude to every individual and organization that helped me in preparing this atlas.

Nothing can be achieved in this world without the blessings of 'God'. I express my sincere and deepest gratitude to Prof Sujata Bhattacharya, *Ex*-Professor and Head, Department of Microbiology, RG Kar Medical College, for inspiring me to undertake such a project and her constant encouragement, valuable opinion and mental support during my hard days of preparing this atlas.

I convey my regards to our Principal, Prof S Batayabal, for giving me permission to carry out this work without affecting the schedule work in the department. I am really thankful to all my teachers from whom I had gathered knowledge and felt the essence of mycology during my postgraduate days.

I am heartily thankful to all faculties in the Department of Dermatology for their kind cooperation and my special regards to Prof Arghya Prasun Ghosh, Professor and Head, Department of Dermatology, at Bankura Sammilani Medical College and Hospital, for his constant support and confidence on my laboratory work during his days at RG Kar Medical College and Hospital.

I also express my gratitude towards all my senior colleagues, Prof Mitali Chatterjee, Prof Manas Kumar Bandopadhya, Prof. Prabir Kumar Mukherjee, Dr Maitreyi Bandopadhya, and Dr Simit Kumar, who helped me in better understanding of various facets in mycology. They always supported me in all my academic, clinical and research endeavours. My special thanks to my junior colleagues, Dr Sanjeev Das, Dr Purnima Mondal, Dr Smita Samanta, Dr Chakradhar Mandi, Dr Abhishek Sengupta and Dr Abhra Banerjee for their constant encouragement and valuable suggestions.

I wish to express my sincere thanks to all my postgraduate students for their helpful cooperation, encouragement and motivation to complete this work. It would have not been possible to gather so many common and uncommon clinical isolates without their sincere work and perseverance.

Last but not the least, I extend my gratitude to Mr Rabindra Nath Mondal, Vice President, and Mr Somenath Batabyal, Senior Marketing Executive and Author Co-ordinator, at CBS Publishers and Distributors for helping forge my vision into reality.

I shall be failing my duties if I do not acknowledge my family members, my husband Prof Tamal Kanti Ghosh, Special Secretary, Government of West Bengal, Department of Health and Family Welfare and my two sons Tamaghna and Rivu.

Words cannot express the feeling I have for my parents in moulding my career at every step, to my husband Prof Tamal Kanti Ghosh, to whom I am really indebted for his valuable suggestions, moral boost up and supervisions in my efforts.

All books, old and new, remain unfinished manuscripts. Regardless of the number of revisions and reprints made, there always remains room for improvement and I request my readership and students to help me strive to further polish, refine and revise this book. Valuable suggestions are welcome at: ghoshreena@hotmail.com

Reena Ray Ghosh

Contents

Superficial Infections

SUPERFICIAL MYCOSIS

The superficial infections include diseases in which cellular response of the host is generally lacking because the organisms are so remote from living tissues, or infection is so innocuous. There is essentially no pathology elicited by their presence and patients may be unaware of their condition.

PITYRIASIS VERSICOLOR

Pityriasis versicolor is a chronic, mild, usually asymptomatic infection of the stratum corneum. The lesions are characterized by a branny or furfuraceous consistency; they are discrete or concrescent and appear as discoloured and depigmented areas (Figs 1.1–1.3) of the skin. A common observation in reviewing a series of cases of pityriasis versicolor is that both hypopigmented and hyperpigmented lesions (Figs 1.4 and 1.5) occur, sometimes on the same patient.

The affected areas are principally on the chest, and to a lesser extent from the back, trunk, limbs, abdomen and occasionally the face and other areas. The etiologic agents are the lipophilic yeasts belonging to the genus *Malassezia*. Several species have been identified till date. They are namely

- *Malassezia furfur*
- *Malassezia ovalis*
- *Malassezia orbiculare*
- *Malassezia pachydermatis*

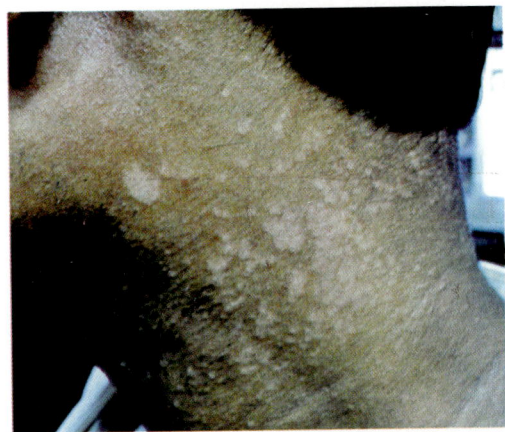

Fig. 1.1: Pityriasis versicolor. Multiple scaling lesions with a fawn discolouration—the most common type of the disease.

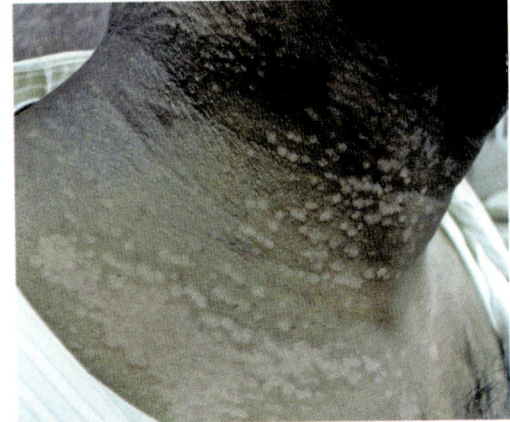

Fig. 1.2: Pityriasis versicolor. Fawn to light brown macules with scaling as a continuous sheath involving the upper part of chest and neck.

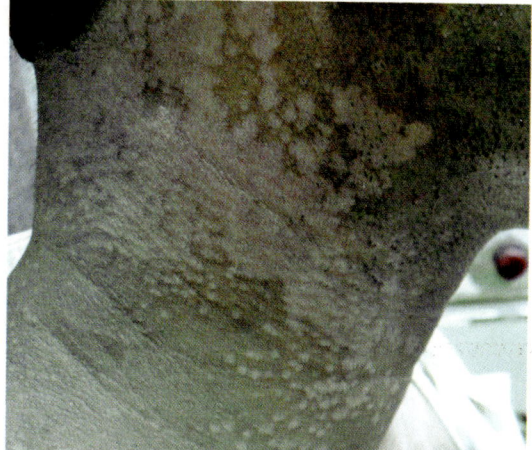

Fig. 1.3: Extensive macular lesions like a continuous sheath is present over the neck region in pityriasis versicolor.

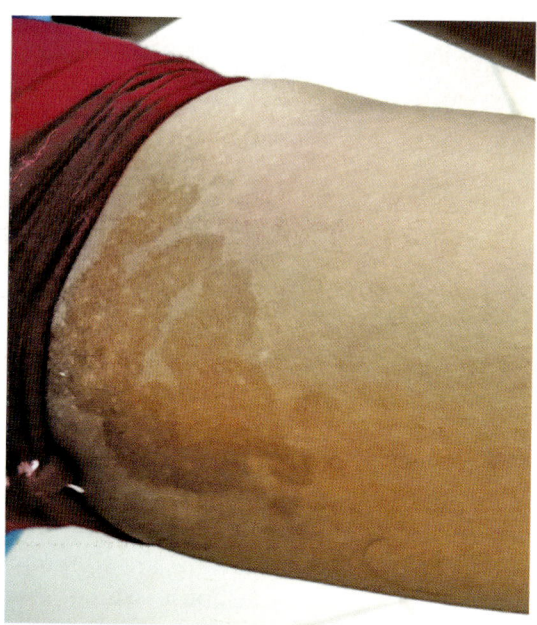

Fig. 1.5: Hyperpigmented macular lesions on the abdomen. Pityriasis versicolor.

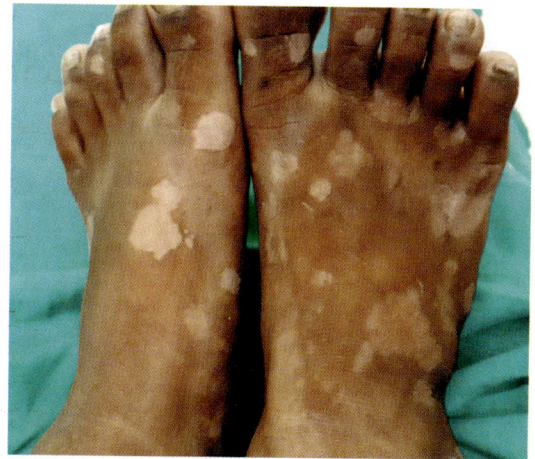

Fig.1.4: Pityriasis versicolor. Unusual site of lesions. Fawn coloured, sharply delineated macules are seen on the dorsum of the feet.

Malassezia furfur **and** *Malassezia ovalis* are part of the normal flora of the skin.

Laboratory Identification

Direct Examination

Direct examination of the skin scrapings is necessary for diagnosis. Scales may be scraped with a scalpel and heated gently on a glass slide in a drop of KOH with or without methylene blue stain. KOH preparation shows pathognomonic cluster of round, budding yeast cells (up to 8 μ) and the short, septate, occasionally branched hyphal fragments 2.5 to 4 mm in diameter (Fig. 1.6). Hyphae may be difficult to find if they are scanty and unstained or if the patient has been using a topical antifungal agent. Hyphae may be abundant in untreated infection (Fig. 1.7). Under rare circumstances either yeast form or hyphal form will predominate. The oval and cylindrical forms can be observed by defatting epidermal scales of the scalp with xylol and staining with methylene blue (Figs 1.8 and 1.9) or with special fungal stains. The oval and cylindrical cells can be seen in clusters and measure 1.5 to 2.5 × 3 to 3.5 mm in diameter.

Isolation of Malassezia Species in Culture

Culturing *Malassezia* is more complicated than the procedures for other yeasts or yeast like fungi, however, **culture is not essential for diagnosis.**

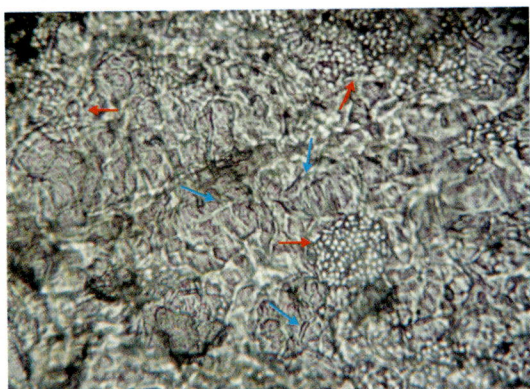

Fig. 1.6: Pityriasis versicolor. Skin scales in KOH preparation shows round budding yeast cells (red arrow) and short septate occasionally branched hyphal fragments (blue arrow) [×400].

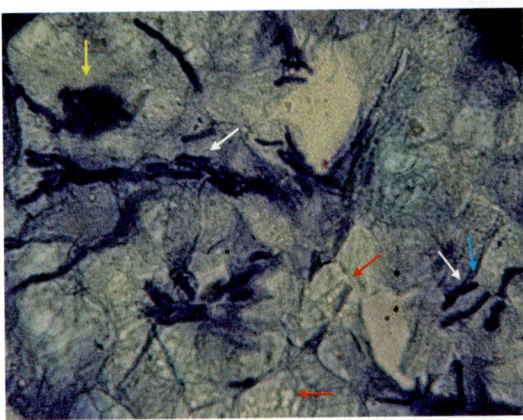

Fig. 1.8: Pityriasis versicolor. Skin scales stained with KOH and methylene blue shows short branched and also unbranched mycelium (white arrow); grouped small yeast cells (yellow arrow); a few unstained yeast (yet to take the stain) cells are seen. (red arrow) [×400].

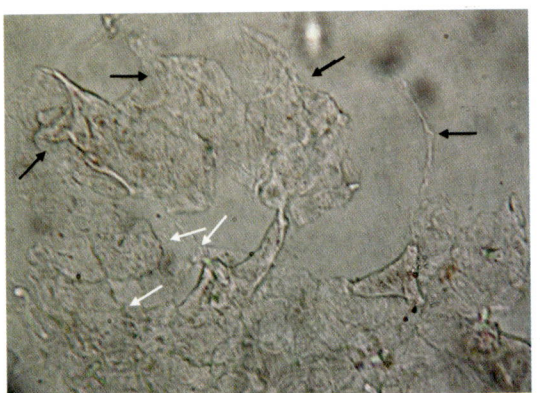

Fig. 1.7: Pityriasis versicolor. KOH preparation of skin scales shows predominance of hyphal forms (black arrow); however, yeast form, budding yeast cells, are also noticed at places in the smear (white arrow) [×400].

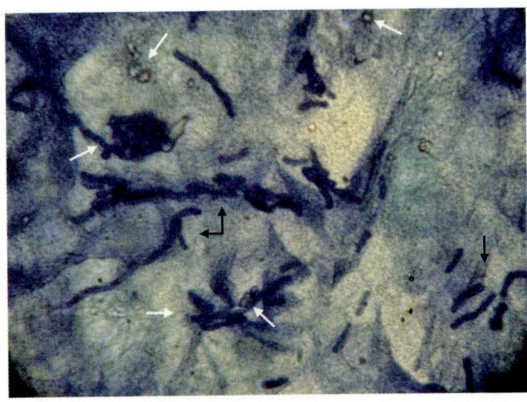

Fig. 1.9: Budding yeast cells and also grouped small yeast cells (white arrow) along with short branched mycelium (black arrow) are diagnostic of this disease. [KOH with methylene blue mount of skin scales ×400].

Malassezia can be isolated from skin scrapings or swabs by inoculating the specimens on Sabouraud's dextrose agar containing chloramphenicol and cyclohexamide (pH 5.5). The surface of the agar after inoculating the specimen should be covered with a thin layer of olive oil and incubated at 37°C for 1 to 2 weeks. **M. pachydermatis** grows readily on Sabouraud's agar without an oil overlay but addition of Tween 80 into media may enhance growth. Modified Dixon agar is used as selective media for isolation of *Malassezia* species (Figs 1.10 and 1.11).

Colony Morphology

Colonies produced on Sabouraud's dextrose agar with olive oil overlay are white to creamy in colour and dry in texture (Fig. 1.12). The

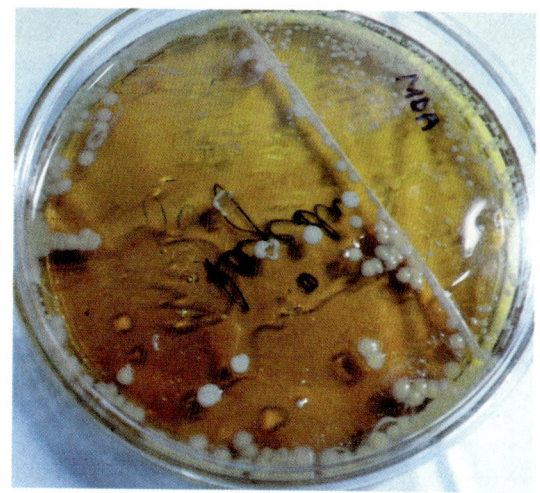

Fig. 1.10: Colony morphology of *Malassezia furfur* grown on modified Dixon agar (MDA) at 37°C for 10 days.

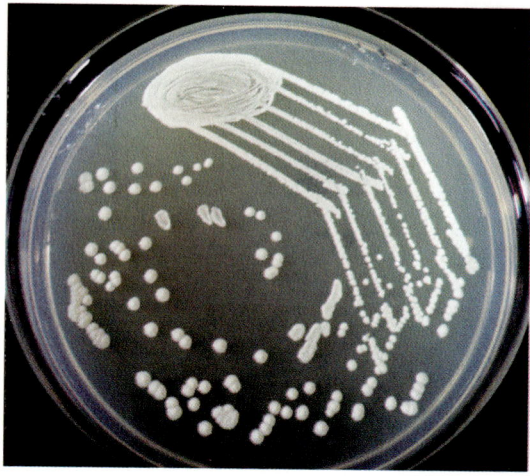

Fig. 1.12: *Malassezia pachydermatis* grown on Sabouraud's dextrose agar with chloramphenicol (SDCA) without an oil overlay. Colonies are white to creamy, dry in texture.

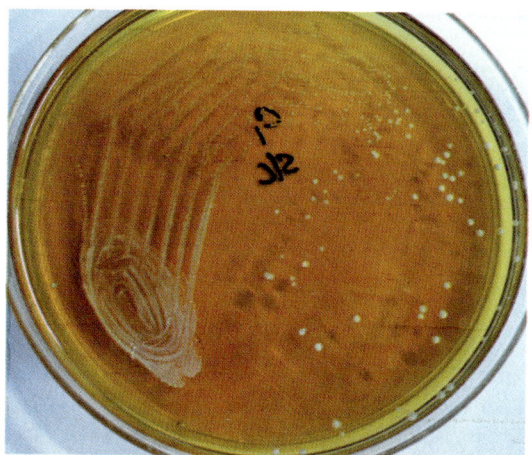

Fig. 1.11: Colonies of *Malassezia* species grown on modified Dixon agar (MDA) with olive oil overlay. White to cream colour pasty, yeast like colonies appeared after 5 days of incubation at 30°C (subculture).

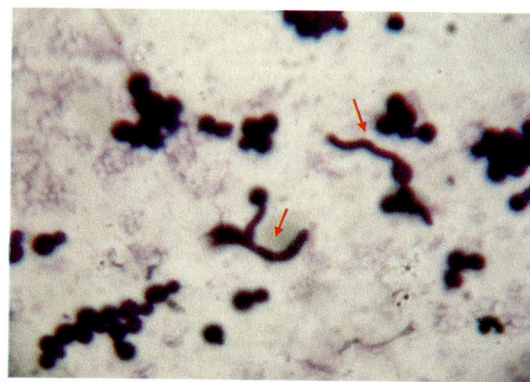

Fig. 1.13: Yeast cells (2 to 8 µ) of *Malassezia furfur* grown on modified Dixon agar at 37°C for 10 days. Rare elongation of yeast cells to form hyphal elements (2 to 3 µ) are also noticed (red arrow) [Gram stained smear ×1000].

colonies consist of yeast cells with a rare elongation to form hyphal elements. The size of the cells varies from 3 to 3.5 mm in diameter in some strains while others may measure 4 to 7 mm (Figs 1.13–1.15). The cells reproduce by unipolar budding and the manner of budding is phialidic, several buds are produced in sequence from the same site on the mother cells. In culture at 37°C yeast cells appear globose at first and are seen to be reduced phialides (Fig. 1.15). **Multiple budding does not occur,** but the cells are often found in clusters because of incomplete detachment.

Some strains are regularly more hyphal in nature, and there is speculation that these strains may be more likely to produce pityriasis versicolor in susceptible patients.

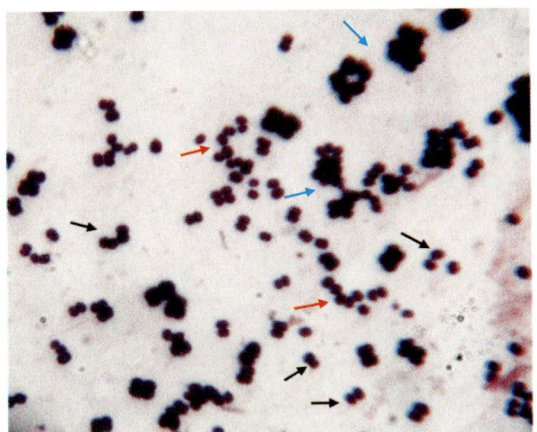

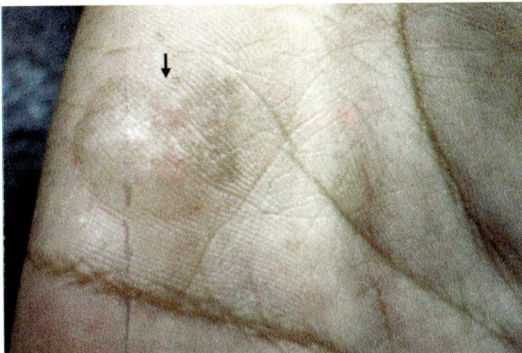

Fig. 1.16: Tinea nigra. Dark, flat lesion with sharp border on the palm.

Fig. 1.14: *Malassezia ovalis*. Gram stained smear prepared from colonies grown on modified Dixon agar at 37°C for 10 days. Yeast cells are 2 to 5 μ in size oval to cylindrical (black arrow) having unipolar budding (phialidic manner) and several buds are produced in sequence from the same site on the mother cells (red arrow). Clusters of cells (blue arrow) are due to incomplete detachment. [×1000].

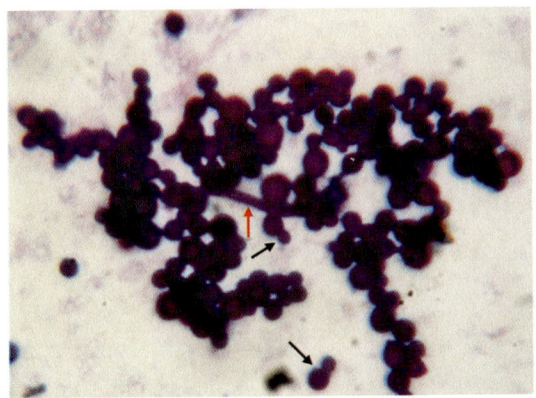

Fig. 1.15: *Malassezia furfur*. Gram stained smear prepared from colony grown on modified Dixon agar at 37°C. Yeast cells are globose to oval with phialidic budding (black arrow). Hyphal forms are occasionally seen (red arrow) [×1000].

TINEA NIGRA

Tinea nigra is a superficial asymptomatic fungus infection of the stratum corneum characterized by brown to black nonscaly macules. The palmar surfaces are most often affected (Fig. 1.16), but lesions may occur on the plantar and other surfaces of the skin. The etiologic agent is *Exophiala werneckii*.

The lesions of tinea nigra are painless macules that are neither elevated nor scaly. They are sharply marginated and usually single. The colour is usually mottled, with deeper pigmentation seen at the advancing periphery.

The most common site of infection is the palmar surface although infection of other areas has been reported including plantar surface, neck and thorax.

Laboratory Identification

Direct Examination

Epidermal scrapings are placed on a microscope slide with a drop of 10% KOH and cleared by heating gently for a minute.

Examination with low power lens reveals brownish to olivaceous, multiple branched septate hyphae and budding cells. Hyphal elements are up to 5 mm in diameter. Terminal portions of the hyphae are usually hyaline (Fig. 1.17). Older sections are twisted and tortuous with numerous septations and thickening of the cell walls that become deeply pigmented. Chlamydoconidia, swollen cells, yeast cells and fragmented hyphae are also seen (Fig. 1.18).

Mycelia of *exophiala werneckii* differs from dermatophyte hyphae in following aspects

- Colour of the hyphae (hyaline/colourless in dermatophyte)

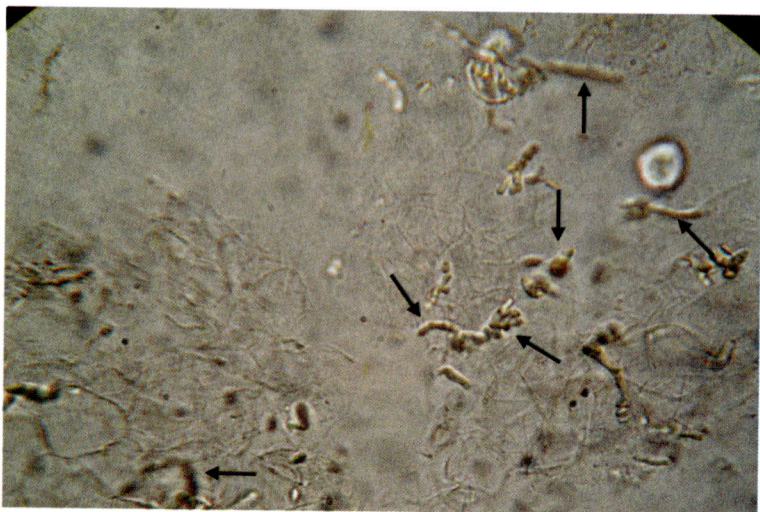

Fig. 1.17: *Exophiala werneckii* in tissue. Hyphae and fragmented cells are seen in a KOH mount of scrapings from a palm lesion (×400).

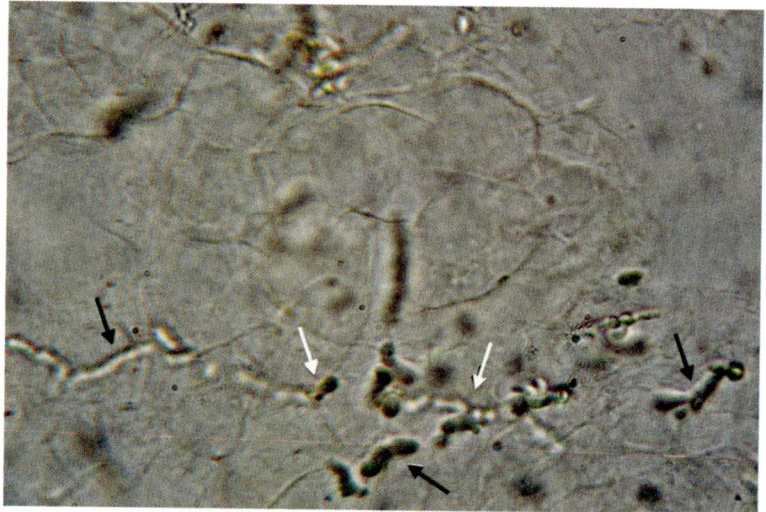

Fig. 1.18: *Exophiala werneckii* in tissue. Hyphae and fragmented cells (black arrow), elongated budding cells (white arrow) are seen in KOH mount of scrapings from a palm lesion (×600).

- Branching (less in dermatophytes)
- Contour of terminal branches (tapering not found in dermatophytes)

Colony of *Exophiala werneckii* grows slowly in Sabouraud's dextrose agar attaining a colony diameter of 0.9 to 1.5 mm in 1 week at 25°C. The colony appears yeast-like at first, and the colour is dirty white to gray or olivish, but quickly changes to greenish black to black. Sometimes the black yeast-like colonies produce a metallic sheen (Fig. 1.19). Soon the colonies are covered with floccose dark grey to greenish gray aerial hyphae. Hyphae (3–10 mm) are brown at first, but become darker and thick walled with age (Fig. 1.20). Reverse is dark brownish black (Fig. 1.21).

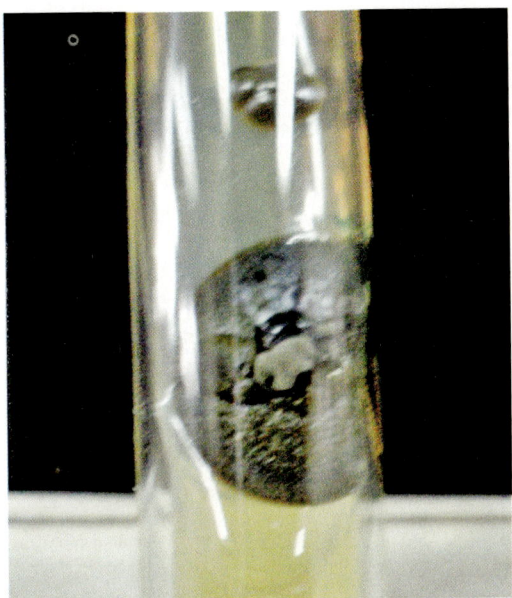

Fig. 1.19: Four weeks old culture of *Exophiala werneckii* grown on Saboraud's dextrose agar with chloramphenicol (obverse).

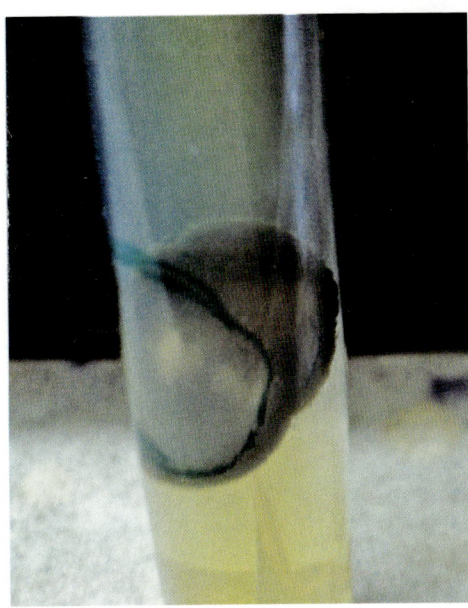

Fig. 1.21: Four weeks old culture of *Exophiala werneckii* grown on Sabouraud's dextrose agar with chloramphenicol (reverse).

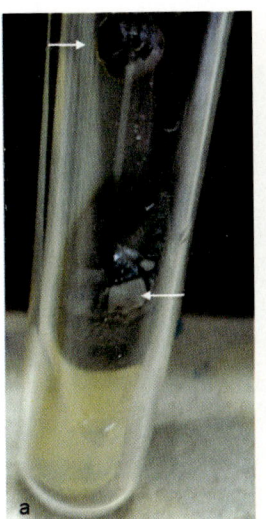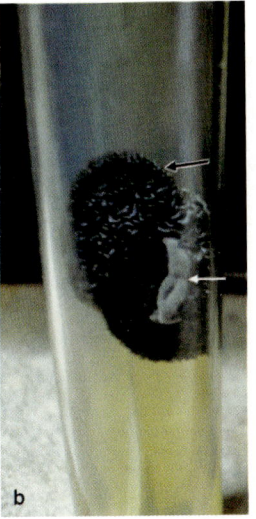

Fig. 1.20: Colony morphology (obverse) of *Exophiala werneckii* grown on SDCA at 28°C; (a) initial growth after 3 weeks of incubation are shiny, moist, adherent, brownish yeast like colony and rapidly becomes olive to shiny black (white arrow); (b) colony after 5 weeks growth on SDCA reveals olive black moist colony is covered by blackish gray mycelium (black arrow).

Microscopic Morphology

Colonies to be composed primarily of two-celled, cylindrical to spindle shaped yeast like cells that taper toward the ends, which bear annellations. They are 3 to 10 mm in diameter. Some of the cells have a central cross wall. As the colony ages, there is development of an elongate mycelium, which is tortuous and has numerous septations. It becomes pigmented and develops a sleeve of conidia from undifferentiated, usually intercalary conidiogenous cells. The conidiogenous cells are annellides. Conidia are produced percurrently. At this stage mycelium may be very thick (up to 7 mm) with thick walled, squarish, pigmented cells in a chain like arrangement (Fig. 1.22). The conidia are numerous and may develop from annellides anywhere on the mycelium. They vary from white elliptical cells to olive coloured are one celled to occasionally two celled (2 to 4 × 20 mm) (Fig. 1.23). As the colony ages, a green-gray to gray-black fuzz develops over it. Sometimes a few chlamydoconidia

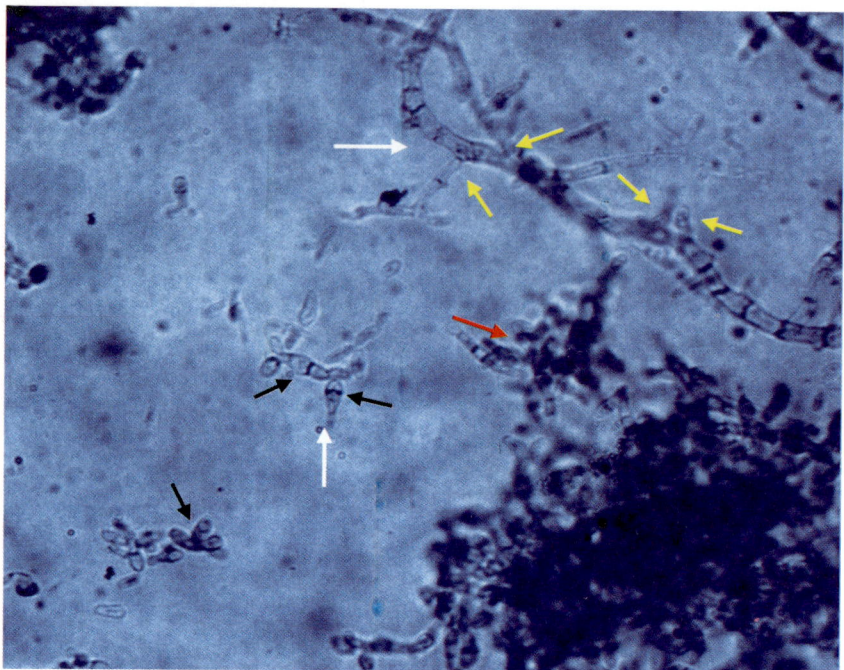

Fig. 1.22: Conidia of *Exophiala werneckii* are produced from intercalary annelides (white arrow) and from short lateral branches (yellow arrow); Seceded conidia are often yeast-like annelides, produce new conidia by polar budding (black arrow), deeply pigmented yeast cells (red arrow) are also seen (×400).

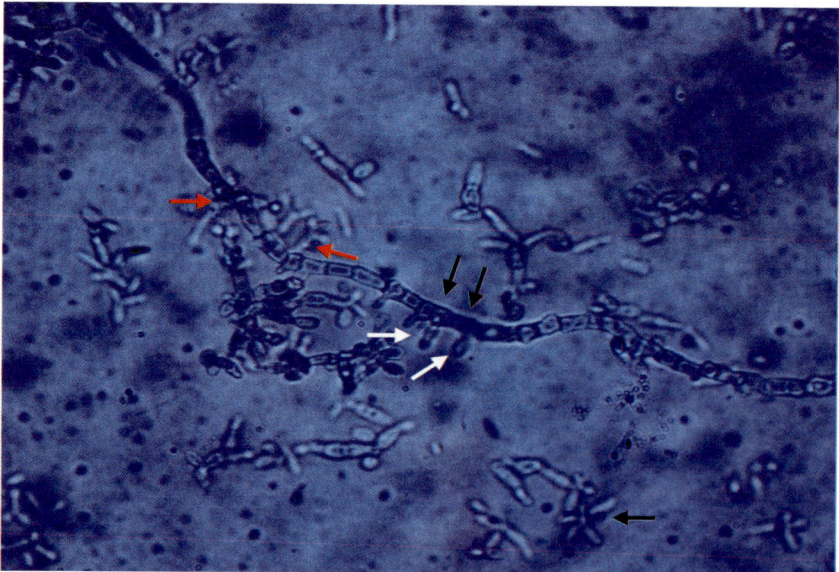

Fig. 1.23: *Exophiala werneckii*. One or two celled ellipsoidal conidia (white arrow) produced from intercalary short, undifferentiated conidiogenous cells (black arrow). Ellipsoidal or elongated conidia are also produced from conidiophores (red arrow; ×600).

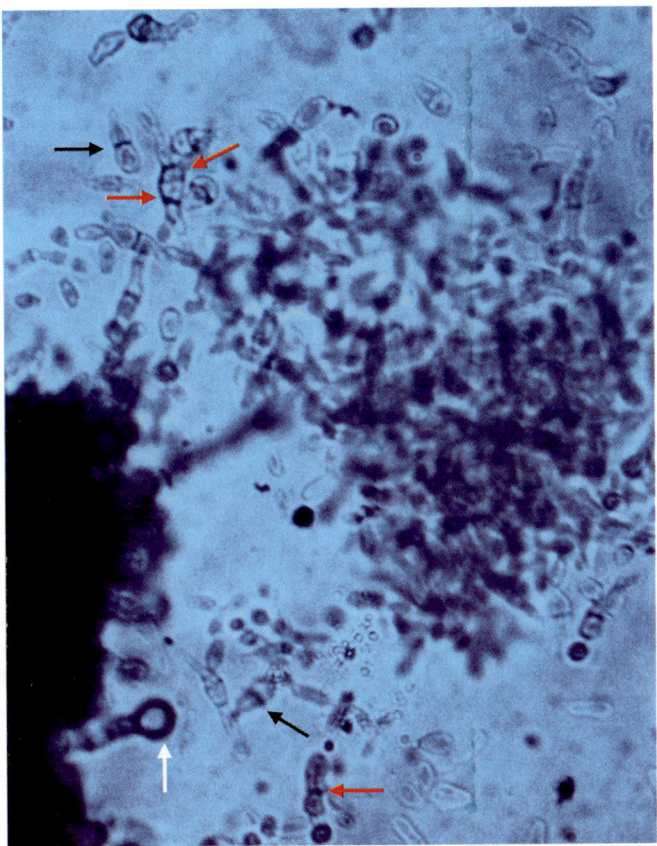

Fig. 1.24: *Exophiala* typical two-celled yeast cells (black arrow) are producing annelloconidia (red arrow). Some of the cells are deeply pigmented. Chlamydoconidia (white arrow) appear in old culture.

(Fig. 1.24) with dark thick walls appear throughout the colony. Such conidia are singular and one or more septations.

PIEDRA

Piedra is a fungus infection of the hair shafts, characterized by the presence of firm irregular nodule. The nodules are composed of fungal elements cemented together anywhere along the hair shaft (Fig. 1.25). Multiple infections of the same strand are common. Two varieties of piedra are recognized, white piedra caused by *Trichosporon beigelii,* and black piedra caused by *Piedraia hortae.*

Direct microscopic examination of infected material (hair shaft nodule) in a 20% KOH preparation can differentiate not only two

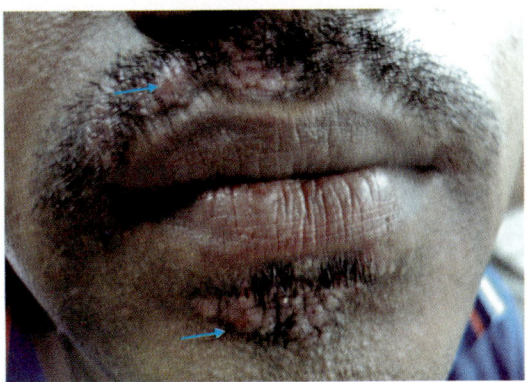

Fig.1.25: Coexistence of both "black piedra" and "tinea barbae" in a 21-year-old man. Extensive folliculitis (blue arrow) is an important feature of "tinea barbae" which is not found in "black piedra". Both *Piedraia hortae* and *Trichophyton tonsurans* were isolated from the lesion.

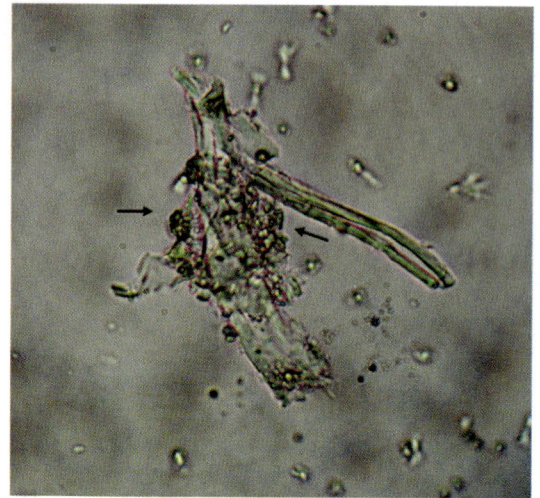

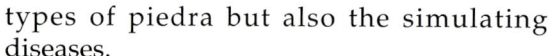

Fig. 1.26: Firmly adherent, black hard gritty nodules composed of a cemented mass of hyphal cells (black arrow) in black piedra. The hyphae are dark brown and frequently segmented to form rectangular arthrospores 4 to 8 µm in size (KOH mount ×600).

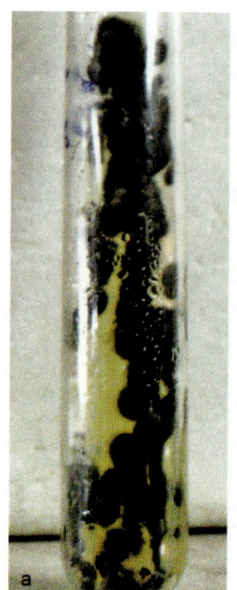
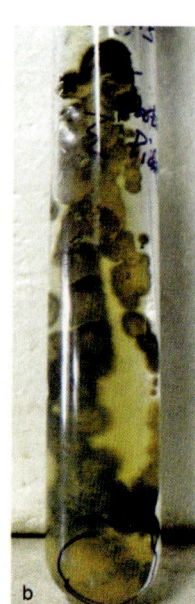

a   b

Fig. 1.27: Colony morphology of *Piedraia hortae* grown on Sabouraud's dextrose agar at 27°C for 3 weeks; (a) obverse, (b) reverse.

types of piedra but also the simulating diseases.

Black piedra is composed of a tightly packed stroma of regularly arranged, thick walled, rhomboid cells (resembling arthroconidia) and dichotomously branched hyphae held together by a cement-like substance. The hyphae and cells are 4 to 8 mm in diameter and there is even pigmentation in the walls (Fig. 1.26).

Colony Morphology

Piedraia hortae grow very slowly at 25°C, developing into small dark brown to black, conical adherent colonies (Fig. 1.27). The centre of the colony is elevated and cerebriform and the periphery is flat. The colony may be glabrous when young but usually develops a short greenish brown aerial mycelium with time. A rusty red pigment may be seen in the media.

Microscopic Morphology

Microscopic morphology reveals thick walled, closely septate hyphae, chlamydoconidia, and swollen irregular cells (Figs 1.28 and 1.29). In the centre of the colony, locules may be found in which asci develop in a manner similar to that seen on the nodules of the hair shaft.

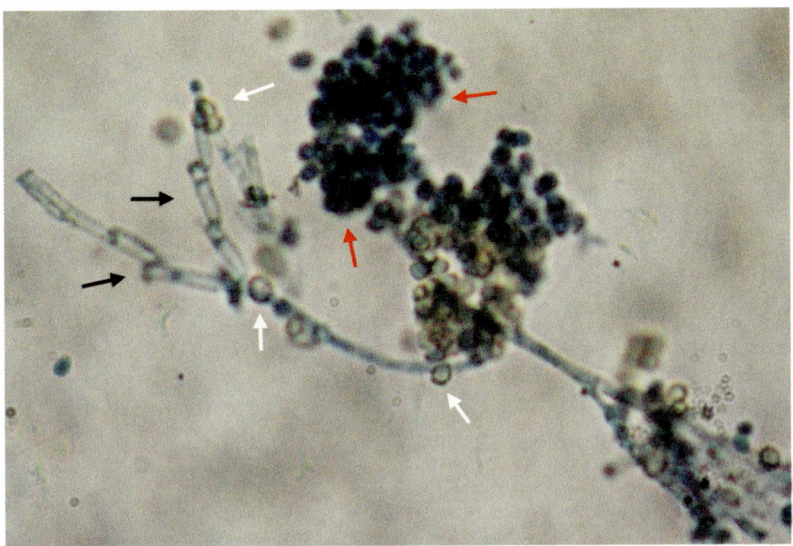

Fig. 1.28: *Piedraia hortae*. Thick-walled, highly septated hyphae (black arrow) that have many chlamydospore-like swollen intercalary cells (white arrow). Locules containing asci and ascospores (red arrow) may be found in the thicker part of the colony (LPCB mount ×600).

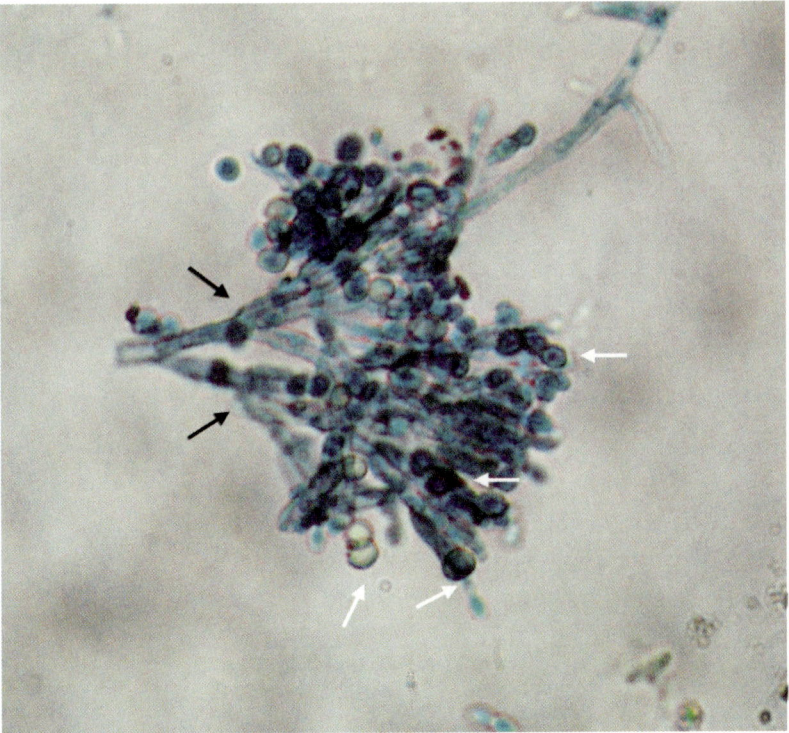

Fig. 1.29: Thick-walled, highly septated hyphae (black arrow) which have chlamydospore-like swollen intercalary cells (white arrow) are characteristic features in *Piedraia hortae*. (LPCB mount ×600).

CUTANEOUS MYCOSIS

The cutaneous infections of man include variety of diseases in which the integument and its appendages, the hair and nail are involved. Infection is generally restricted to the nonliving cornified layers, but a variety of pathologic changes occur in the host because of the presence of the infectious agent and its metabolic products.

The majority of these infections are caused by a homogenous group of keratinophilic fungi called the dermatophytes.

THE DERMATOPHYTES

Dermatophytosis is colonization by a dermatophytic fungus of the keratinized tissues—the nails, the hair and the stratum corneum of the skin.

Dermatophytosis includes several distinct clinical entities, depending on the anatomic sites and the etiologic agent. The severity of the disease depends on the strain or species of the dermatophyte and the sensitivity of the host to that (Flowchart 1.1).

Clinical Manifestations

Tinea Capitis

Tinea capitis is a dermatophyte infection of the scalp, eyebrows and eyelashes caused by species of the genera: *Microsporum* and *Trichophyton*. The disease varies from a benign scaly noninflamed subclinical colonization to an inflammatory disease characterized by the production of a scaly erythematous lesions and by alopecia that may become severely inflamed with the formation of deep, ulcerative kerion eruptions. This often results in keloid formation and scarring, with permanent alopecia. The type of disease elicited is dependent on the interaction of host and the etiologic agent.

Fungi involved

The commoner types of ringworm are classified according to the site of formation of their arthroconidia.

Flowchart 1.1: Ecology of human dermatophyte species

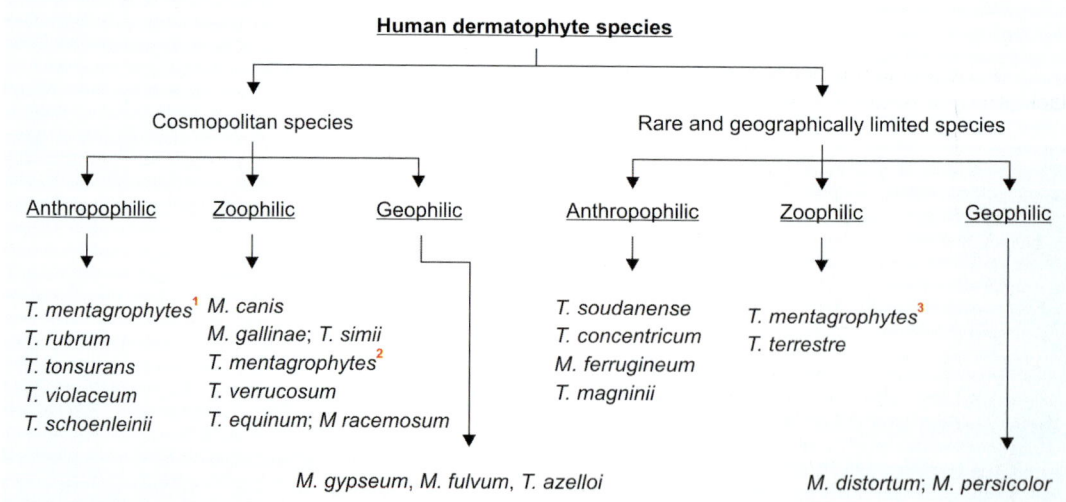

¹ *var. interdigitale*
² *var. mentagrophyte*
³ *var. quinckeanum*

Ectothrix infection is defined as fragmentation of the mycelium into conidia around the hair shaft or just beneath the cuticle around the hair with destruction of the cuticle (Fig. 1.30). The classical causative agents are:

*Anthropophilic—**M. audouinii**, **M. ferrugineum**.*

*Zoophilic—**T. mentagrophyte**[2], **T. verrucosum**, **M. canis**.*

*Geophilic—**M. gypseum**, **M. fulvum**.*

In **endothrix** infections arthroconidia formation occurs by fragmentation of hyphae within the hair shaft without destruction of the cuticle (Figs 1.31 and 1.32).

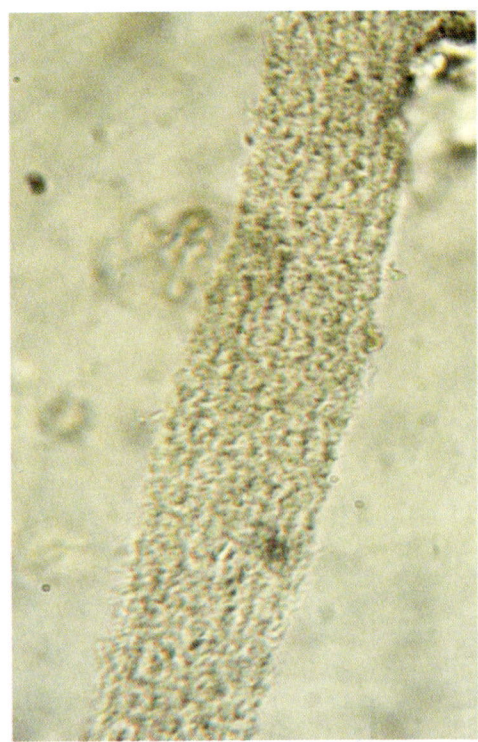

Fig. 1.32: Hyphae within the hair showing characteristic channeling (KOH mount ×400).

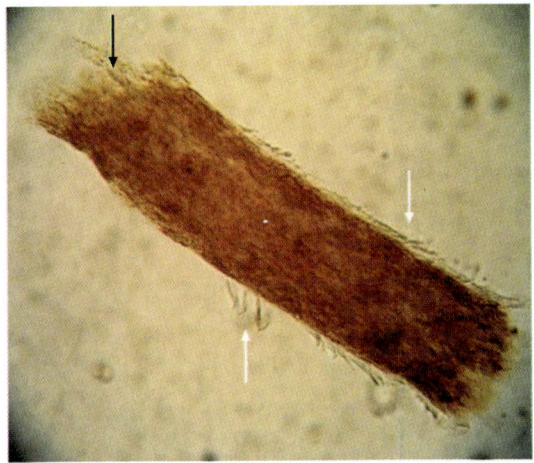

Fig. 1.30: Both ectothrix (white arrow) and endothrix (black arrow) invasion of hair (×400).

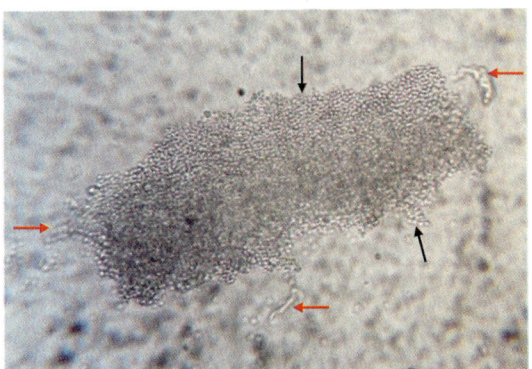

Fig. 1.31: Ectoendothrix arthroconidiation. Chains of arthroconidia are found in the medulla of the hair shaft as well as around the cortex.

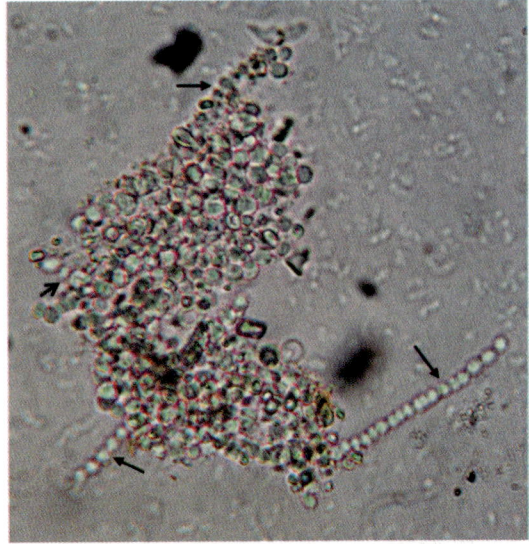

Fig. 1.33: Dermatophyte in scalp scraping. Chains of conidia (black arrow) of *Microsporum audouinii* [KOH mount ×200].

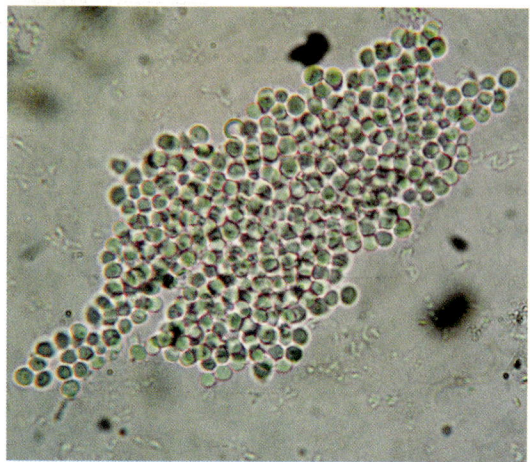

Fig. 1.34: Hair stubs and scalp scrapings from a case of 'Tinea capitis' in KOH preparation. Conidia in mosaic masses are seen. *Microsporum audouinii* was isolated in pure culture [×400].

Fig. 1.36: Tinea capitis. Multiple kerions and patchy alopecia in scalp infected by *Microsporum canis*. The large kerion consisting of crusts, exudate, scalp debris.

Small spored (conidia) ectothrix organisms include *M. audouinii*, *M. canis*, *M. ferrugineum*. Masses of conidia (1–3) μ are produced in a mosaic pattern (Fig. 1.31).

The principal organism producing endothrix infections are *T. tonsurans*, *T. violaceum*.

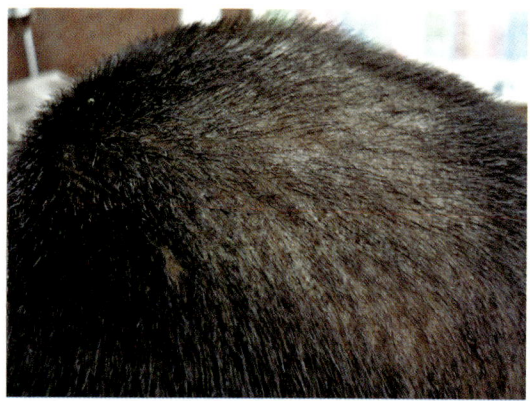

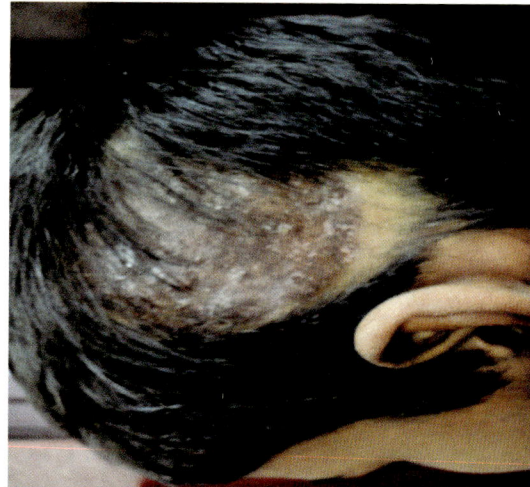

Fig. 1.37: Tinea capitis. Suppurative folliculitis with severe inflammatory reaction produced by *T. violaceum*. Patchy alopecia at the infection site and scarring noticed.

Fig. 1.35: Tinea capitis. Severe inflammatory reaction and suppurative folliculitis produced by *T. tonsurans*.

Tinea Favosa

Favus is a clinical entity characterized by the occurrence of dense masses of mycelium and epithelial debris which form yellowish, cup-shaped crusts, called scutula. The scutulum develops in a hair follicle, with the hair shaft in the centre of the raised lesion (Fig. 1.38).

Tinea Corporis

Tinea corporis is a dermatophyte infection of the glabroua skin most commonly caused by species of the genera *Trichophyton* and

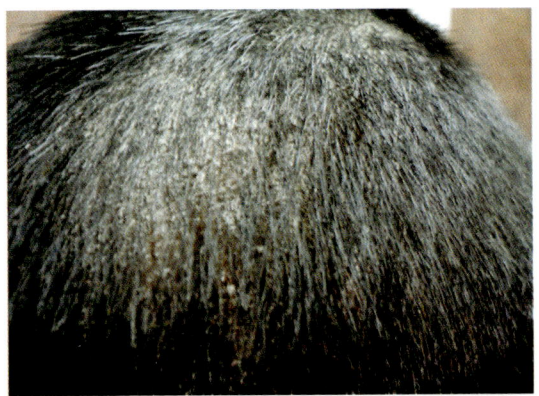

Fig. 1.38: Tinea favosa. The infected hair is gray, whereas normal hair is pigmented. Middle stage of the disease. Large crusts and scutula covering most of the area of the scalp.

Microsporum. The infection is generally restricted to the stratum corneum of the epidermis. The clinical symptoms are a result of the fungal metabolites acting as toxins and allergens. Lesions vary from simple scaling, scaling with erythema and vesicles to deep granulomata. Hair follicles often act as a reservoir for recrudescence of the disease.

Two types of lesions are most commonly encountered. One is dry and scaly *annulare*

(annular patches) (Fig. 1.39) and the other *vesiculare* (iris form) (Figs 1.35; 1.64 and 1.65).

Organisms involved

All species of dermatophytes are able to produce lesions of the glabrous skin, even though some species are more commonly associated with other types of infections.

In contrast to tinea capitis, there is a little tendency for geographic dominance of a particular species in tinea corporis.

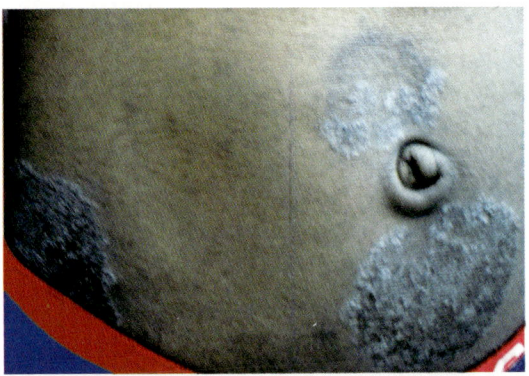

Fig. 1.40: Tinea corporis. Psoriasiform lesion. Infiltrated maculopapular area are covered by silvery scales. Some vesicles are evident in several places on the surface.

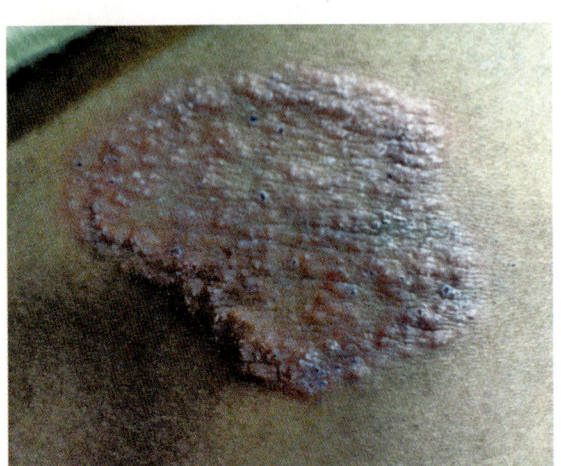

Fig. 1.39: Psoriasiform lesion in 'tinea corporis'. Maculopapular area is covered with silvery scales, many vesicles are prominent on the surface but the overlying epidermis has many wrinkles and folds.

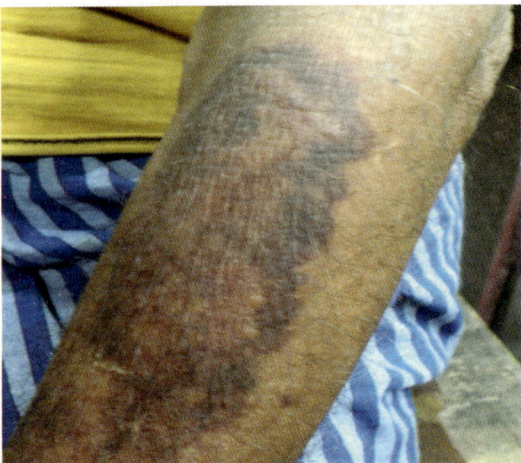

Fig. 1.41: Tinea corporis. Plaque-like lesion. The outer ring is infiltrated and has a red rolled border with a few vesicles. The remaining surface of the lesion is smooth, firm, infiltrated and plaque like.

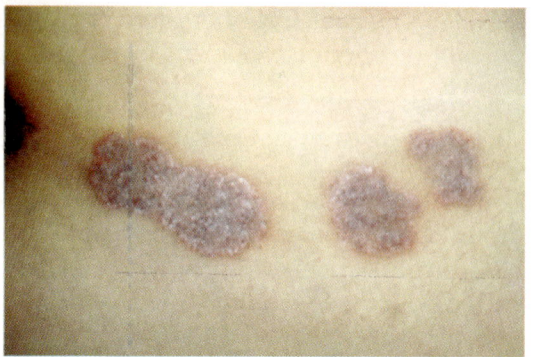

Fig. 1.42: Tinea corporis on right lateral aspect of abdomen. Lesions are raised and erythematous caused by *Trichophyton mentagrophytes* var *quinckeanum.*

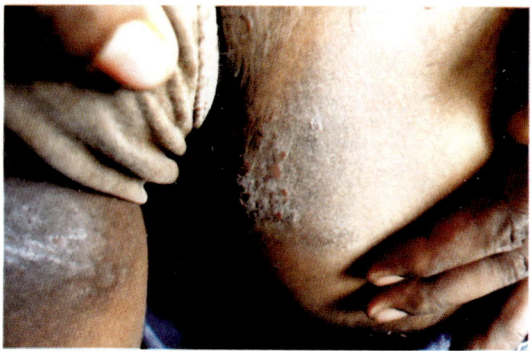

Fig. 1.44: Tinea cruris. Serpiginous lesion on thigh and scrotum.

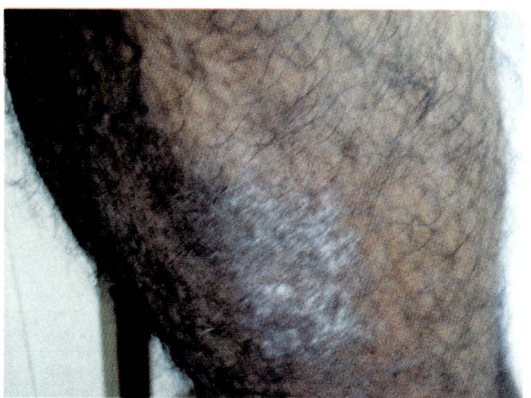

Fig. 1.43: Tinea corporis. Granulomatous reactions around hair follicles resembling Majocchi's granuloma.

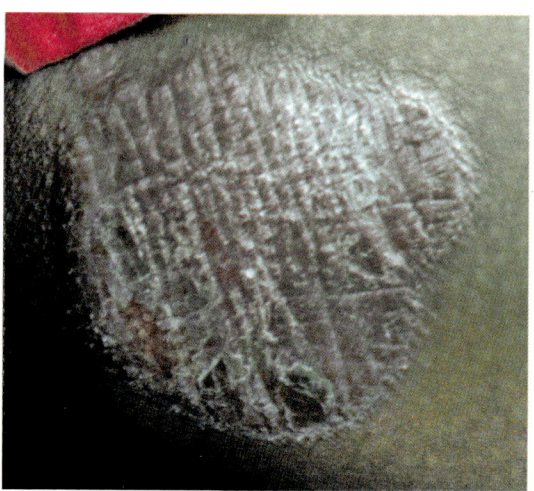

Fig. 1.45: Tinea cruris. Serpiginous lesion of the left thigh in contact with scrotum. The lesion looks similar to eczema marginatum. The infection is due to *T. rubrum.*

The most universally encountered species is probably **T. rubrum**, followed in frequency by **T. mentagrophytes.**

An outbreak of tinea capitis in children owing to **M. canis** and **M. audouinii** will manifest itself in an associated adult population as tinea corporis.

Tinea Cruris

Tinea cruris is a dermatophyte infection of the groin, perineum and perianal region which is acute or chronic and generally severely pruritic. The lesion is characteristically sharply demarcated, with a raised, erythematous margin and thin dry epidermal scaling (Fig. 1.44).

T. rubrum appears to be the predominant species throughout the world. Among other dermatophytes **E. floccosum** and **T. mentagrophytes** are also important. **Trichophyton mentagrophytes** is associated with the more pustular type of tinea cruris.

Tinea Unguium

Tinea unguium is an invasion of the nail plates by a dermatophyte. The term onychomycosis refers to an infection of the nails caused by nondermatophytic fungi and yeasts.

The disease, tinea unguium is clinically classified into four types.

1. Distal lateral subungual onychomycosis (DLSO) (Fig. 1.46)
2. Proximal subungual onychomycosis (PSO) (Fig. 1.47)
3. White superficial onychomycosis (WSO) (Fig. 1.48)
4. Total dystrophic onychomycosis (TDO) (Fig. 1.49)

Almost all species of dermatophytes have been isolates from ringworm of the nail. The etiologic agents are usually those which are common or endemic in the population.

Tinea unguium of the fingernail is most commonly due to *T. rubrum*. Other common species causing fingernail infection are *T. tonsurans, T. mentagrophytes, T. schoenleinii, T. megninii* and *E. floccosum*.

Toenail may be infected by a variety of dermatophyte species. Nail involvement associated with tinea corporis and tinea pedis occurs most commonly with *T. rubrum, T. mentagrophytes, T. verrucosum* and *E. floccosum*.

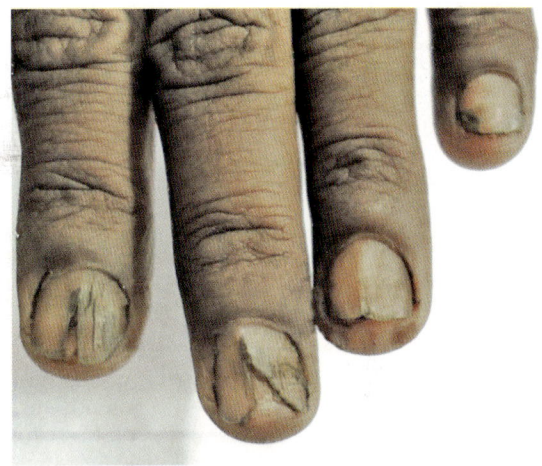

Fig. 1.46: Tinea unguium. Clinical type—distal lateral subungual onychomycosis (DLSO).

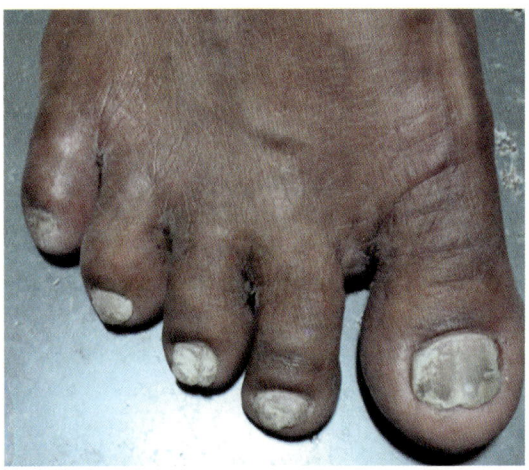

Fig. 1.48: Tinea unguium. Clinical type—white superficial onychomycosis (WSO).

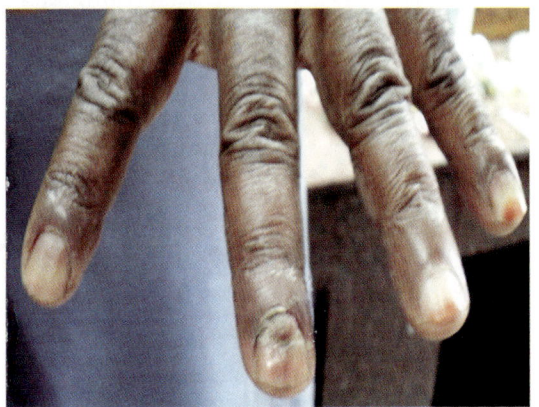

Fig. 1.47: Tinea unguium. Clinical type—proximal subungual onychomycosis (PSO).

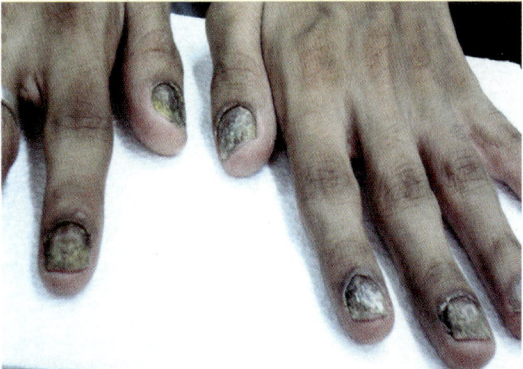

Fig. 1.49: Tinea unguium. Advanced disease involving several nails. Clinical types—total dystrophic onychomycosis (TDO).

Rarely encountered species include *M. audouinii, M. gallinae, M. canis, T. soudanense.*

Tinea unguium associated with tinea capitis and tinea favosa are due to *T. tonsurans* and *T. violaceum*.

T. concentricum, a causative agent of tinea imbricata, have been isolated in our laboratory from a patient with tinea unguium residing in suburban Kolkata (Fig. 1.50). Another interesting case of tinea unguium is noteworthy where *M. gallinae* have been isolated from a 19 years old male, an inhabitant of North 24 Parganas district in West Bengal (Figs 1.51 and 1.52).

Tinea Manuum

Tinea manuum refers to those infections in which the interdigital areas and the palmar surfaces are involved and show characteristic pathologic features (Fig. 1.57).

Almost all dermatophytes are potential invaders of the hand. Majority of the infections are caused by *T. rubrum, T. mentagrophytes* and *E. floccosum*. Tinea manuum is always associated with tinea pedis, so that the flora of the latter is usually the etiologic agent of the hand infections.

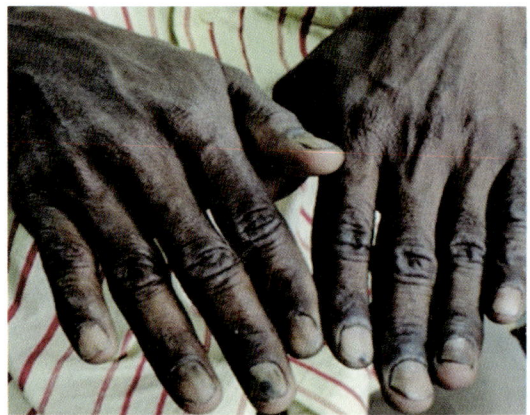

Fig. 1.50: Tinea unguium. Several nails are involved. Brown to black patchy lesions are seen at the proximal part of the nail plate but gradually the complete nail involvement (in few nails) is noticed in advanced disease. *Trichophyton concentricum* is the causative fungi isolated in this case.

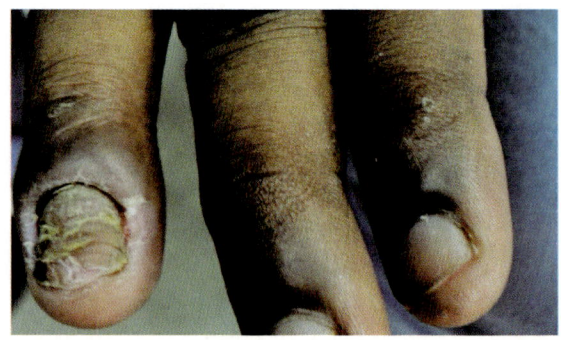

Fig. 1.51: Tinea unguium of a 21-year-old student, a part-time worker in his father's fish business. His toe nails are also involved (as shown in Fig.1.52). *Microsporum gallinae* and *Trichophyton violaceum* were isolated from all lesions involving different nails.

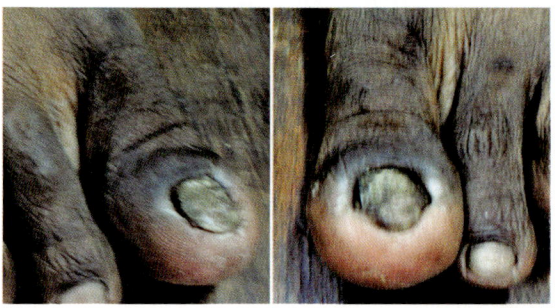

Fig. 1.52: Tinea unguium involving toe nails (great toes only) in the same patient as shown in Fig. 1.51. The infection is chronic and of more than two years duration but all other toe nails remain uninfected.

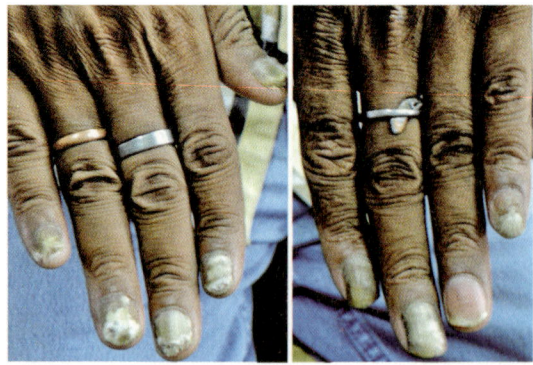

Fig. 1.53: Tinea unguium. Leukonychia mycotica. Multiple white irregular lesions on surface of nail. Both *Trichophyton mentagrophytes* and *Microsporum persicolor* were isolated in this case and considered as involvement of dual fungal pathogen producing lesions.

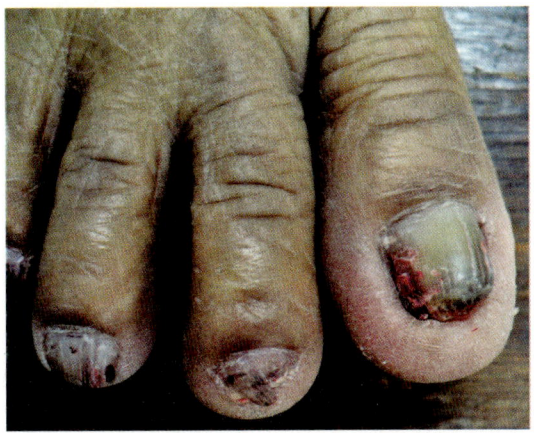

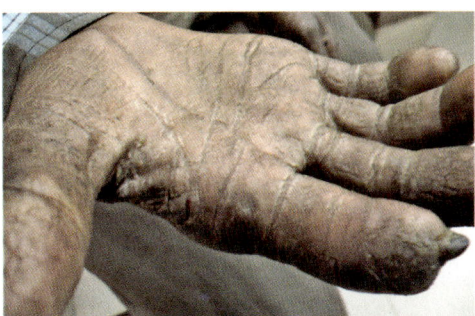

Fig. 1.57: Tinea manuum. Diffuse hyperkeratosis of palm and finger. In this chronic infection only the palmar surface was involved; the dorsum was spared. The patient had tinea pedis due to same etiology.

Fig. 1.54: Tinea unguium. Advanced disease showing grooved dark brown colouration. The infection is chronic and of many years' duration. *T. verrucosum.*

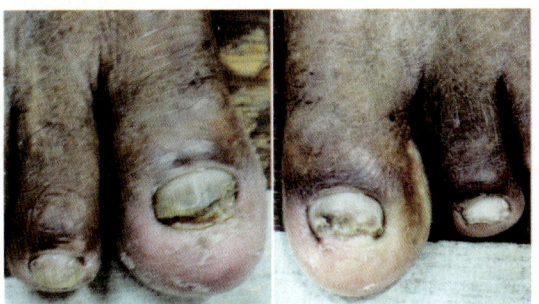

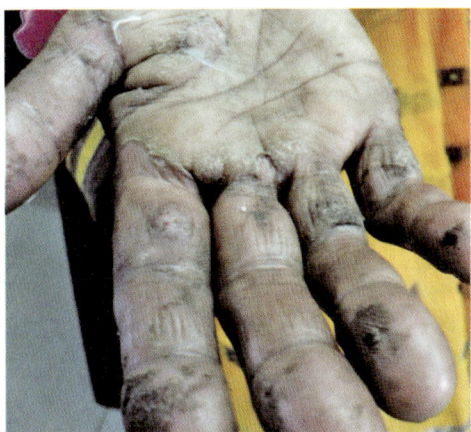

Fig. 1.55: Tinea unguium. Advanced disease of many years' duration. Infection started at the distal edge of nail plate. *Trichophyton rubrum.*

Fig. 1.58: Tinea manuum. Exfoliating skin lesions with patchy hyperkeratosis are present.

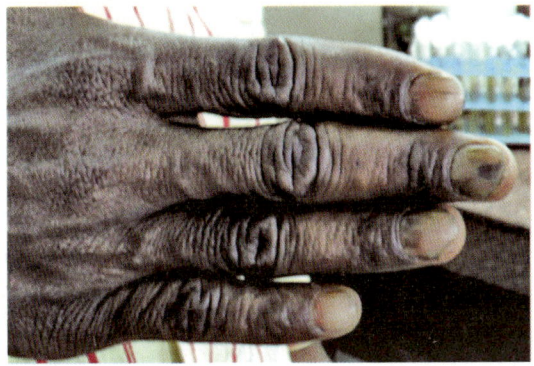

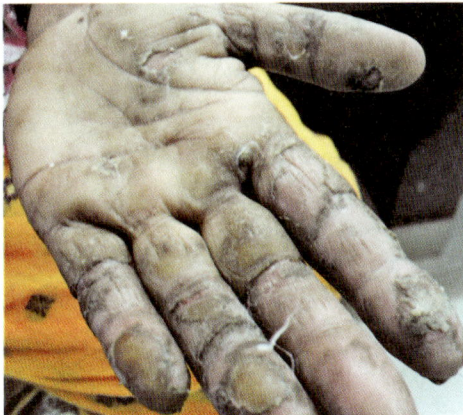

Fig. 1.56: Tinea unguium caused by *Trichophyton concentricum.*

Fig. 1.59: Vesicular lesion with circumscribed patches in 'tinea manuum'. This condition is caused by *Trichophyton mentagrophytes.*

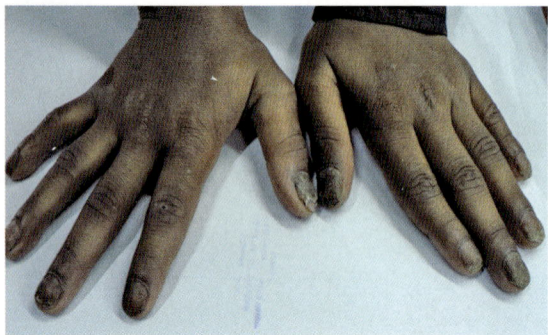

Fig. 1.60: 'Twenty nail syndrome' in a 14-year-old boy. All finger and toe nails involvement in an infection by *Aspergillus flavus*.

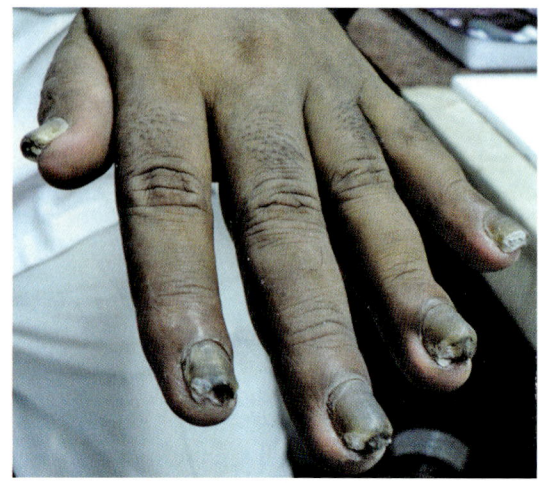

Fig. 1.62: A 40-year-old male, a professional tailor, suffering from onychomycosis for more than 16 years.

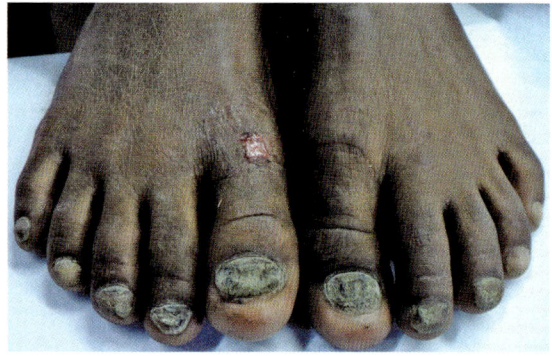

Fig. 1.61: Tinea unguium involving almost all toe nails. The infection is due to *Aspergillus terreus*.

Tinea Pedis

Tinea pedis is a dermatophyte infection of the feet involving the toe webs and soles. The lesions are of several types, varying from mild, chronic and scaling to an acute, exfoliative, pustular and bullous disease (Figs 1.63–1.66).

Laboratory Diagnosis

Direct Microscopy

Diagnosis of dermatophytosis can be readily made with potassium hydroxide (KOH) preparation of the infected specimens such as hair stumps, skin and nail scrapings. The size and morphology of hyphae in these preparations permit easy differentiation of dermatophytes from other fungi causing superficial infections.

In tinea capitis and tinea barbae only infected hair stumps should be selected for examination. When infected hairs are a few in number or the characteristics of hair are not apparent, Wood's lamp (ultraviolet) may be used to detct the invaded hairs.

For microscopical examination, a few hair stubs are pulled out with the help of a fine forceps (Fig. 1.69) placed on a slide with a drop of KOH and covered with a coverslip. The slide can be gently heated before examination. Alternatively hair samples may be dipped into a vial containing small amount of KOH and kept overnight. One drop from the vial is put on a slide and a coverslip is placed on it to examine under microscope. In order to observe the true position of the fungus (as to endothrix ectothrix), the outer walls of the hair should not be damaged during this preparation. The position of the fungus in or out of the hair offers a reliable clue to its identity.

In tinea pedis, the white macerated skin from the interdigital space should be cleaned by rubbing it with a gauge sponge with 70% alcohol before stripping the epidermal scales from the edge of the lesion (Fig. 1.70). The epidermal scales can be stripped with forceps

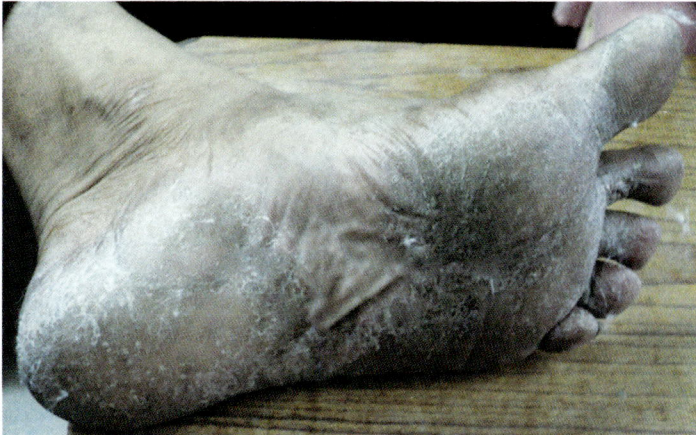

Fig. 1.63: Tinea pedis. Intertriginous form involving plantar aspect of foot.

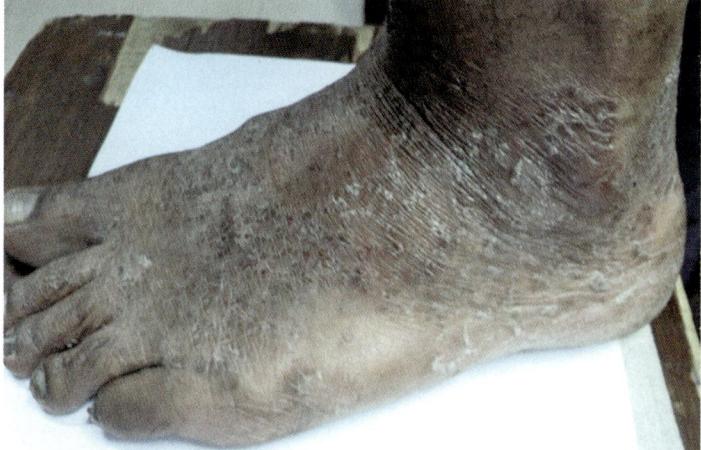

Fig. 1.64: Tinea pedis. Vesicular type involving dorsum of the foot.

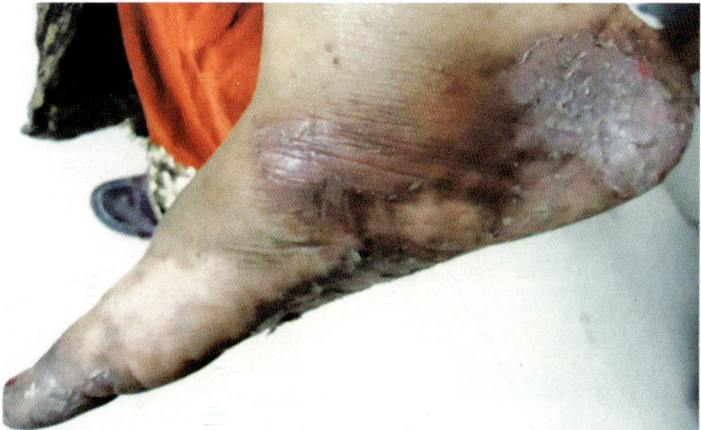

Fig. 1.65: Tinea pedis. Vesicular form involving intertrigo and instep.

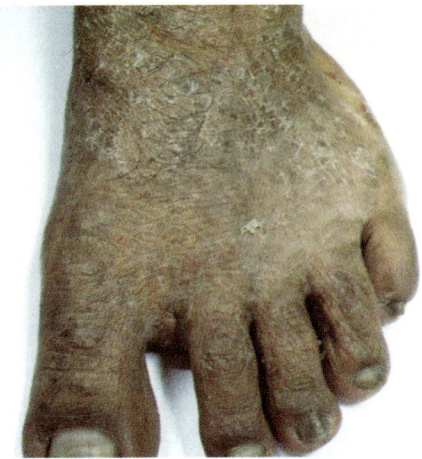

Fig. 1.66: Eczematoid vesiculopustular lesion in tinea pedis.

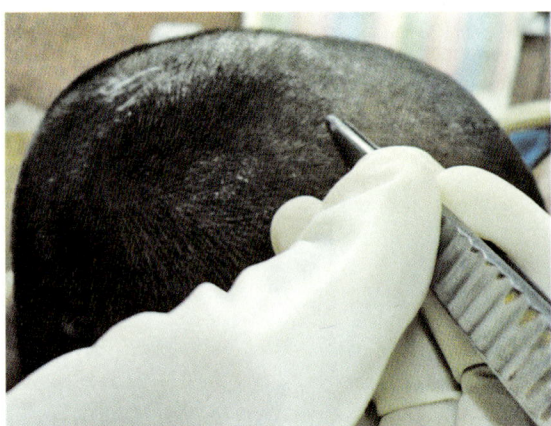

Fig. 1.69: Epilating hair sample from the affected area in tinea capitis.

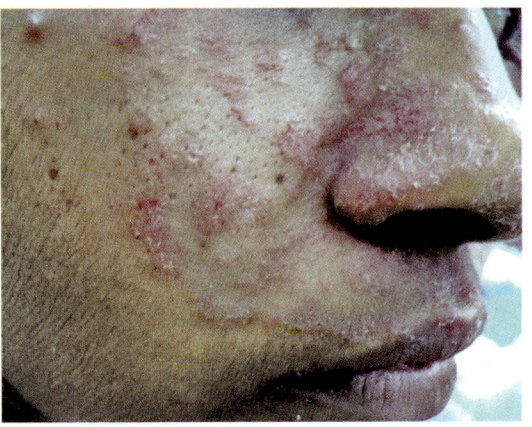

Fig. 1.67: Tinea faciei. Vesicular type lesion.

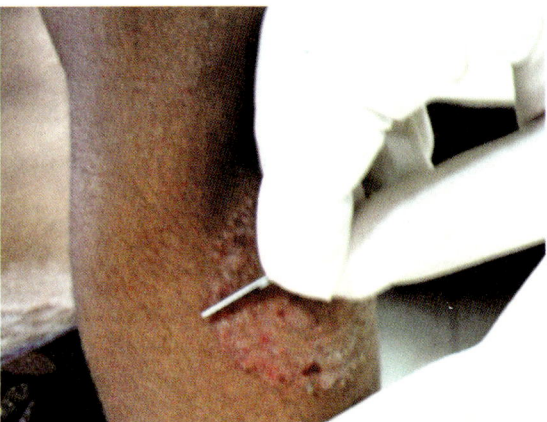

Fig. 1.70: Skin scrapings is being taken from the active margin of the lesion.

and fine scissors. When vesicles are present, the upper part of the vesicles can be clipped off and used for KOH plus calcofluor white preparation.

Care should be taken not to overheat the slide because boiling precipitates KOH crystals.

Young hyphae are seen as long undulate branching threads; older hyphae are seen with numerous septations or barrel-shaped arthroconidia (Fig. 1.71). These conidia are the results of fragmentation at each septum and are the infectious propagules in disseminating the disease to another host.

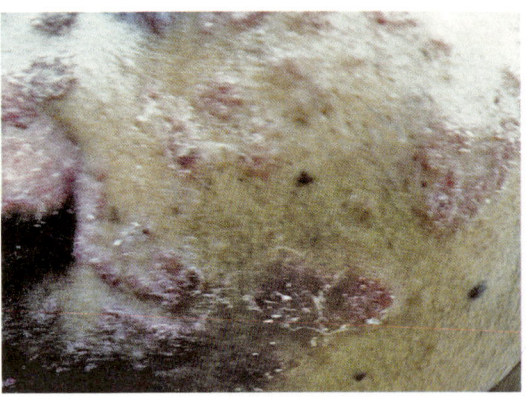

Fig. 1.68: Tinea faciei. Vesicles and crusts are seen. *Trichophyton rubrum* was isolated from lesions.

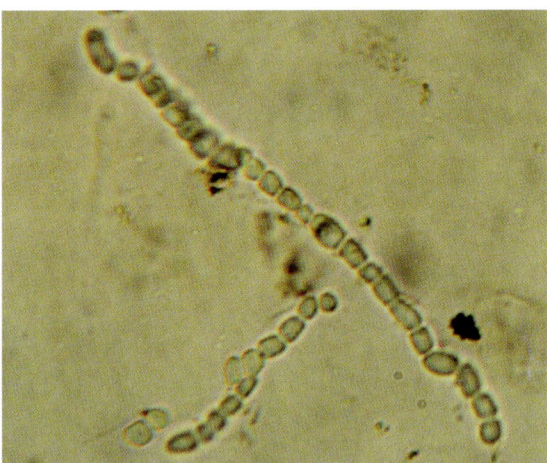

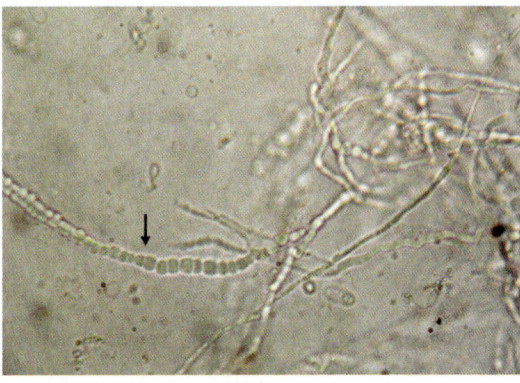

Fig. 1.73: KOH preparation of nail sample of a 4-year-old male child suffering from tinea unguium involving almost all fingernails. Chains of arthroconidia (black arrow) and hyphae with regular septation are noticed. *Trichophyton mentagrophytes* (nodular varient) was the causative agent isolated from the lesions [×400].

Fig. 1.71: Dermatophyte in nail. *Trichophyton soudanense*. Chains of arthoconidia are seen (KOH mount ×400).

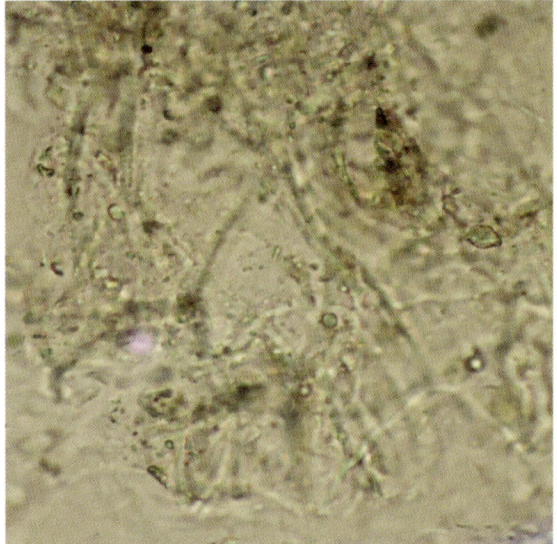

Fig. 1.72: Entangled mass of hyphae are noticed in skin scrapings (KOH mount ×400).

Fibres of cotton or other fabrics and the network of material from host tissue including cholesterol crystals should not be mistaken as hyphae (Fig. 1.74).

Under a high power microscope, **fungal hyphae can be differentiated from such debris** by their:

- Manner of septation,
- Uniform thickness of walls
- Branching of hyphae

Epidermal scales from tinea corporis can be processed similarly, except that it is not necessary the superficial material before obtaining the scales. In case of tinea unguium, the upper portion of the infected nail is scraped away before obtaining specimens from deeper layer of nails. A scalpel can be used to scrape off deeper layers of nail and collect them on slide for the KOH preparation.

Key to Direct Examination of Hair

Wood's lamp
1. Bright yellow green: *Microsporum audouinii, Microsporum canis, Microsporum ferrugineum.*
2. Dull bluish white: *Trichophyton schoenleinii.*
3. No fluorescence: All other dermatophytes.

KOH mount
1. Ectothrix hairs (Fig. 1.30).
   - Small spores, 2 to 3 μm (in diameter), in mosaic masses on the outside of hair shaft: **M. audouinii, M. canis, M. ferrugineum.**
   - Small spores, 3 to 5 μm, forming sheath or in isolated chains on the surface of hair shaft: **Trichophyton mentagrophytes, M. praecox (rare).**

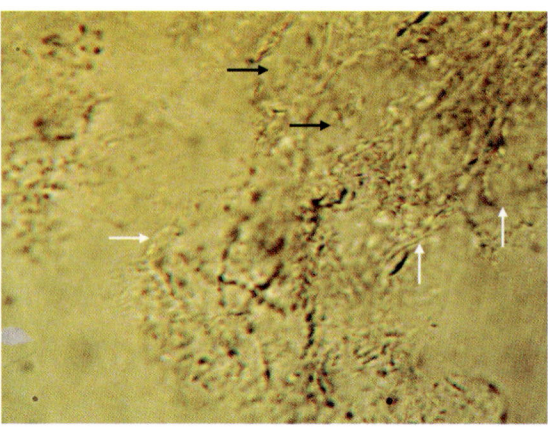

Fig. 1.74: 'Mosaic fungus'; cholesterol crystals (white arrow) among the edge of squames (black arrow). [KOH mount ×400].

- Large spores, 5 to 8 µm, in sparse chains inside and outside of hair shaft: *M. gypseum, M. fulvum, M. nanum, M. gallinae, M. vanbreuseghemii.*
- Large spores, 5 to 8 µm, forming sheath or in isolated chains on the surface of hair shaft: *T. equinum, T. magninii, T. rubrum (rare).*
- Large spores, 8 to 10 µm, forming sheath or chains on surface of hair shaft: *T. verrucosum.*

2. Endothrix hairs (Fig. 1.31).
   - Chains of spores, 5 to 8 µm, packed inside the hair shaft, hairs thickened, twisted and broken off short: *T. violaceum, T. soudanense, T. gourvilli, T. rubrum (rare).*
3. Favic hairs (Fig. 1.32)—hyphae without spores inside throughout hair length, fat droplets commonly seen in the empty areas where hyphae have degenerated: *Tichophyton schoenleinii.*
4. Hair not invaded: *Epidermophyton floccosum, T. concentricum, M. persicolor.*

Direct Culture

It is essential to isolate a dermatophyte in culture because direct examination does not allow species identification and the prognosis and therapy may vary depending on the species.

Dermal and nail lesions should be cleaned with 70% alcohol and specimens are removed as described above. Now the collected samples are placed directly on Sabouraud's dextrose agar containing chloramphenicol (SDCA) and Sabouraud's dextrose agar containing both chloramphenicol and cyclohexamide (SDCCA). The use of a medium containing gentamicin is recommended for specimens heavily contaminated with bacteria.

Dermatophyte test medium (DTM) is widely used in the laboratory. Dermatophytes turn the medium red by producing alkaline pH while growing on the medium. A few green and black molds also turn DTM red, but they can readily be differentiated from dermatophytes on the basis of colony morphology without microscopic examination.

Final identification of dermatophytes should be made from the microscopic examination of the purified culture, because certain white molds , such as *Histoplasma capsulatum,* also turn DTM red.

Incubation of culture is at 25°C to 30°C for at least 4 weeks. When colonies appear, a small agar block containing hyphal tips may be cut out and transferred to fresh medium to avoid contamination by other microorganisms associated with the specimens. Some dermatophytes sporulate within 5 days, whereas others take longer and seldom produce spores. Nutritional tests are needed for the cultures that seldom produce spores or distinctive pigments.

Nutritional Tests

Various dermatophytes require thiamine, inositol, histidine or nicotinic acid for good growth. To test the requirements, vitamin free casamino acid is used as the basal medium to which the vitamin solutions are added. For the amino acid requirement, ammonim nitrate agar is the basal medium. The basal medium without additives are used as controls. The inoculum size should be very small (pinhead size) to avoid carryover from the medium in which the inoculum has been grown.

Hair Perforation Test (in vitro)

Hair perforation test is useful in differentiating *Trichophyton rubrum* from *Trichophyton mentagrophytes*. The isolates of *Trichophyton mentagrophytes* produce hair perforating organs that penetrate hair readily and cause wedge-shaped perforation. Isolates of *Trichophyton rubrum* grow on the hair and disintegrate it without perforation.

Test procedure

To observe hair perforation, short strands of human hair are placed in petri dishes with 20 ml of distilled water and autoclaved. Two to three drops of 10% sterilized yeast extract are added to the petri dishes and hair strands are inoculated with small fragments of test fungi grown on Sabouraud's agar. Incubation is at 25°C and the hair strands are examined periodically over a period of 4 weeks. The hair strands covered with mycelium can be examined under microscope by mounting in lactophenol cotton blue. Wedge-shaped perforations may be more readily detected when the slide is gently heated.

Trichophyton mentagrophytes

Colony morphology

Obverse: The anthropophilic form grows as a flat, downy thallus with white edges and a cream tinted central area. Zoophilic isolates produce a flat, rapidly growing granular colony that is cream, yellowish buff to tan or reddish brown in colour. Mycelium is usually sparse and the powdery appearance is due to quantities of microconidia. The edges are often ray like. Numerous variations of colony morphology occur (Figs 1.75–1.77).

Reverse: Pigmentation is variable; colourless, yellow-brown, brown and a deep wine red resembling *T. rubrum* is seen. In differentiating pigmented colonies from *T. rubrum*, both species are inoculated onto potato dextrose agar (PDA) and cornmeal 1% glucose agar where *T. rubrum* produces a red pigment, while *T. mentagrophytes* does not.

Almost all strains of T. mentagrophytes are urease positive except the var. erinacei, which is negative. T. rubrum is urease negative.

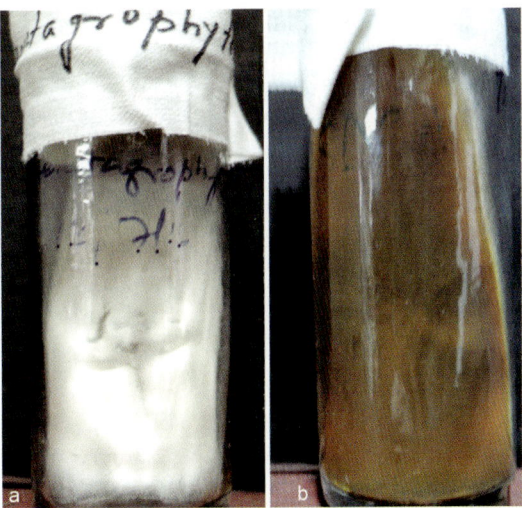

Fig. 1.75: *Trichophyton mentagrophytes.* Flat granular colony with light cream colour in the central area are observed when grown on SDCA. Reverse is brown; (a) obverse, (b) reverse.

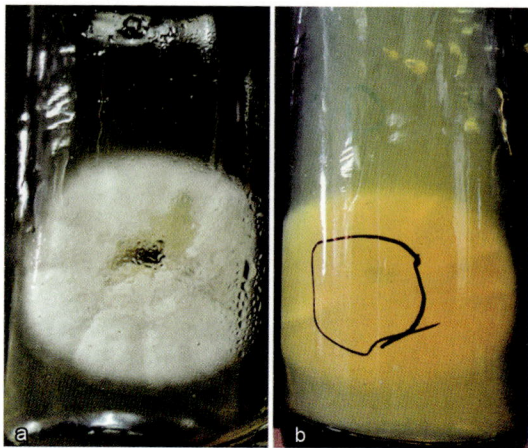

Fig. 1.76: *Trichophyton mentagrophytes var. mentagrophytes.* On SDCA colony appears as flat gently folded in the centre with radial forrows and the surface is white in colour, felt or seudelike. Reverse is light yellowish brown; (a) obverse, (b) reverse.

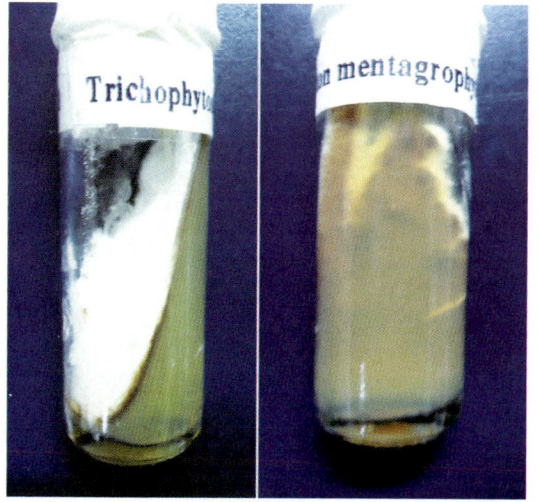

Fig. 1.77: White floccose colony of *Trichophyton mentagrophytes var. interdigitale*. Reverse is brown; (a) obverse (b) reverse.

Microscopic morphology

The most consistent feature of **T. mentagrophytes** is the production of globose microconidia in grapelike clusters (*en grappe*). These are most abundant in zoophilic granular strains, and less so in downy strains. In downy strains the conidia are more clavate shaped and resemble those of **T. rubrum.** Macroconidia are thin-walled, smooth, and variable in shape. Their size ranges from 4 to 8 × 20 to 50 μ and they have three to five cells. They are generally cigar shaped with a narrow base (Figs 1.78 to 1.80). **The typical picture of T. mentagrophytes seen under microscope is massed microconidia, some macroconidia, and several spiral hyphal cells, all in clusters on the vegetative hyphae.**

Structure like peridial hyphae, antlerlike hyphae, arthroconidia, nodular bodies, racquet mycelium and chlamydoconidia are also seen.

The variety designated as *quinckeanum* (mouse favus) has a gently folded thallus and lateral clavate microconidia (Figs 1.84 and 1.85).

Hair perforating organs are formed which is absent in T. rubrum.

In some strains , presence of nodular bodies are numerous but microconidia are a few in number (Figs 1.87–1.89).

Trichophyton rubrum

T. rubrum is anthropophilic and has become the most common and widely distributed dermatophyte causing human infection. It is very rarely isolated from animal and never from soil. It is extremely variable in its

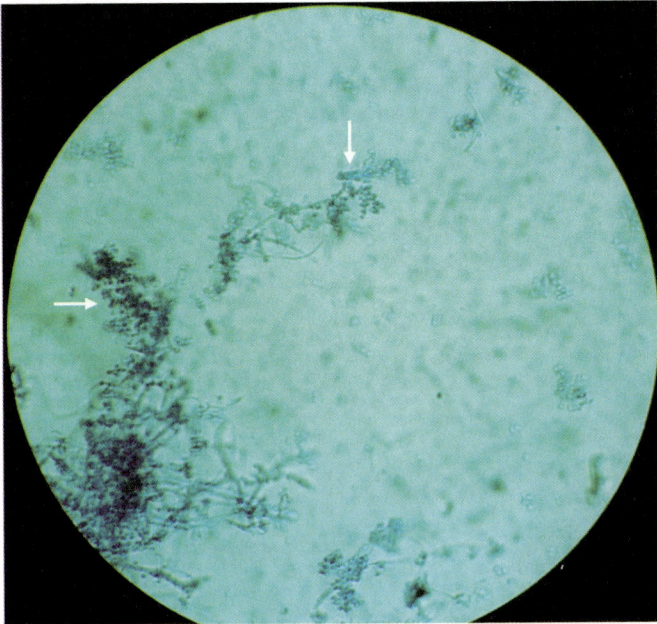

Fig. 1.78: *T. mentagrophytes.* Abundant microconidia (black arrow) and infrequently found macroconidia (white arrow) from *T. mentagrophytes* var. *mentagrophytes* [LPCB mount ×100].

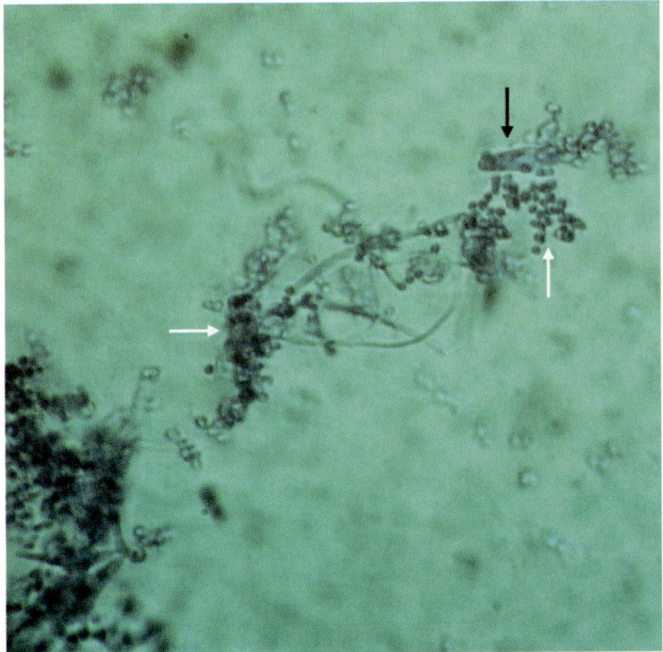

Fig. 1.79: Same microphotograph as in Fig. 1.78; Clusters of microconidia, 'en grappe' (white arrow), a single macroconidia (black arrow) [LPCB mount ×400].

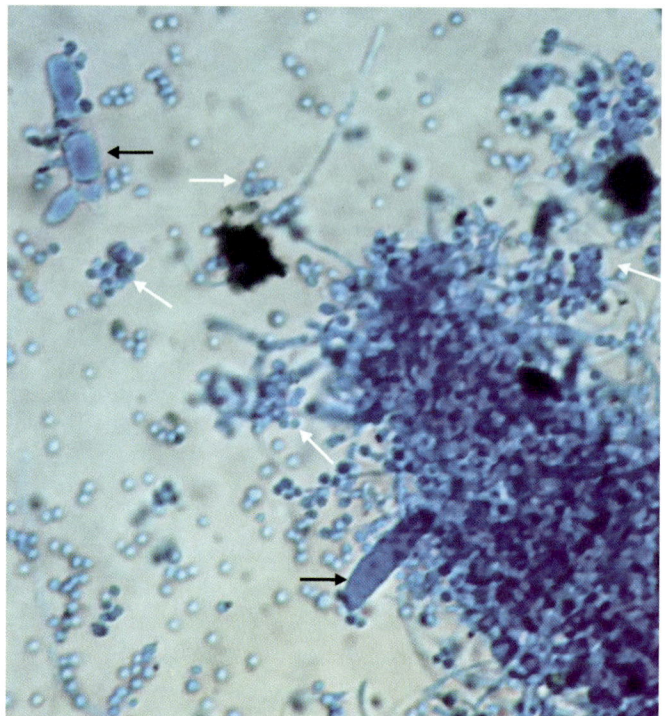

Fig. 1.80: *Trichophyton mentagrophytes.* Abundant globose microconidia in clusters (en grappe, white arrow) and two cigar-shaped macroconidia (black arrow) are seen [LPCB mount ×400].

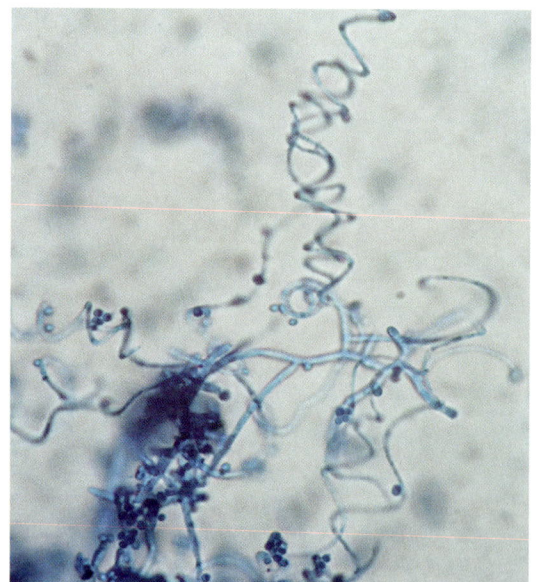

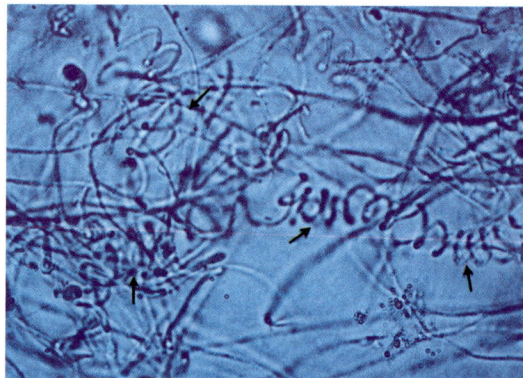

Fig. 1.82: *Trichophyton mentagrophytes.* Only the spiral hyphae (white arrow) are predominant in this strain [LPCB mount ×400].

morphology. Scalp infections are uncommon and hair is rarely invaded. In scalp infection involving hair, ectothrix and endothrix conidia are important features which are nonfluorescent as well.

Fig. 1.81: *T. mentagrophytes.* Presence of spiral hyphae is characteristic [LPCB mount ×400].

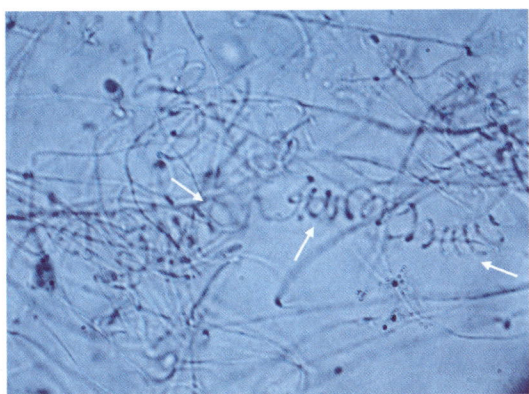

Fig. 1.83: *Trichophyton mentagrophytes* var. *mentagrophytes*. Spiral hyphae (white arrow) are the prominent feature observed in this strain [LPCB mount ×400].

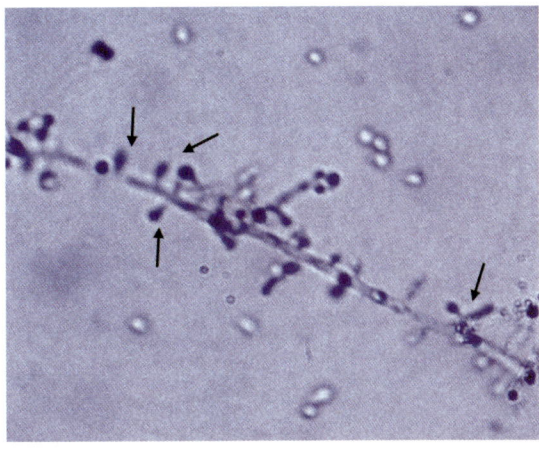

Fig. 1.85: *Trichophyton mentagrophytes* var. *quinckeanum*. Clavate microconidia (2–3 × 3–5 μ; black arrow) are produced lateral to the hyphae [LPCB mount ×400].

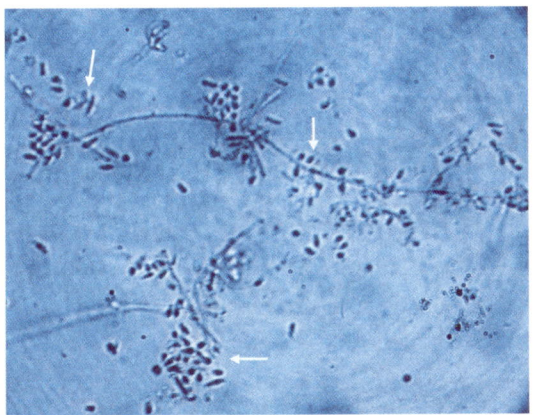

Fig. 1.84: *Trichophyton mentagrophytes* var. *quinckeanum*. Numerous clavate microconidia (white arrow) produced lateral to the hyphae [LPCB mount ×200].

Colony morphology

Obverse: Typical thallus is slow growing, downy white, generally devoid of conidia, and pigmented on the reverse. Other isolants are less cottony, less pigmented and produce numerous macroconidia. The conidiating strains usually come from inflammatory tinea corporis, tinea capitis, and granulomatous lesions (Figs 1.94 and 1.95).

Reverse: The typical pigment is an intense, nondiffusing, port wine or venous blood red.

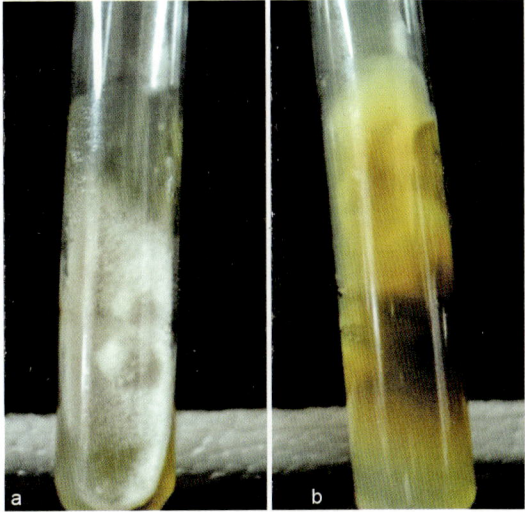

Fig. 1.86: Colony morphology of *Trichophyton mentagrophytes* (nodular variant) grown on SDCA after 2 weeks of incubation at 28°C; (a) obverse, (b) reverse.

Pigment is slow in developing and is usually first noted on the edge of the colony in agar slants where the media is dried. Some strains, particularly those from patients on griseofulvin therapy, fail to show pigment.

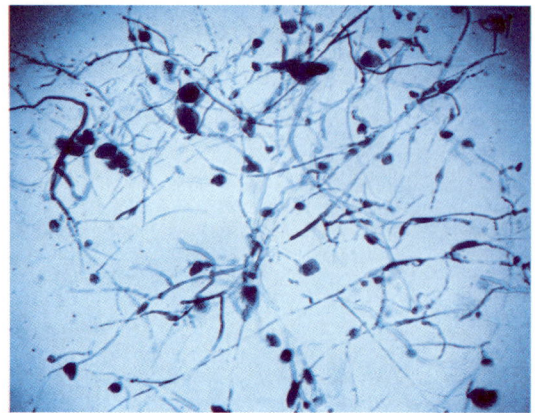

Fig. 1.87: *Trichophyton mentagrophytes* (nodular variant). Nodular bodies of varied size and shapes are seen in clusters or in discrete manner on the vegetative hyphae [LPCB mount ×200].

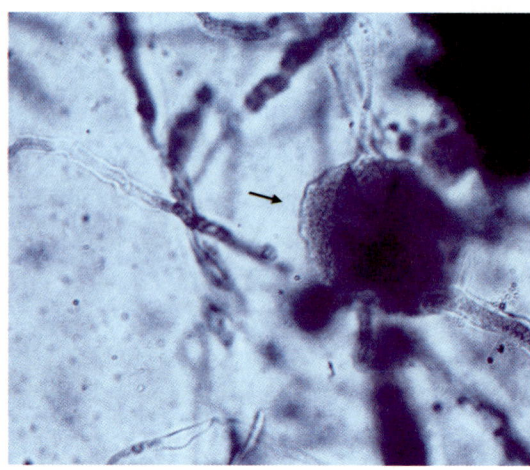

Fig. 1.89: A magnified view of 'nodular body' (black arrow) produced on the vegetative hyphae in *Trichophyton mentagrophytes* (nodular variant) [LPCB mount ×600].

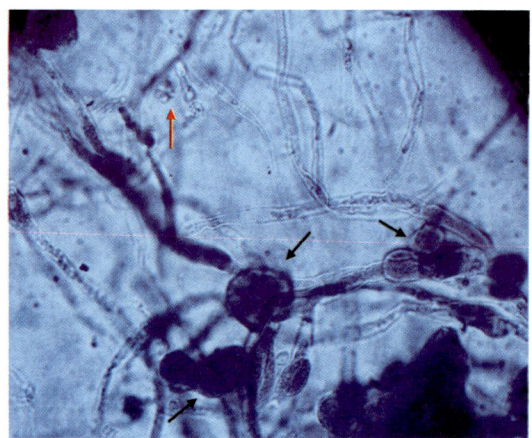

Fig. 1.88: Nodular variant of *Trichophyton mentagrophytes*. Several nodular bodies (knot-like structures; black arrow) are formed on the vegetative hyphae. Globose microconidia are produced in grape-like clusters (en grappe; red arrow) occasionally, which is the most consistent feature of *T. mentagrophytes*. Other features of this species are absent in this type [LPCB mount ×400].

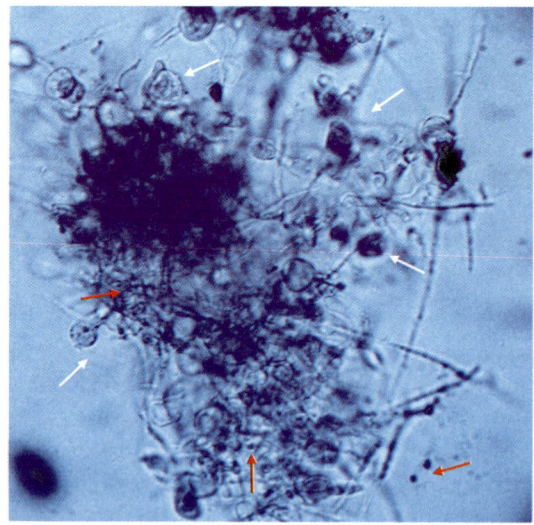

Fig. 1.90: *Trichophyton mentagrophyte* var *interdigitale*. Abundant chlamydoconidia are produced (white arrow). Massed microconidia (red arrow) are also seen but macroconidia are usually absent [LPCB mount ×400].

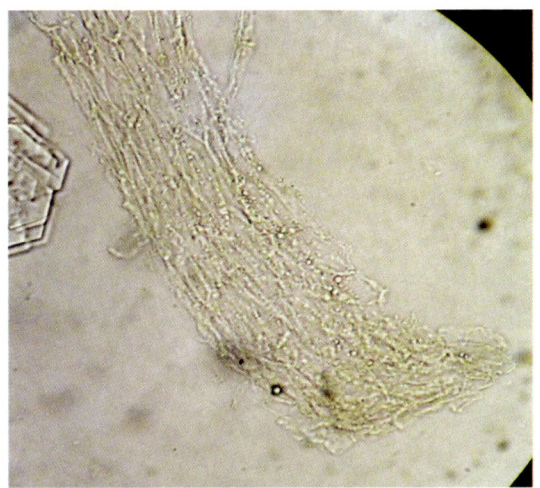

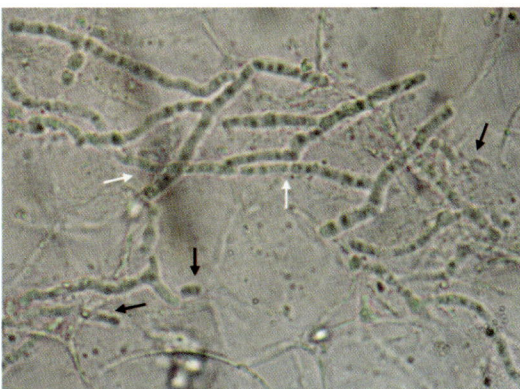

Fig. 1.91: Potassium hydroxide mount of nail from tinea unguium. Refractile, branching, septate hyphae are seen. *T. rubrum* ×400.

Fig. 1.93: Dermatophyte in epidermis. Older hyphae with numerous septations (white arrow) and barrel-shaped arthroconidia (black arrow) of *Trichophyton rubrum* are seen (KOH mount ×600).

Pigment production on special media, negative urease test and lack of *in vitro* hair perforating organs differentiates *T. rubrum* from *T. mentagrophytes.* Potato dextrose agar or cornmeal agar are superior to Sabouraud's agar for the observation of red pigment in *T. rubrum.*

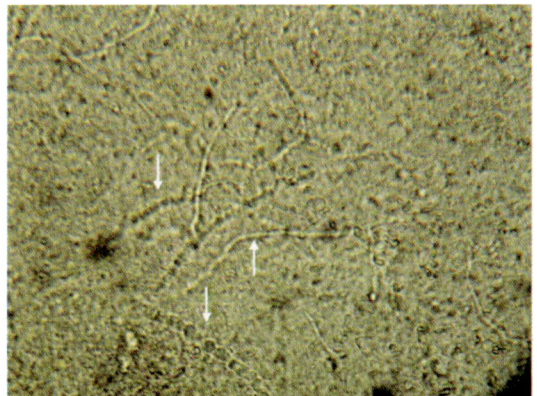

Fig. 1.92: Invasion of epidermis by dermatophytes. *Trichophyton rubrum.* Characteristic septate hyphae (white thin arrow) and arthroconidia (white thick arrow) are seen [KOH mount ×400].

Microscopic morphology

The common isolants of *T. rubrum* produce a few conidia. There are clavate "tear drop" microconidia (2 to 3 × 3 to 5 μ) produced lateral to the hyphae (Figs 1.95 and 1.96). Clusters of conidia in an arborescent or "pine tree" arrangement are seen (Fig. 1.97). Macroconidia are absent or rare except in granular conidiating strains. These macroconidia are long, narrow, fusiform (pencil shaped) multicelled and often develop in groups directly from hyphae.

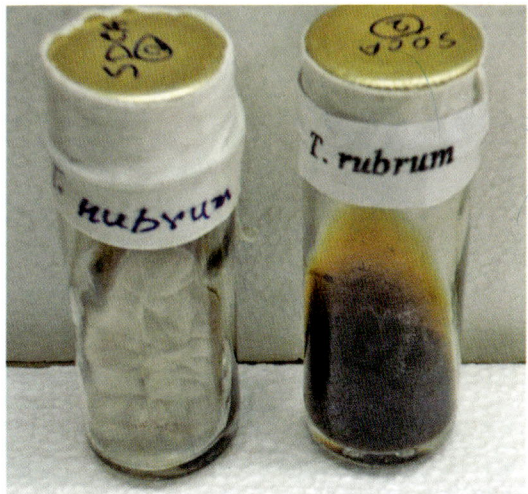

Fig. 1.94: Colony morphology of *T. rubrum* grown on Sabouraud's agar for 3 weeks at 30°C (both obverse and reverse).

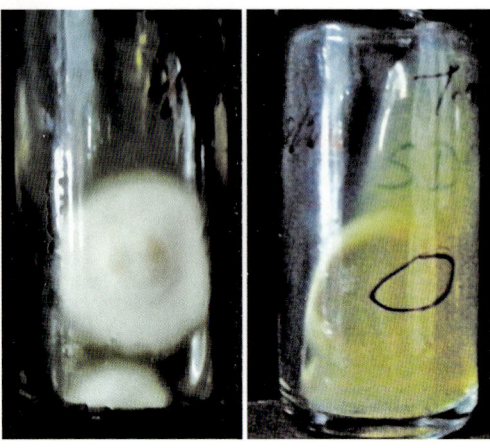

Fig. 1.95: a. Obverse: *Trichophyton rubrum* showing fluffy white mycelium; b. Reverse: *T. rubrum* showing reverse demonstration of wine red pigment.

Trichophyton tonsurans

This is another species that varies particularly in colour, texture and morphology of the thallus. It is anthropophilic, endothrix, and nonfluorescent in infected hair.

Colony morphology

Obverse: There are four common colonial forms: Crateriform, cerebreform, plicatile and flat. Most frequently isolated strains show a flat growth initially which is powdery and yellow tinged. The colony develops into a folded thallus (plicate), with a grayish to buff

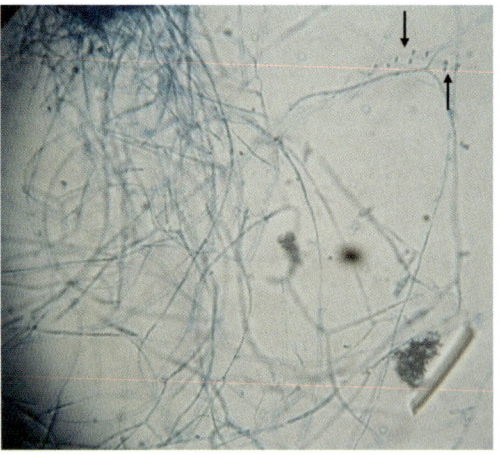

Fig. 1.96: *T. rubrum*. Clavate (tear drop) *macroconidia* are produced lateral to the hyphae [LPCB mount ×200].

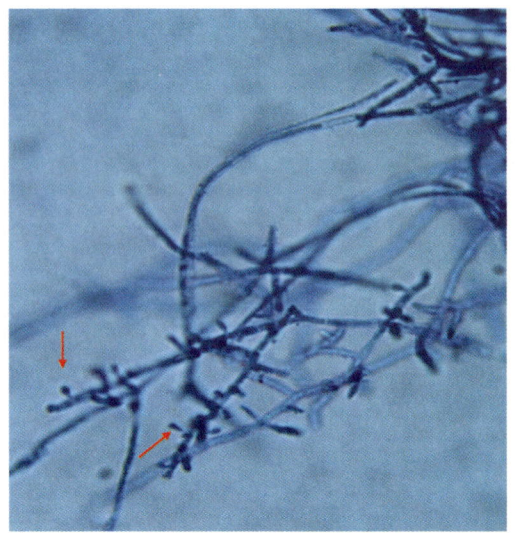

Fig. 1.97: *T. rubrum*. Clavate (tear drop) microconidia are produced lateral to the hyphae [LPCB ×400].

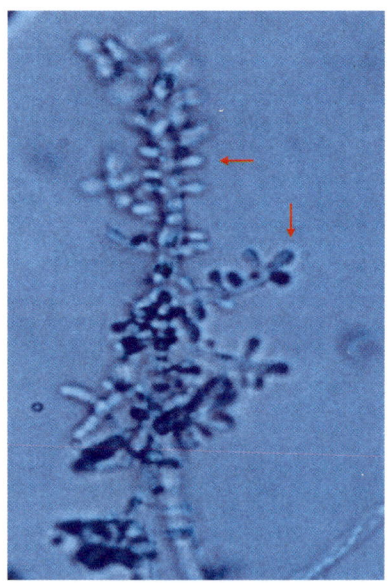

Fig. 1.98: *T. rubrum*. Clusters of 'pear-shaped' microconidia in an arborescent arrangement [LPCB mount ×400].

suedelike surface. The most common type among the isolates of rural Bengal is buff colour granular colonies (Fig. 1.99).

Reverse: The colony reverse is most frequently yellow brown to reddish brown. *Trichophyon*

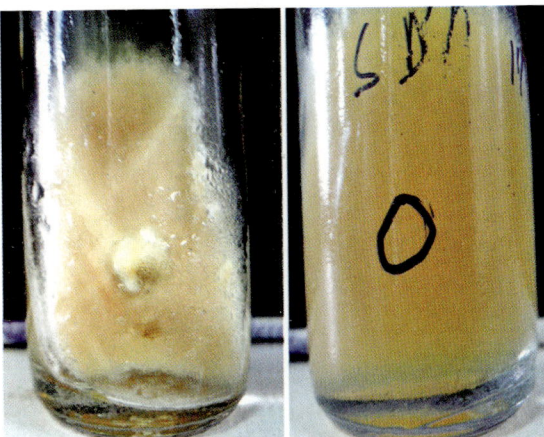

Fig. 1.99: *Trichophyton tonsurans.* Colony grown on Sabouraud's dextrose agar is light buff to tan or white in colour, flat, granular and with spreading margin. The reverse is colourless to pale yellow.

tonsurans unlike *Trichophyton rubrum* does not produce deep colour on cornmeal agar or potato dextrose agar.

Microscopic morphology

Trichophyton tonsurans produce abundant clavate to tear drop shaped microconidia that vary greatly in size. Their size is 2 to 5 × 3 to 7 μ. They are produced laterally on undifferentiated hyphae or on simple conidiophores. A characteristic feature is the tendency of some microconidia to enlarge and appear like clustered balloons (Fig. 1.104). A few macroconidia, irregular in shape and with thick walls may be produced (Fig. 1.103). Chlamydoconidia and large arthroconidia may also be seen.

Trichophyton schoenleinii

Trichophyton schoenleinii is an anthropophilic species and typically causes favus, which is characterized by large inverted cones of hyphae and arthrospores in the mouth of hair follicles (scutula) and inepidermal crusts. Favus in the scalp causes permanent alopecia in the scarred areas. Favus may occur on any part of the body, including the nails. Hair invasion is endothrix type, and the longitudinal tunnels it produces within the hair shaft are filled with air bubbles after

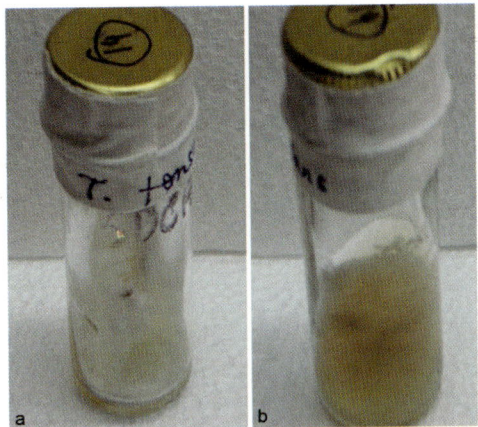

Fig. 1.100: Colony morphology of *Trichophyton tonsurans* grown on Sabouraud's dextrose agar at 30°C for 3 weeks; (a) obverse, (b) reverse.

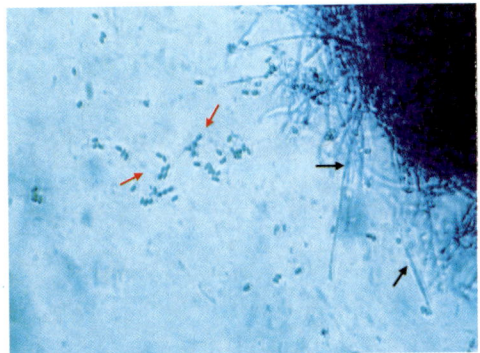

Fig. 1.101: *Trichophyton tonsurans.* Abundant clavate to tear shaped microconidia are produced that vary greatly in size (red arrow). Hyphae are usually thin (white arrow). [LPCB mount ×200]

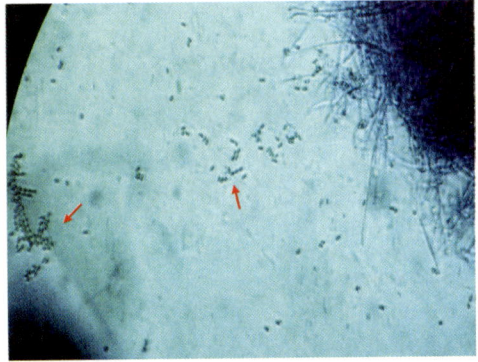

Fig. 1.102: Clusters of tear-shaped microconidia (red arrow) are seen. *Trichophyton tonsurans* [LPCB mount ×400].

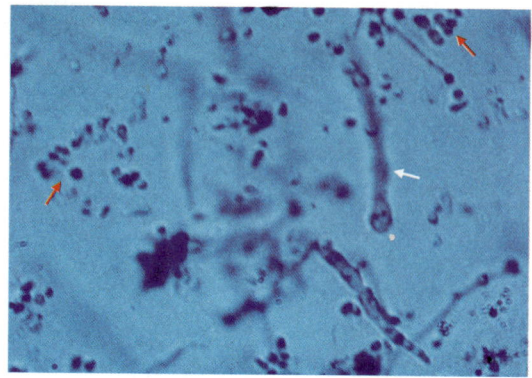

Fig. 1.103: *Trichophyton tonsurans.* Some micro-conidia enlarge to produce 'clustered balloons' (red arrow). A few macroconidia, irregular in shape, having thick walls may be produced in some strains (white arrow) [LPCB mount ×400].

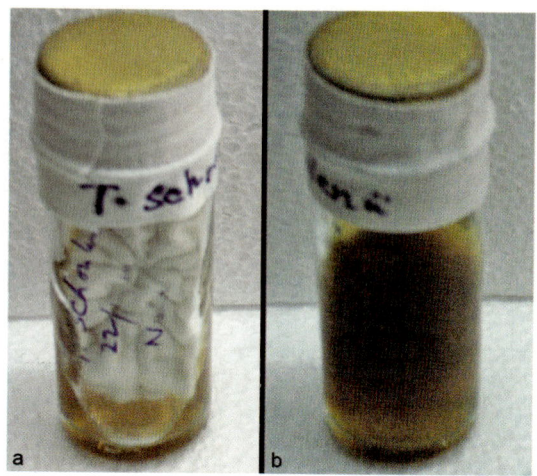

Fig. 1.105: Colonies of *Trichophyton schoenleinii* grown on Sabouraud's dextrose agar at 30°C for 5 weeks; (a) obverse (b) reverse.

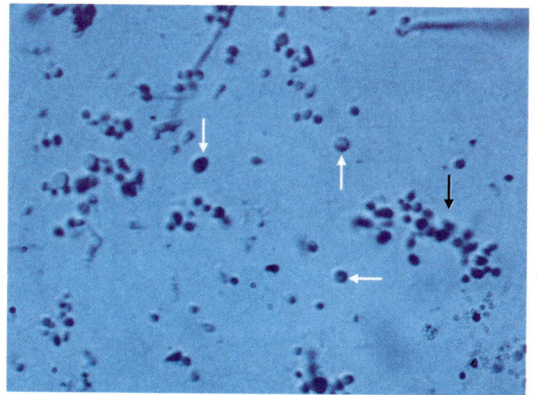

Fig. 1.104: *T. tonsurans.* Some microconidia show balloon swelling (white arrow); clustered balloons (black arrow) are characteristic feature of *T. tonsurans* [LPCB mount ×400].

degeneration of the hyphae. Arthroconidia are a few or absent within the hair shaft.

T. schoenleinii grows well at 37°C and does not require special nutritional factors for growth.

Colony morphology

Obverse: *Trichophyton schoenleinii* grows slowly and produces glabrous to waxy or suedelike off-white colonies with raised centres (1 to 4 µm) and irregularly folded surface (Fig. 1.104). There are gentle folds

(faviform) but the colony may become very distorted and convoluted, rising off the agar surface or into it, causing cracking and splitting. Freshly isolated strains may produce almost yeast like colonies but become more mycelial and downy when maintained in the laboratory. The margin of the colony mostly consists of submerged mycelium.

Reverse: The underside is usually colourless to light yellow.

Microscopic morphology

Macro and microconidia are not produced but characteristic antler-like terminal hyphal branching (**favic chandelier**) is seen in the submerged growth. The antler-like hyphae are also observed in other slow growing dermatophytes. The characteristic of *T. schoenleinii* is the swollen hyphal tips (**nail head**) (Figs 1.106—1.108).

Trichophyton verrucosum

Colony morphology

Obverse: The colony is very slow growing, slightly folded, heaped, glabrous, gray white (Fig. 1.109). This morphology is referred to as the var. *album*, yellow, glabrous colony and var. *discoides* has a flat gray white thallus. Growth is enhanced at 37°C and also when

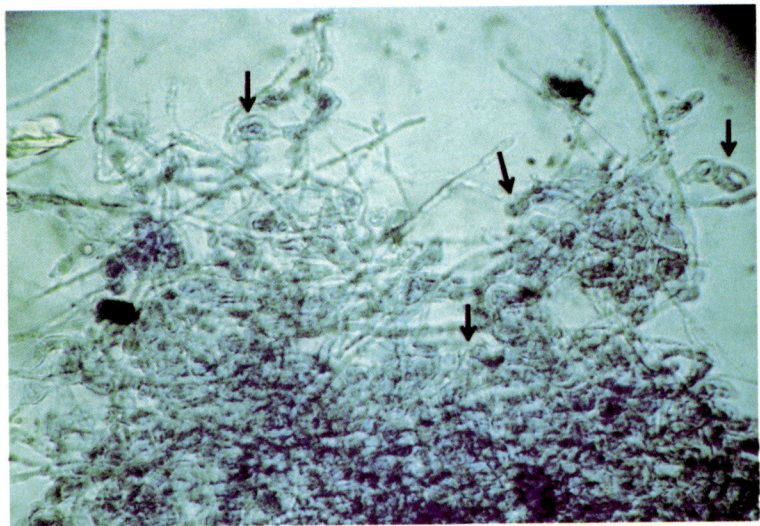

Fig. 1.106: *Trichophyton schoenleinii*. Macro or microconidia are not produced. Swollen hyphal tips (nailhead hyphae; black arrow) are characteristic of *T. schoenleinii* [LPCB mount ×400].

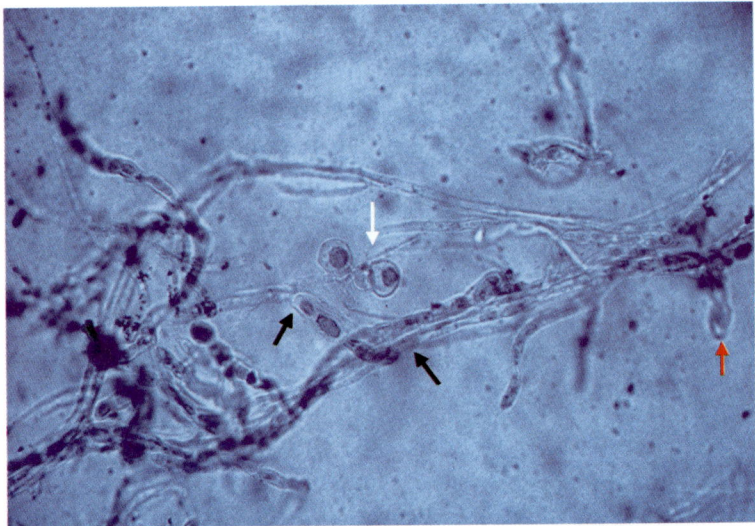

Fig. 1.107: *Trichophyton schoenleinii*. Irregular hyphal swelling (black arrow), swollen hyphal tips (red arrow) and chlamydoconidia (white arrow) are quite characteristic [LPCB mount ×600].

medium is enriched with thiamine and inositol.

Reverse: No characteristic pigment is produced on the reverse.

Microscopic morphology

On unenriched media, distorted hyphae are seen with some suggestions of antler-like branching similar to that of *T. schoenleinii*. No conidia are produced. On enriched media clavate macroconidia and rarely elongate fusiform or the characteristic 'rat tail' macroconidia are produced (Fig. 1.110). These have 3 to 5 cells and sometimes are shaped like a string beans. **At 37°C the fungus grows as a chain of chlamydoconidia** (Figs 1.112 and 1.113).

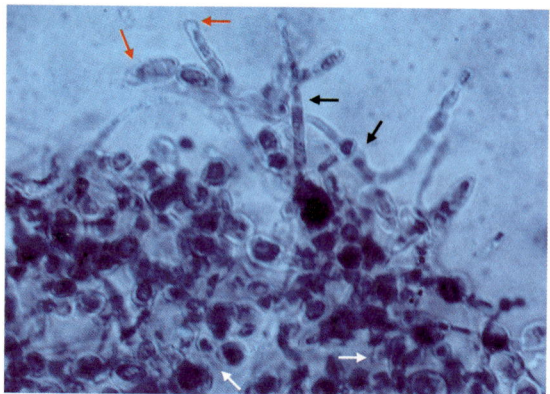

Fig. 1.108: *T. schoenleinii.* Abundant chlamydoconidia (white arrow) are produced in old culture. Swollen hyphal tips (nail head; red arrow) and irregular hyphal swelling (black arrow) are characteristics of this species [LPCB mount ×600].

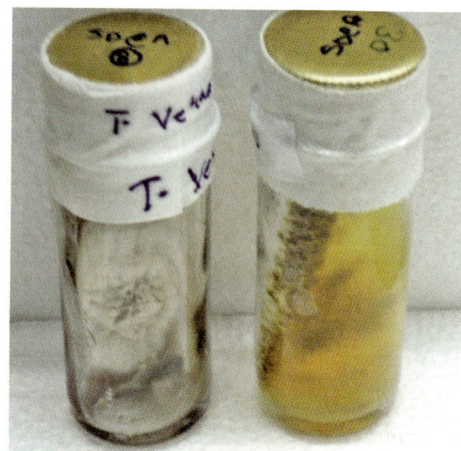

Fig. 1.109: Colony morphology of *Trichophyton verrucosum* grown on Sabouraud's agar for 4 weeks at 30°C (both obverse and reverse).

Trichophyton soudanense

Trichophyton soudanense is an anthropophilic species. ***T. soudanense*** mainly causes tinea capitis and associated tinea corporis. Invasion of hair is endothrix type.

Colony morphology
Obverse: *T. soudanense* produces slow-growing, yellow to apricot coloured, flat-to-folded colonies with fringed or raylike radiating margins. The surface texture of the colony is leathery and readily develops cottony tufts (Fig. 1.114).

It does not survive refrigeration and does not require any growth factors.

Reverse: Usually deep yellow but there is also a violet variant.

Microscopic morphology
Round chlamydoconidia, short, segmented hyphae (arthroconidia), reflexive or right-angle

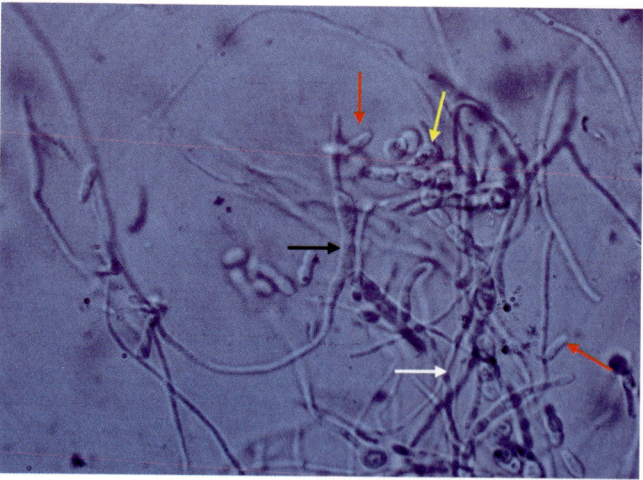

Fig. 1.110: *Trichophyton verrucosum.* Elongate to fusiform characteristic 'Rat tail macroconidia' (white arrow) are produced. Sometimes these are shaped like a 'string bean' (black arrow). Clavate microconidia (red arrow) are produced on enriched medium. Chains of chlamydoconidia are also noticed (yellow arrow) [LPCB mount ×600].

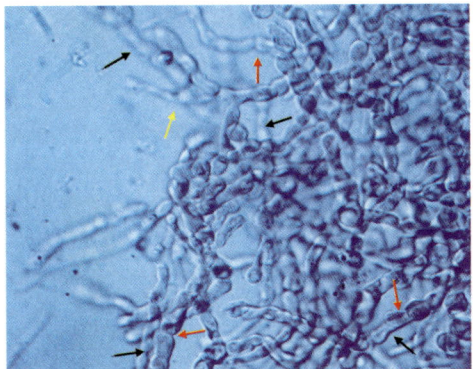

Fig. 1.111: Peridial hyphae of *Trichophyton verrucosum*. Hyphae are dichotomously branched (green arrow) and the cells are constricted at the septa (red arrow) and also constriction are seen at the centre of each cell (black arrow) [LPCB mount ×600].

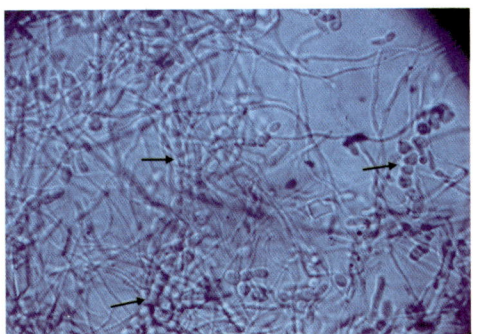

Fig. 1.112: *Trichophyton verrucosum*. Chains of chlamydoconidia (black arrow) are produced at 37°C [LPCB mount ×600].

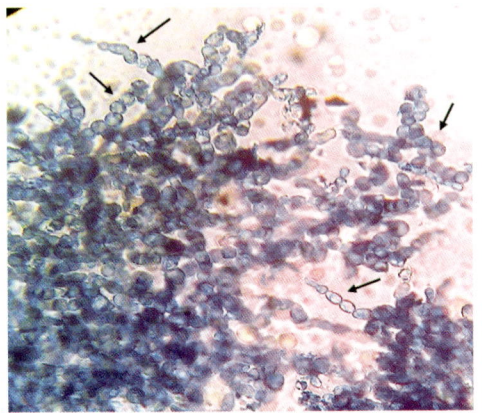

Fig. 1.113: *Trichophyton verrucosum*. Chains of chlamydoconidia are produced (in a different strain shown here) at 37°C [LPCB mount × 600].

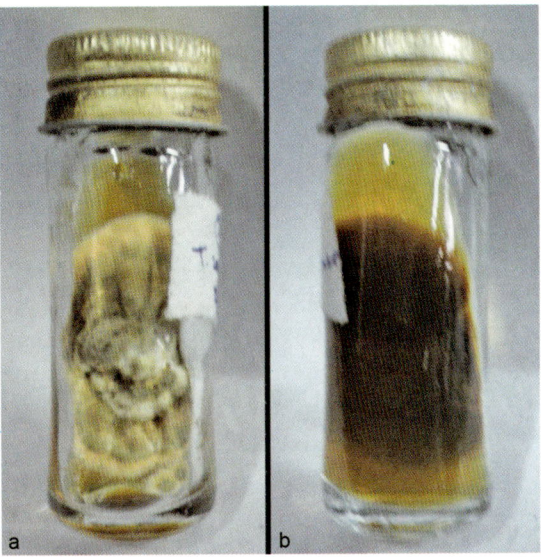

Fig. 1.114: Colony morphology of *Trichophyton soudanense* grown on Sabouraud's dextrose agar at 30°C for 3 weeks; (a) obverse, (b) reverse.

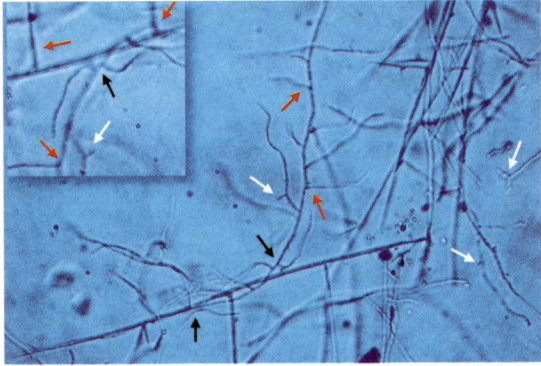

Fig. 1.115: *Trichophyton soudanense*. Macroconidia are not produced. Microconidia may be found directly on the hyphae (white arrow). Reflexive (backward growing; black arrow) or right angle branching hyphae (red arrow) and segmented hyphae are diagnostic features of this species [LPCB mount ×400].

branching mycelium that are branched into bushlike bundle are seen on microscopic examination. Pyriform microconidia are formed laterally on the mycelium occasionally (Fig. 1.115).

Trichophyton violaceum

Trichophyton violaceum is an anthropophilic fungus that primarily causes tinea capitis. It also causes tinea corporis and tinea unguium. Invasion of hair is endothrix type, and abundant arthroconidia inside the hair shaft causes the hair to curl, burst, or crumble. The broken hairs produce black dots or a 'chicken skin' effect on the scalp.

T. violaceum grows better when **thiamine** is added to the medium. **Cultures do not survive in the refrigerator.**

Colony morphology

Obverse: *T. violaceum* is very slow growing, a conical or verrucous (faviform) thallus that is heaped up, folded, glabrous or waxy, and deep violet in colour (Fig. 1.116). The organism rapidly becomes pleomorphic, sectoring as pale to white mycelia that quickly overgrow the original colony. Old stock cultures become flat, white and fluffy (Fig. 1.117).

Reverse: The purple pigment that stains the mycelium is also found on the underside.

Microscopic morphology

Distorted hyphae and the lack of conidia are typical of strains grown on the usual media. The hyphae contains cytoplasmic granules (Figs 1.118 and 1.119). The aerial hyphae may show thick-walled elements that resemble the macroconidia of *T. rubrum*. Clavate macroconidia are a few in number and pyriform microconidia may be produced on media enriched by the addition of thiamine.

Trichophyton concentricum

Trichophyton concentricum is a strictly anthropophilic species with restricted geographic distribution. It causes tinea imbricata (tokalau). Tinea imbricata is chronic and the lesions are characterized by concentric rings of epidermal scales attached along the proximal edges. *T. concentricum* does not invade hair. The growth *in vitro* is stimulated by the addition of

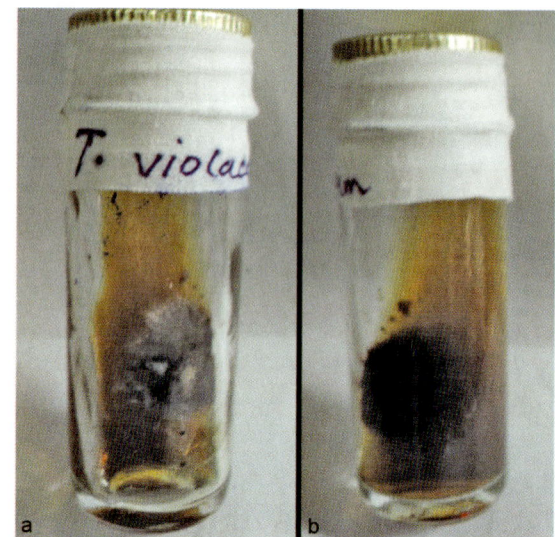

Fig. 1.116: Colonies of *Trichophyton violaceum* grown on neutral Sabouraud's agar at 30°C for 2 weeks; (a) obverse, (b) reverse.

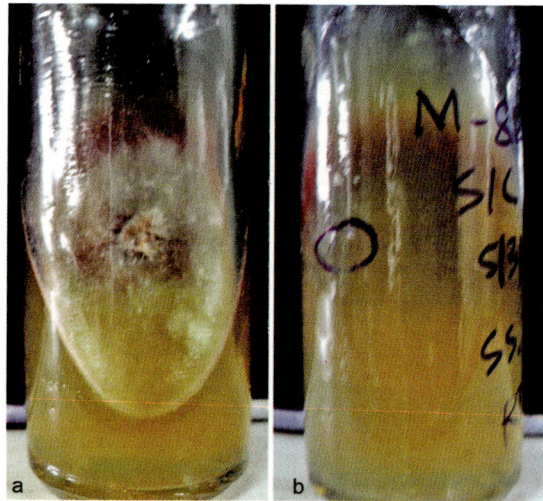

Fig. 1.117: *Trichophyton violaceum*. Colony becomes pleomorphic with ageing, sectoring as pale to white mycelia occurs which quickly overgrow the original colony; (a) obverse, (b) reverse.

thiamine to the medium in about 50% of the isolates.

Colony morphology

Obverse: *Trichophyton concentricum* grows slowly on Sabouraud's dexrtose agar and

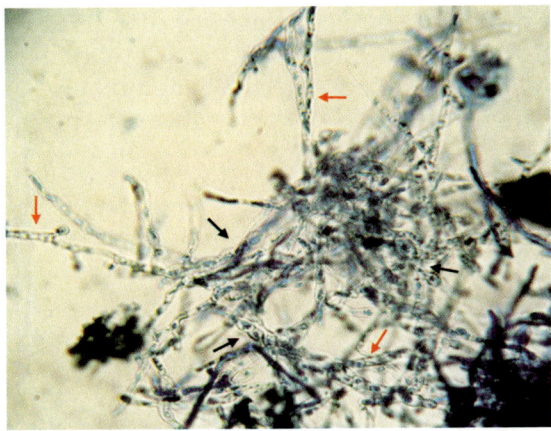

Fig. 1.118: *Trichophyton violaceum*. Distorted hyphae (black arrow) and lack of conidia are typical of *T. violaceum*. The hyphae contains cytoplasmic granules (red arrow) [LPCB mount ×400].

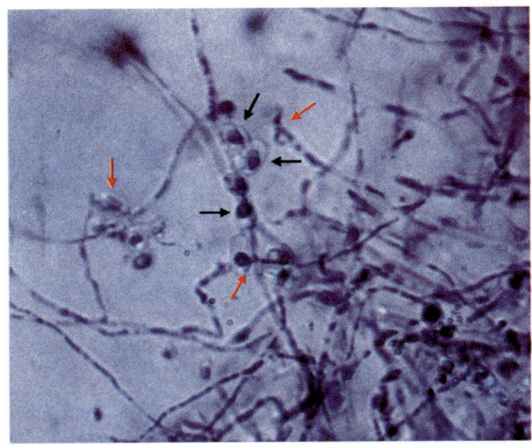

Fig. 1.120: Hyphal distortion (red arrow) and cytoplasmic granules (black arrow) are seen. *Trichophyton violaceum* [LPCB mount ×400].

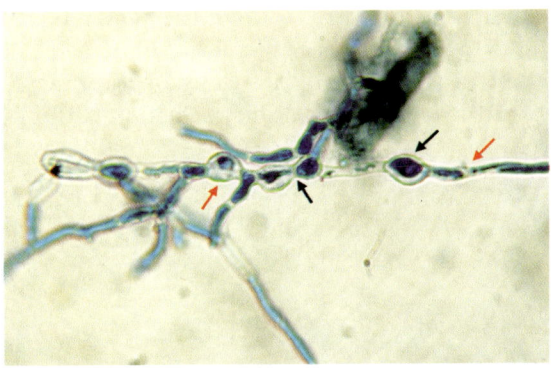

Fig. 1.119: *Trichophyton violaceum*. Distorted hyphae (black arrow) and hyphal cytoplasmic granules (red arrow) are characteristics of *T. violaceum* [LPCB mount ×400].

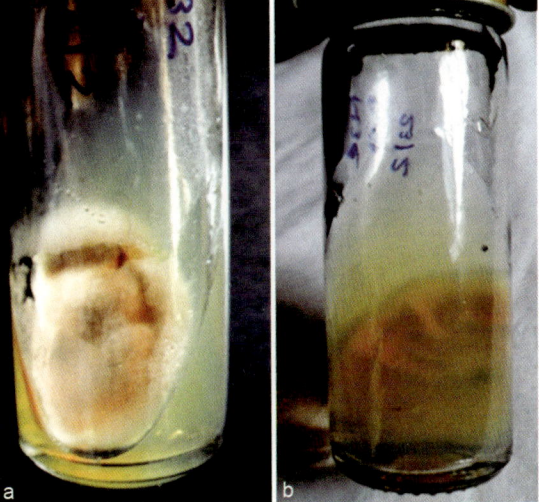

Fig. 1.121: Colonies of *Trichophyton concentricum* grown on Sabouraud's dextrose agar at 30°C for four weeks. Colonies are white and glabrous at first, gradually become deeply folded, convoluted and the colour changes to cream, amber to orange-brown. The reverse is yellowish brown; (a) obverse, (b) reverse.

produces a heaped up highly folded colony covered with a short gray hyphae. The colour of the colony is white, yellowish brown to orange brown. A fuzzy or velvety growth of aerial mycelium may occur (Fig. 1.121).

Reverse: The underside of the colony is usually yellowish brown in colour.

Microscopic morphology
Tangled or highly branching hyphae are seen without macro or microconidia. The terminally branching hyphae usually lack swollen nailhead ends which are typical of *T. schoenleinii*. Chlamydoconidia appears in clusters in old culture (Figs 1.122 and 1.123).

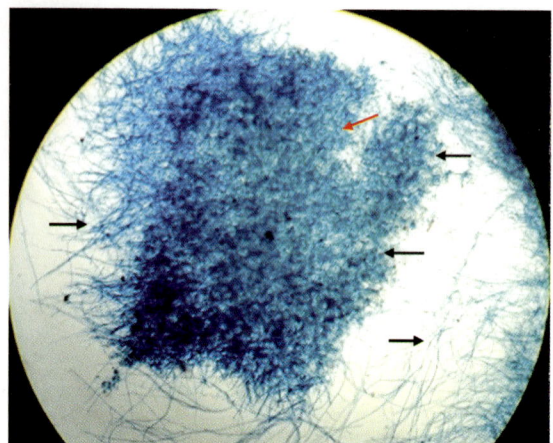

Fig. 1.122: *Trichophyton concentricum.* Microscopic morphology shows thin, highly branching and tangled hyphae (white arrow) without any macro or microconidia. Numerous chlamydoconidial found in clusters (black arrow) and sheets (red arrow) are produced in old culture [LPCB mount ×200].

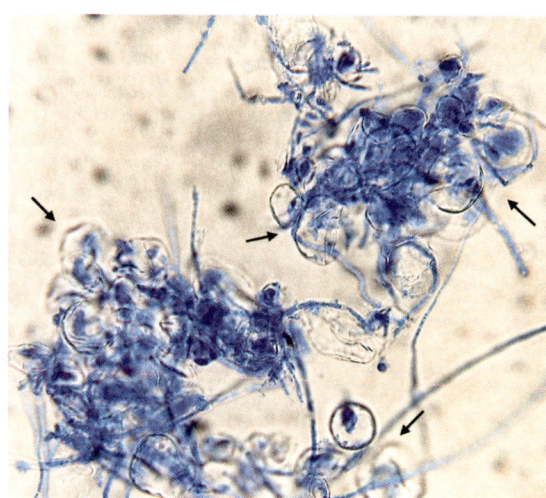

Fig. 1.123: *Trichophyton concentricum.* Macroconidia and microconidia are usually absent but chlamydoconidia (black arrow) appears in clusters in old culture. [LPCB mount ×400].

Trichophyton simii

Trichophyton simii is a geophilic species that is a frequent cause of ringworm in monkeys, chickens and other animals in India. It causes occasional tinea corporis in humans who

contract this fungus from infected animals. It has been isolated regularly from soil and small mammals. It causes an ecto-endothrix type of hair invasion.

Colony morphology

Obverse: The fungus grow rapidly, a flat granular colony with a central umbo. Buff is the usual colour, but it varies from cream to white (Figs 1.124 and 1.125).

Reverse: In time the colony may have a pigmented undersurface. The colour is usually vinaceous (red brown), but may range from yellow to madder rose.

Microscopic morphology

Macroconidia are usually produced in great abundance. They are thin-walled, smooth and clavate, cylidriform or fusiform in shape and have four to ten septa. Conidia often occur in clusters (Fig. 1.126). The cells of the macroconidia frequently enlarge, become thick-

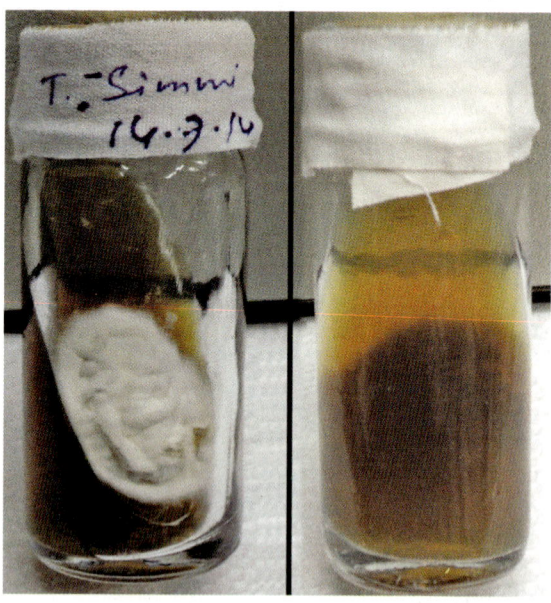

Fig. 1.124: *Trichophyton simii.* Colonies grown on SDCA are flat granular with central umbo. Colour of the colony varies from buff to cream to white. The undersurface is pigmented and usually vinaceous (red-brown).

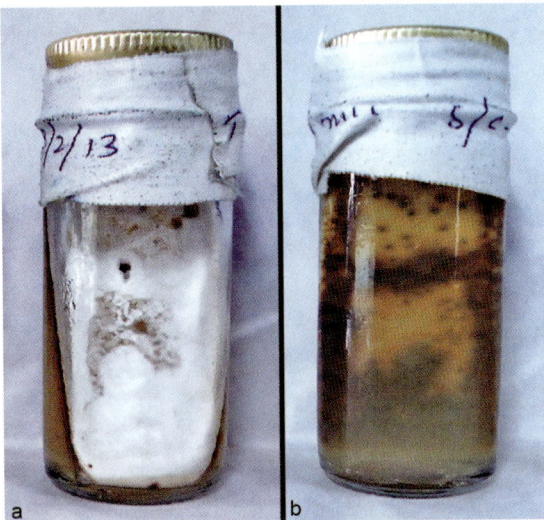

a   b

Fig. 1.125: *Trichophyton simii*. Flat, granular surface, white colonies with central umbo are produced on Sabouraud's dextrose agar at 30°C. Reverse is reddish brown pigmented.

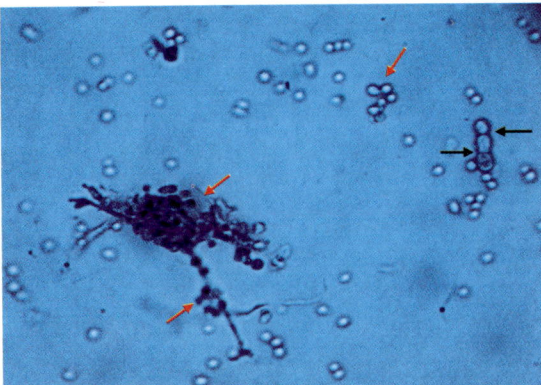

Fig. 1.127: *Trichophyton simii*. Macroconidia are thin walled, smooth and have prominent constriction at the septa (black arrow). Microconidia (red arrow) are clavate, elongate, pyriform or peg-shaped produced laterally on hyphae [LPCB mount ×400].

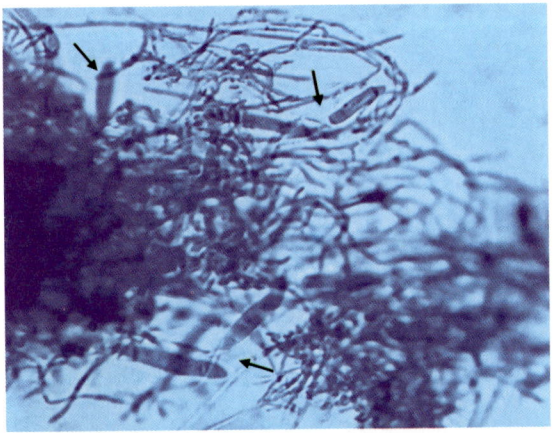

Fig. 1.126: *Trichophyton simii*. Macroconidia (black arrow) are produced in great abundance. They are thin walled, smooth and clavate, cylindriform or fusiform in shape and have three to ten septa. Macroconidia often occur in clusters [LPCB mount ×400].

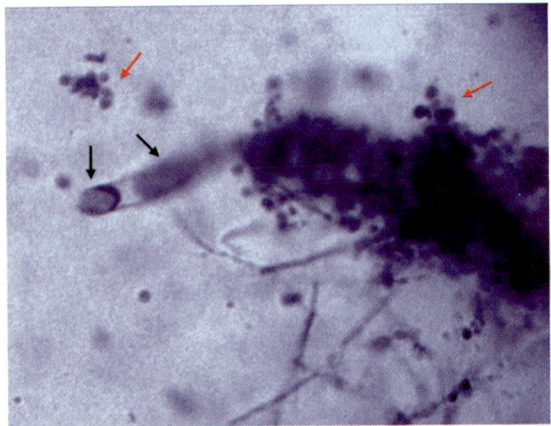

Fig. 1.128: *Trichophyton simii*. Macroconidia with endochlamydoconidia (black arrow). The cells of macroconidia enlarge, become thick-walled and termed 'endochlamydoconidia'. The cell between endochlamydoconidia are empty and ruptures. Microconidia (red arrow) are pyriform, clavate or peg-shaped [LPCB mount ×400].

walled and are termed **endochlamydoconidia.** The cells between the enlarged chlamydoconidia are often empty and rupture, causing fragmentation of the macroconidia. Clavate, elongate, pyriform or peg-shaped microconidia are produced laterally on hyphae (Figs 1.127 and 1.128).

Trichophyton equinum

Trichophyton equinum is a cosmopolitan zoophilic species frequently causing infection in horses and rarely in man. The isolates require nicotinic acid for growth. But isolate obtained in our laboratory grew on SDCA with normal environmental conditions without any nutritional supplement.

Colony morphology
The thallus is fluffy, resembling the var. *interdigitale* of *T. mentagrophytes*. Growth is rapid and flat but the colony may develop gentle folds. The colour is cream white to yellow. The revese is bright yellow changing to dark brown. This pigment may diffuse into the media (Fig. 1.129).

Microscopic morphology
Thin elongate to pyriform stalked micro-conidia are formed lateral along the hyphae (Figs 1.130 and 1.131). Macroconidia are similar to those of *T. mentagrophytes* and are rarely seen in cultures. They are fusiform or clavate.

Trichophyton ajelloi (Vanbreuseghem)

It is a very common soil keratinophilic fungus. It has been isolated rarely from 'tinea corporis'

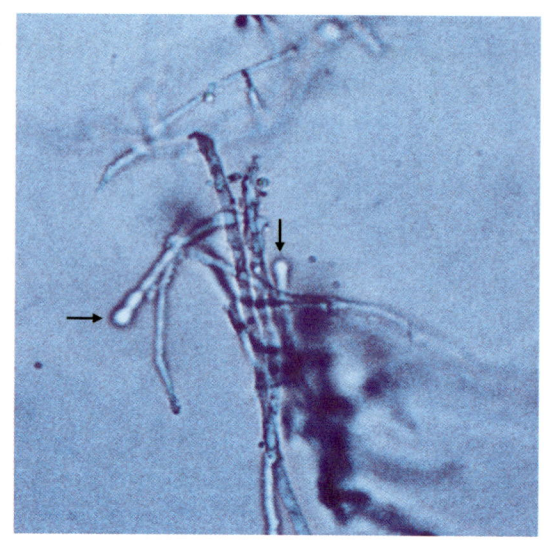

Fig. 1.130: *Trichophyton equinum.* Microconidia are thin, elongate to pyriform, formed laterally along the hyphae (black arrow). Macroconidia are rarely seen in culture [LPCB mount ×400].

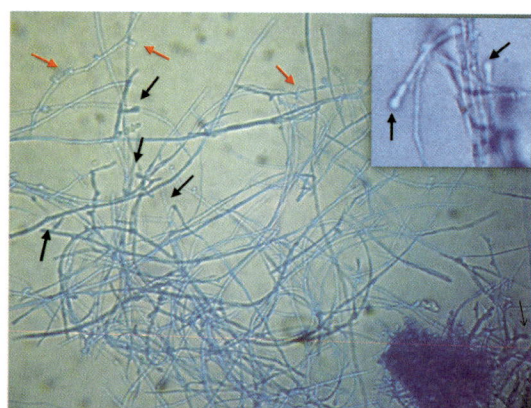

Fig. 1.131: *Trichophyton equinum.* Thin elongate to pyriform stalked microconidia are found laterally along the hyphae (black arrow). A few sessile microconidia are also seen (red arrow) but macroconidia are usually absent [LPCB mount ×200].

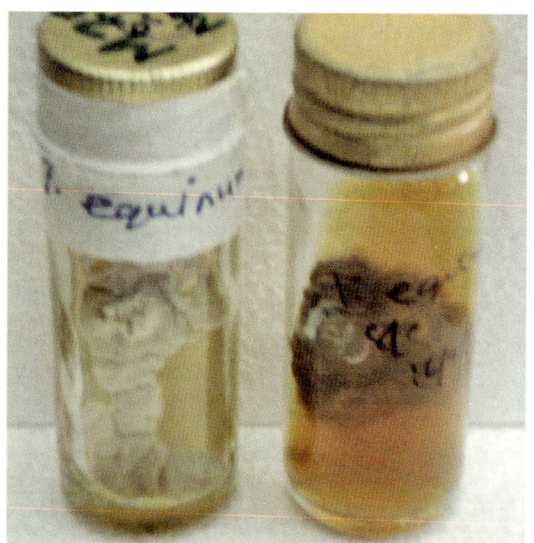

Fig. 1.129: Colony morphology of *Trichophyton equinum* grown on Sabouraud's agar for 3 weeks at 30°C (both obverse and reverse).

cases as documented in the literature. We had isolated it once from a 62 years old farmer, who was suffering from extensive tinea corporis for last two months. The lesions produced are often chronic and resemble psoriasis.

Colony morphology

The colony grows rapidly, producing a flat, thin powdery to downy, cream to yellowish orange thallus (Fig. 1.132). The reverse is usually colourless to light yellow.

Microscopic morphology

Thick walled, smooth macroconidia are numerous. They are fusiform to cylindrical in shape, elongate containing five to ten cells (Figs 1.133 and 1.134). Pyriform sessile microconidia are usually abundant.

Epidermophyton floccosum

This is an anthropophilic species. Chronic infections are uncommon so for maintenance of the species, rapid transmission within the population group is necessary. It is found particularly in tropics and subtropics.

Colony morphology

Colony grows slowly and it is frequently grainy, lumpy and sparse on initial isolation. The colony becomes folded, fuzzy or suede-like in texture when fully developed. The colour of the colony is characteristically khaki chartreuse in colour. Yellowish brown and white varients are also present. The underside is colourless to deep yellow (Figs 1.135 and 1.137).

Microscopic morphology

Characteristic macroconidia are beaver tail shaped or clavate, smooth thin walled and ususlly have two to three septa. The distal end of the macroconidia are round. These are produced abundant. Microconidia are absent (Figs 1.138 and 1.139).

Microsporum audouinii

Colony morphology

Obverse: *M. audouinii* grows slowly on modified Sabouraud's agar producing a flat, spreading, dense colony with a silky, furry, matted consistency and radiating edges (Fig. 1.142). The colour is white or gray to tan or rust buff.

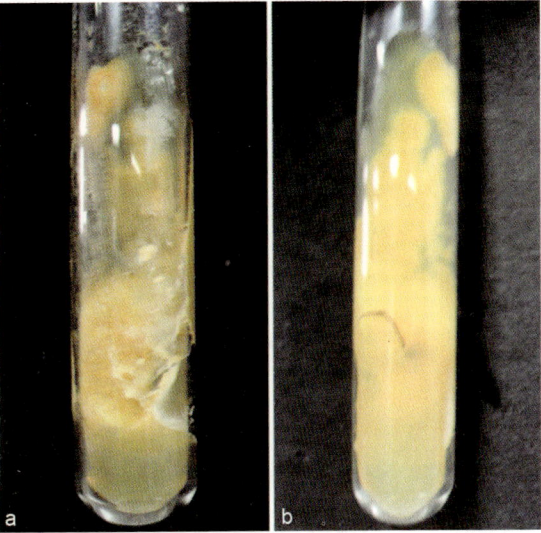

Fig. 1.132: *Trichophyton ajelloi.* Colonies grown on Sabouraud's dextrose agar are thin powdery to downy, cream to light yellowish initially and gradually changes to orange colour. Reverse is colourless to light yellow-orange; (a) obverse, (b) reverse.

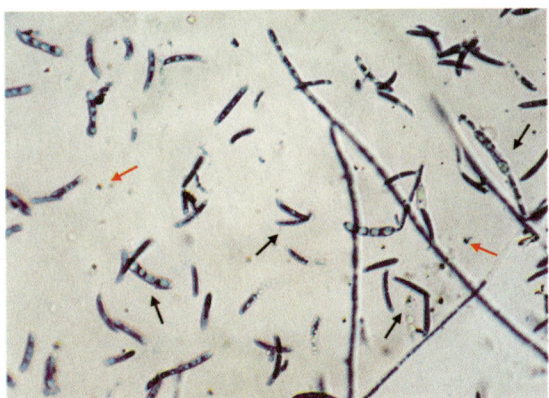

Fig. 1.133: Microscopic morphology of *Trichophyton ajelloi* shows numerous macroconidia (black arrow) which are fusiform to cylindrical in shape with thick, smooth walls. Microconidia (red arrow) are pyriform and fewer in number in this strain [LPCB mount ×200].

Reverse: Salmon rust or peach colour pigment is characteristically produced by *M. audouinii*. Many isolants, however, have a little or no pigment.

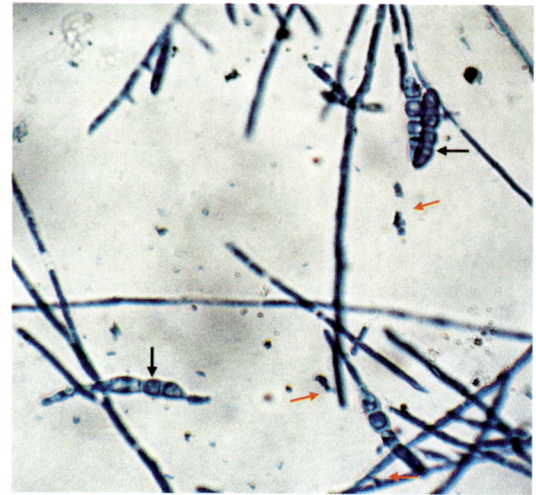

Fig. 1.134: *Trichophyton ajelloi.* Macroconidia (black arrow) are fusiform to cylindrical in shape, thick walled and smooth. Microconidia (red arrow) are pyriform or sessile but are not produced abundantly in this strain [LPCB mount ×400].

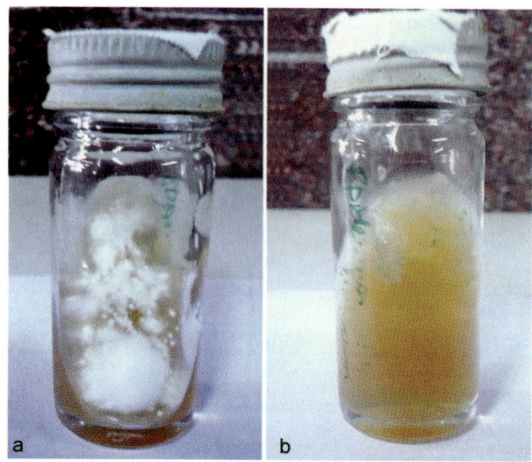

Fig. 1.136: *Epidermophyton floccosum.* Colonies grown on SDCA are white grainy, lumpy and sparse on initial isolation but become fuzzy when developed, in some strains. The reverse is colourless; (a) obverse, (b) reverse.

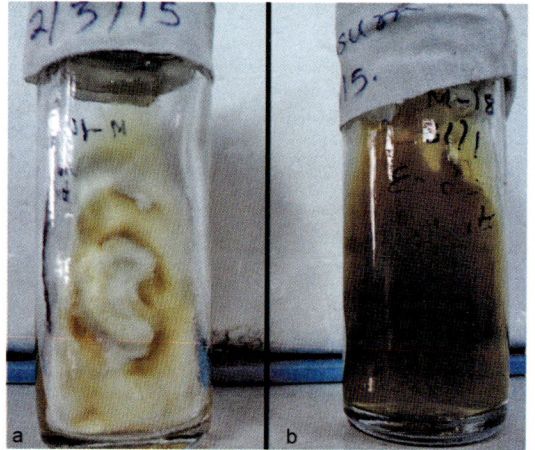

Fig. 1.135: *Epidermophyton floccosum.* Colony is gently folded, fuzzy or suede-like texture and is characteristically khaki in colour. White pleomorphic growth is seen to cover the surface. The underside is deep yellow-brown; (a) obverse, (b) reverse.

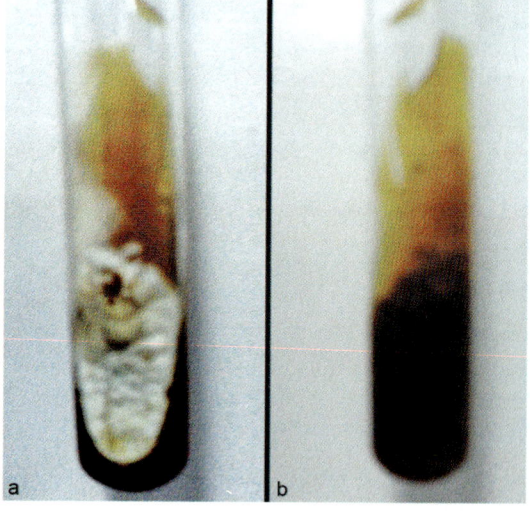

Fig. 1.137: Colony morphology of *Epidermophyton stockdaleae* grown on SDCA at 30°C for three weeks. The colony is gently folded, suede-like in texture and is white to khaki in colour. Reverse is deep yellow brown; (a) obverse, (b) reverse.

Microscopic morphology

Generally a few conidia are seen (Fig. 1.143). The usual microscopic examination shows thick-walled terminal or intercalary chlamydo- conidia that are fairly characteristic and permit identification of the culture. Terminal chlamydo-spores with a short nipple-like structure are

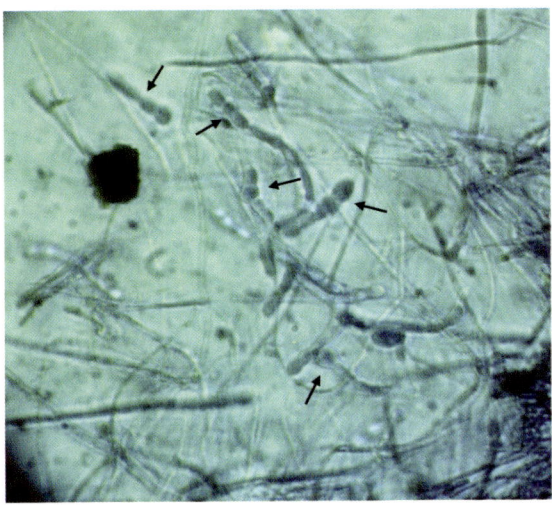

Fig. 1.138: *Epidermophyton floccosum*. Characteristic beaver tail-shaped, thin-walled macroconidia (black arrow) are usually abundant but microconidia are absent [LPCB mount ×400].

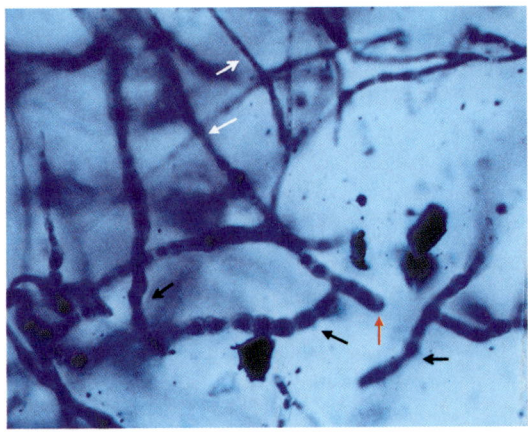

Fig. 1.140: *Epidermophyton stockdaleae*. Macroconidia (black arrow) are club-shaped with round ends (red arrow) and larger in size compared to *Epidermophyton floccosum*. These macroconidia have up to nine septa which are only two to three in *E. floccosum*. Microconidia are absent, white arrow shows normal hyphae [LPCB mount ×400].

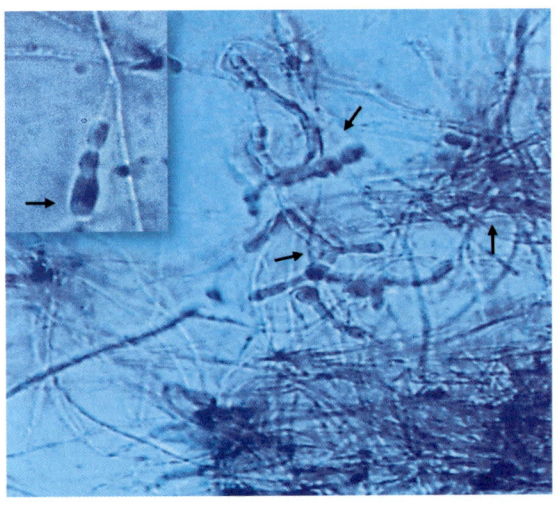

Fig. 1.139: *Epidermophyton floccosum*. Abundant macroconidia (black arrow) are produced which have broad base and round distal ends with smooth outer walls. Microconidia are not produced [LPCB mount ×400].

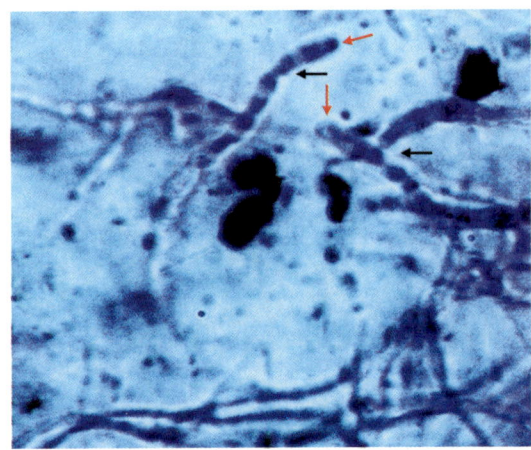

Fig. 1.141: Microscopic morphology of *Epidermophyton stockdaleae* showing macroconidia (black arrow) which are large club shaped, thin walled, having five to nine septa and ends are round (red arrow) [LPCB mount ×400].

usually present and serve as helpful diagnostic criteria (Figs 1.144 and 1.145). Racquet hyphae (hyphal cells with one end swollen), pectinate bodies (hyphal end resembling a comb) and rarely some irregular microconidia may be present. The macroconidia, if seen, are irregular spindle shaped or crooked, elongate, thick walled, and echinulate with a few or no septa (Fig. 1.146).

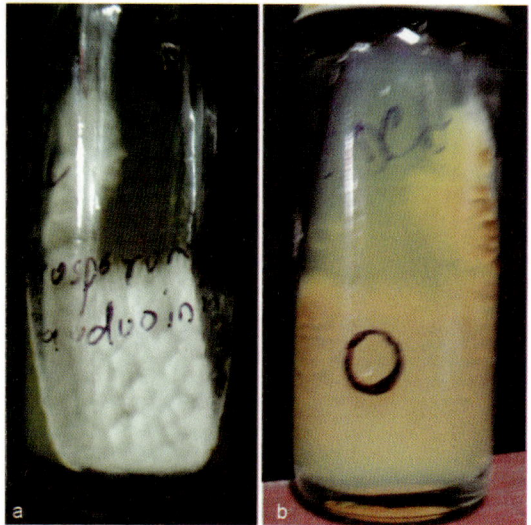

Fig. 1.142: *Microsporum audouinii.* Silky flat growth with pleomorphic tufts appear on SDCA. The reverse is salmon colour.

Microsporum ferrugineum

Colony morphology

Obverse: The growth is slow, forming a heaped folded, glabrous, reddish-yellow to orange-yellow thallus with a waxy surface. A fine velvety white overgrowth may occur occasionally.

Reverse: No characteristic pigment is seen.

Microscopic morphology

Distorted mycelium without conidia is the usual microscopic picture. Faviform, abnormal mycelial elements and coure hyphae with prominent crosswalls (bamboo hyphae) are seen (Figs 1.148–1.150).

Microsporum gypseum

Colony morphology

Obverse: Colonies grow rapidly, producing a flat, spreading, powdery surface that is rich cinnamon-buff to brown, occasionally with overtones of violet. The powder consists of masses of

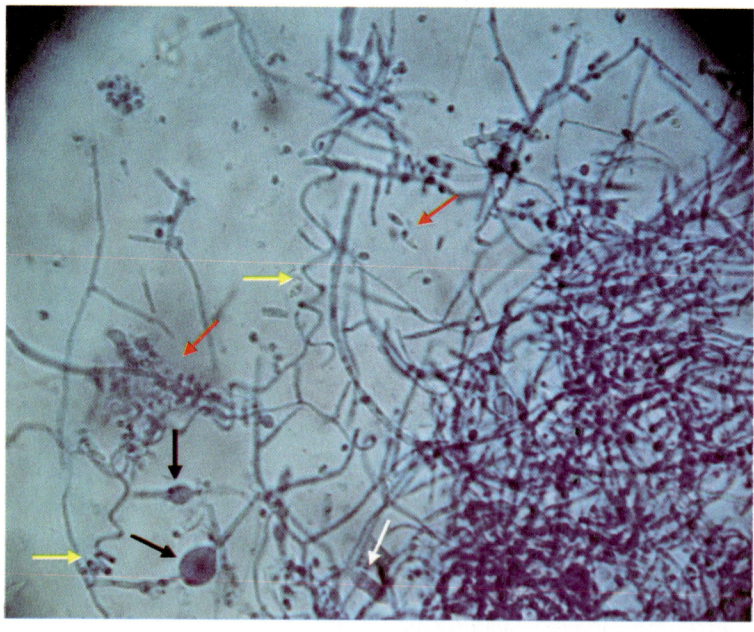

Fig. 1.143: *Microsporum audouinii.* Microscopic view showing hyphae and intercalary chlamydoconidia (black arrow), macroconidia (white arrow), spiral hyphae (yellow arrow) and plenty of microconidia (red arrow) [LPCB mount ×400].

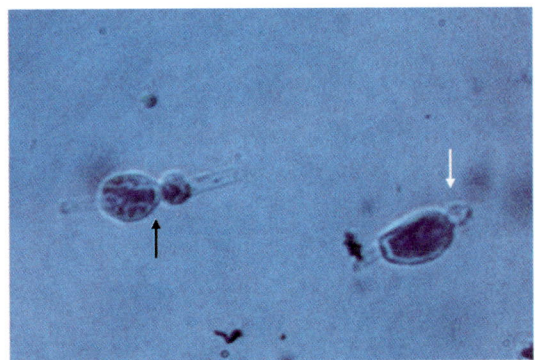

Fig. 1.144: Terminal chlamydoconidia with a short nipple-like structure (white arrow) and intercalary chlamydoconidia (black arrow) of *M. audouinii* (LPCB mount ×600).

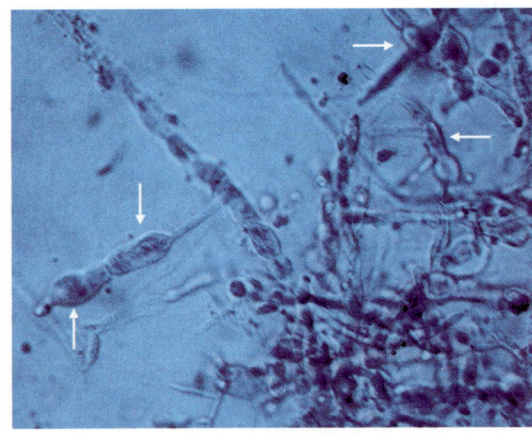

Fig. 1.146: *M. audouinii*, irregular crooked tip macroconidia (white arrow) are characteristic feature (LPCB mount ×800).

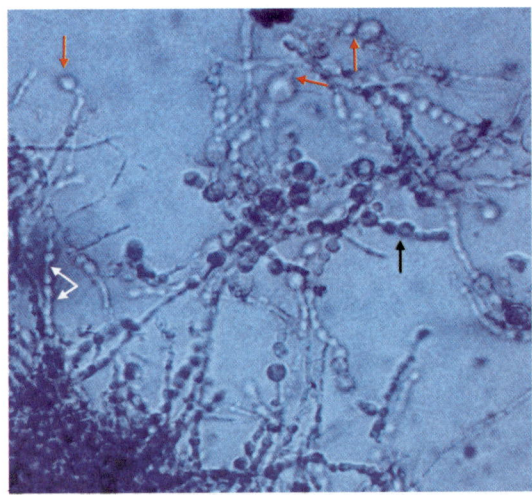

Fig. 1.145: *M.audouinii*. Numerous terminal chlamydoconidia with characteristic 'beaking' (red arrow), peridial hyphae (white arrow) and irregular crooked macroconidia (black arrow) are predominant in this strain [LPCB mount ×400].

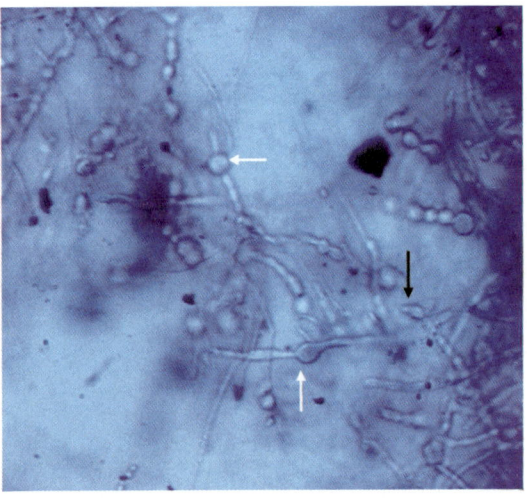

Fig. 1.147: Intercalary chlamydoconidia (white arrow) and nipple-like projection (beaking) of terminal chlamydoconidia (black arrow) are characteristic feature of *M. audouinii* (LPCB mount ×400).

macroconidia. The edges of the colony are entire to scalloped or ragged (Figs 1.151 and 1.152).

Reverse: A variety of pigments or none are produced.

Microscopic morphology

Macroconidia are produced in great abundance. They are thin walled, 8 to 16 × 20 to 60 μ, roughened and have 4 to 6 septa (Fig. 1.153). The usual variety of other conidia including microconidia are also seen. Hair perforation organs are produced.

M. gypseum is geophilic and abundant in soil throughout the world. It is ectothrix but produces a few arthroconidia (Figs 1.154 and 1.155). It is usually associated with an inflammatory disease and cause a kerion formation.

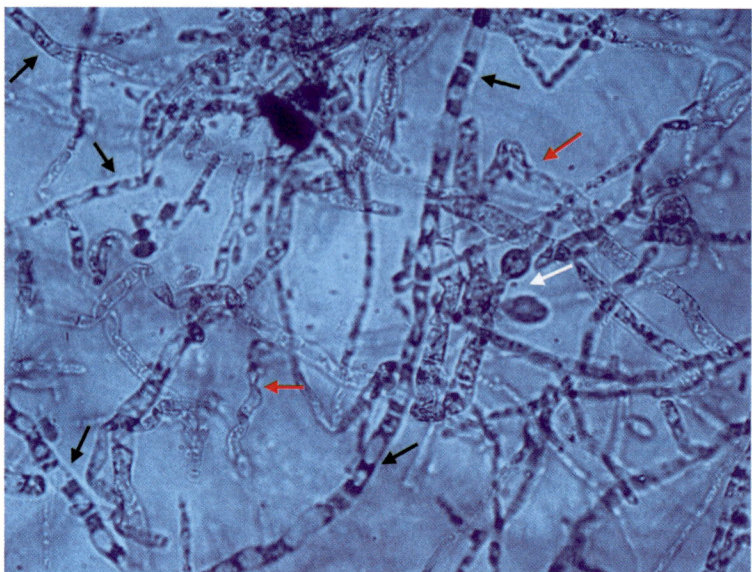

Fig. 1.148: *Microsporum ferrugineum.* Microscopic morphology reveals distorted mycelium (red arrow) without conidia production. But occasional chlamydoconidia (white arrow) may be seen. Faviform, abnormal mycelium (black arrow) and coarse hyphae with prominent cross walls (bamboo hyphae; not shown in this picture) are characteristic features of this species [LPCB mount ×400].

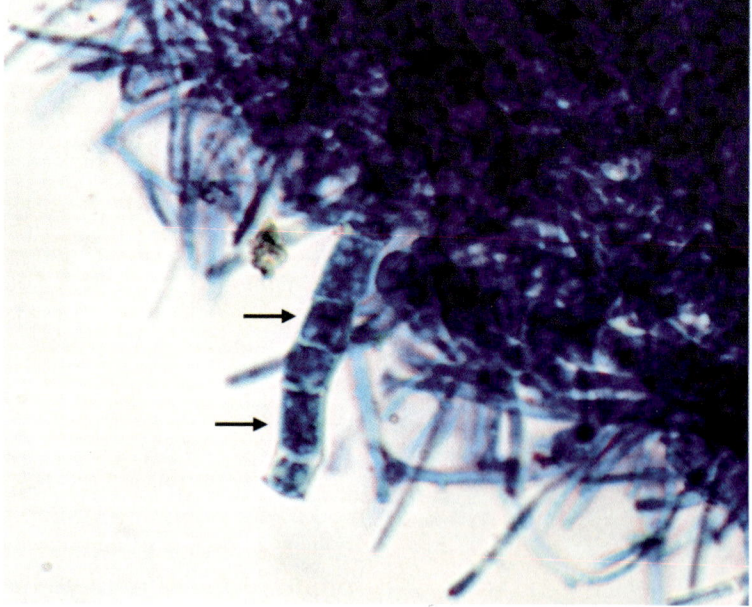

Fig. 1.149: 'Bamboo hyphae' which are thick coarse hyphae with prominent cross walls (black arrow) are seen in *Microsporum ferrugineum* [LPCB mount ×400].

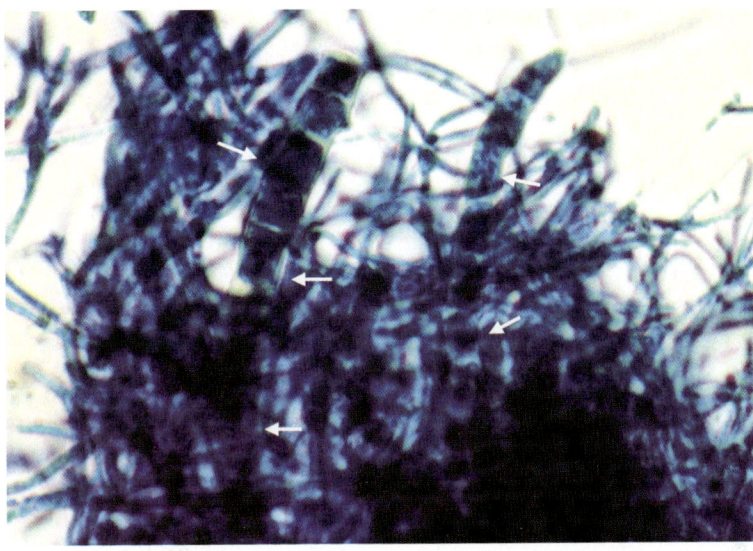

Fig. 1.150: *Microsporum ferrugineum*. Bamboo hyphae (white arrow) are shown here [LPCB mount ×600].

Microsporum canis

Colony morphology

Obverse: The growth is rapid, producing a wooly or cottony, white to yellowish, flat to sparsely grooved colony with radiating edges (Fig. 1.156).

Reverse: The underside of the colony is characteristically a deep chrome yellow. This is best viewed in young growth.

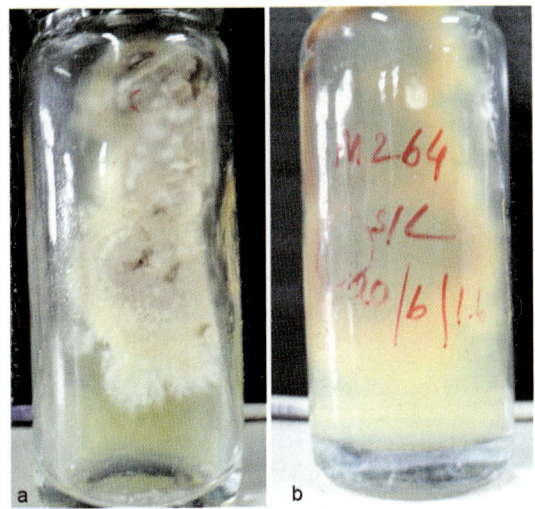

Fig. 1.151: *Microsporum gypseum*. Colonies are flat, spreading, powdery surface and *cinnamon buff* in colour; occasionally violet tinge may appear. The edges of the colony are scalloped or ragged. Diffuse pleomorphism is noticed. Reverse is pigmented; (a) obverse and (b) reverse.

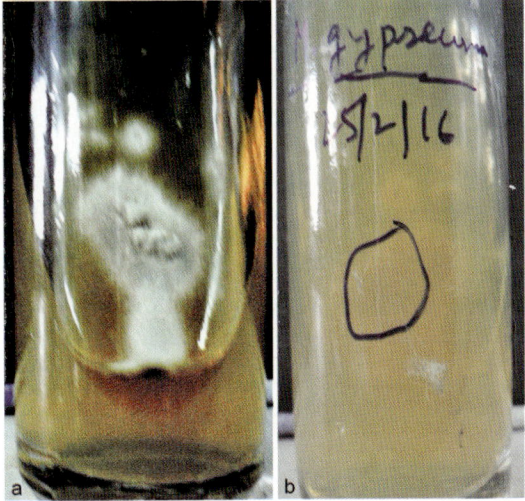

Fig. 1.152: Colony morphology of *Microsporum gypseum* grown on Sabouraud's dextrose agar at 30°C. Colonies grow rapidly and flat, spreading, granular to powdery surface is produced. The centre of the colony becomes heaped up as the colony ages. The reverse is unpigmented; (a) obverse, (b) reverse.

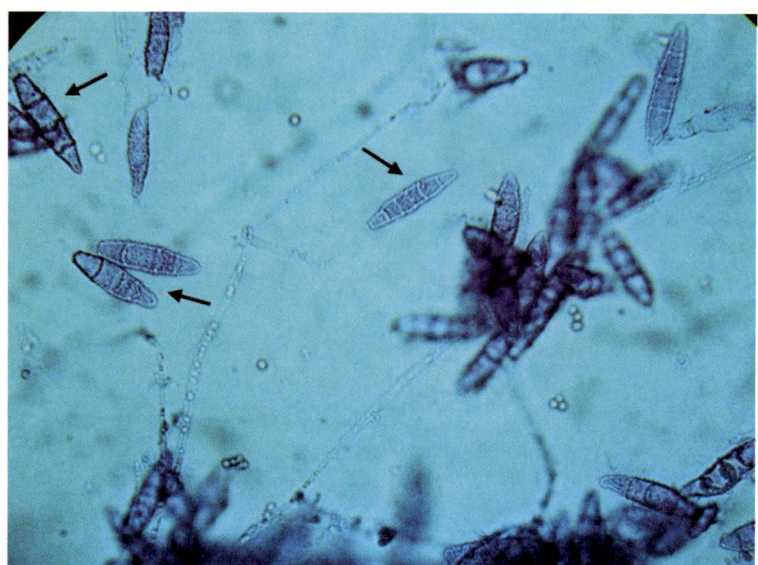

Fig. 1.153: *Microsporum gypseum*. Macroconidia are produced in great abundance. Macroconidia are thin walled, roughened and have four to six septa [LPCB mount ×400].

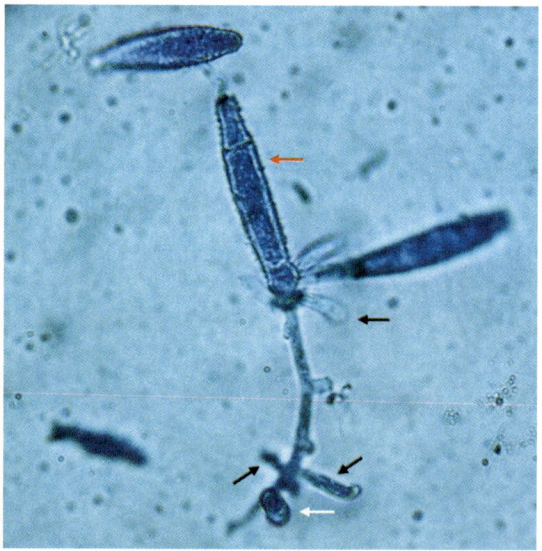

Fig. 1.154: *Microsporum gypseum*. Macroconidia are spindle shaped, rough walled, having 4 to 6 septa (red arrow), clavate-shaped microconidia (black arrow) and chlamydoconidia (white arrow) are also produced [LPCB mount ×400].

Microscopic morphology

The large macroconidia (8 to 20 × 40 to 150 µ) are produced in abundance (Figs 1.157 and 1.158). They have thick walls (2 µ), up to 15 septa and are spindle shaped and echinulate or pitted. Curved or hooked ends are seen (Figs 1.159–1.161). The microconidia are slender and clavate, similar to many other

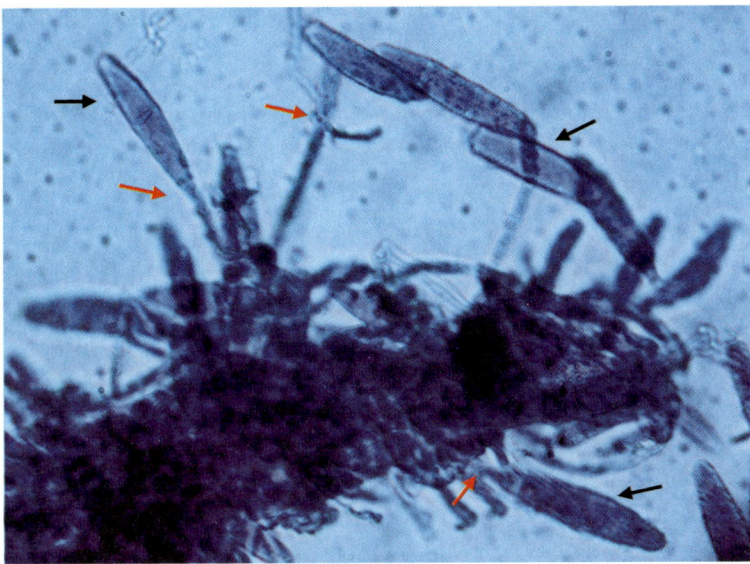

Fig. 1.155: *Microsporum gypseum.* Abundant macroconidia (black arrow) are produced. Macroconidia are broadly spindle shaped with four to six septa and the conidial wall is moderately thick with finely rough. Rattail like filament may be seen at the end of the macroconidia (red arrow) [LPCB mount ×400].

species. Racquet hyphae, pectinate bodies, nodular bodies and chlamydoconidia are seen.

Microsporum fulvum

Colony morphology

Obverse: Although it resembles *M. gypseum* complex, the colony is more floccose and tawny buff in colour. The periphery is often white.

Reverse: A dark red undersurface is occasionally seen; otherwise it is colourless to yellow brown.

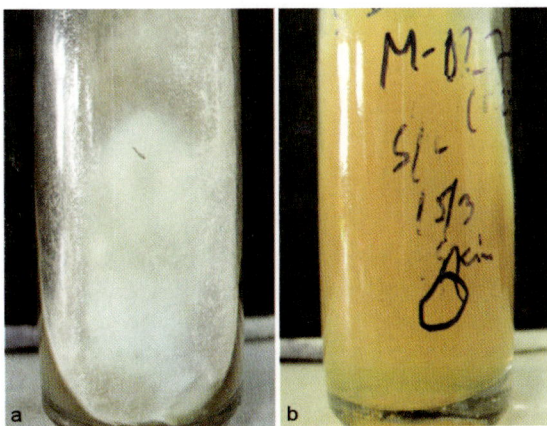

Fig. 1.156: Colony morphology of *Microsporum canis* grown on Sabouraud's dextrose agar at 30°C for 2 weeks; (a) obverse, (b) reverse.

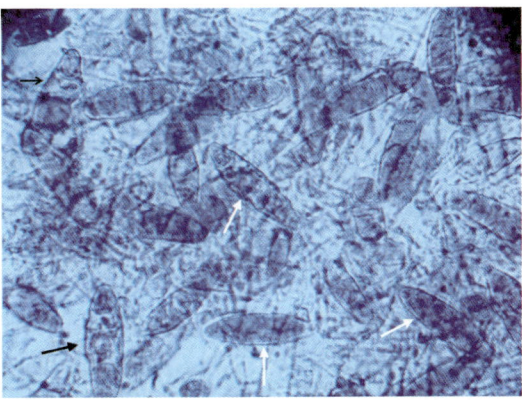

Fig. 1.157: *Microsporum canis.* Macroconidia are spindle shaped (white arrow), thick walled, some are distorted (black arrow) and produced in abundance (LPCB ×600).

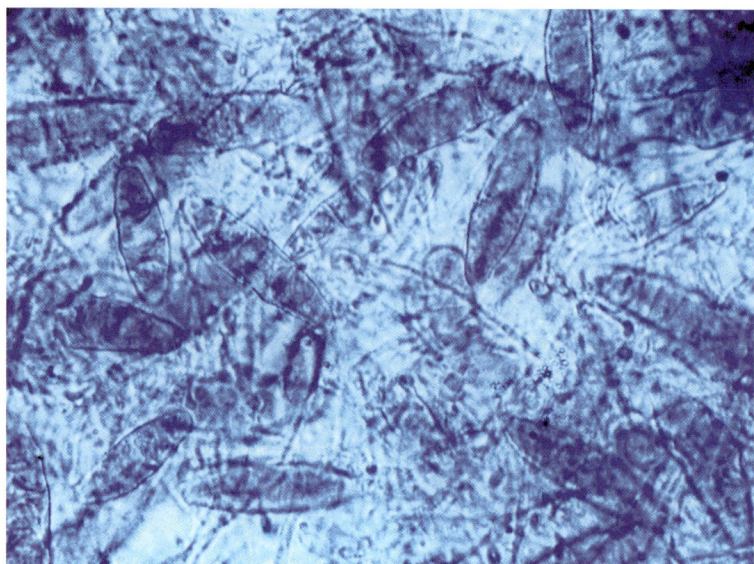

Fig. 1.158: Macroconidia are spindle shaped have close resemblance with that of *M. gypseum* but varied size and shapes of macroconidia with 4 to 10 septa are distinguishing feature. *Microsporum canis* [LPCB mount ×400].

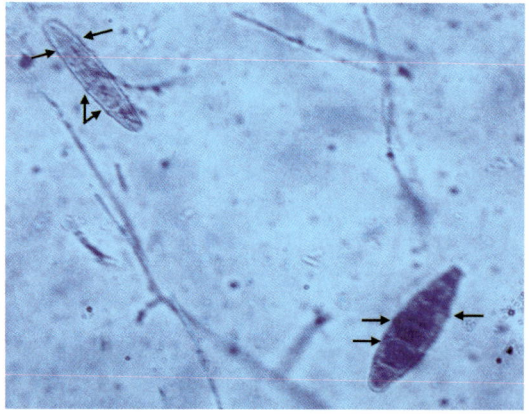

Fig. 1.159: Macroconidia of *Microsporum canis*. These are spindle shaped having rough echinulated surface (black arrow) [LPCB mount ×400].

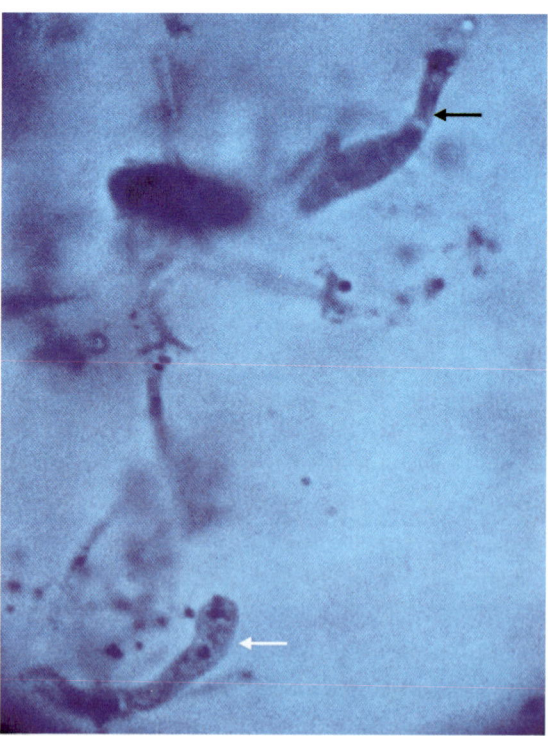

Fig. 1.160: Distorted (white arrow) and crooked (black arrow) macroconidia of *M. canis*.

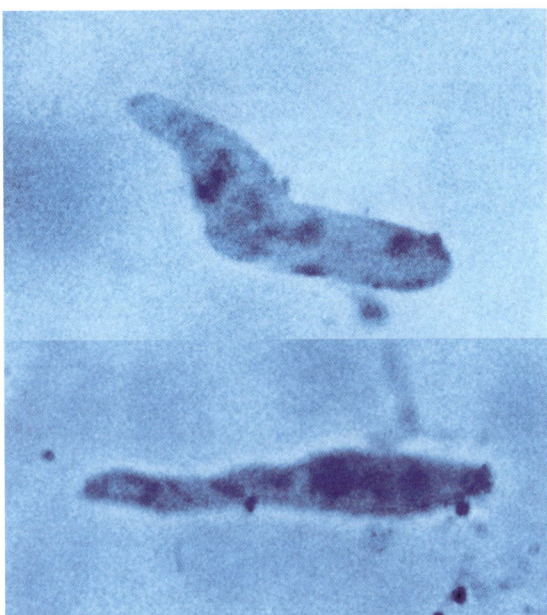

Fig. 1.161: Distorted macroconidia of *M. canis.*

Microscopic morphology

The macroconidia of *M. fulvum* are more clavate, cylindrical or bullet-shaped and are less often in large clusters than those of *M. gypseum*. Microconidia 2 to 3.5 × 3 to 8 μ are produced but these are indistinguishable from those of other species (Fig. 1.162). Numerous spiral hyphae, which are often branched, are seen. Hair perforation organs are produced.

Microsporum gallinae

Colony morphology

Obverse: This species grows rapidly, producing a conical, slightly folded, downy to satiny white colony with an entire to slightly scalloped edge. Sometimes the mycelium may be stained pink.

Reverse: A diffusible pigment is produced within a few weeks. Initially it is yellow, but

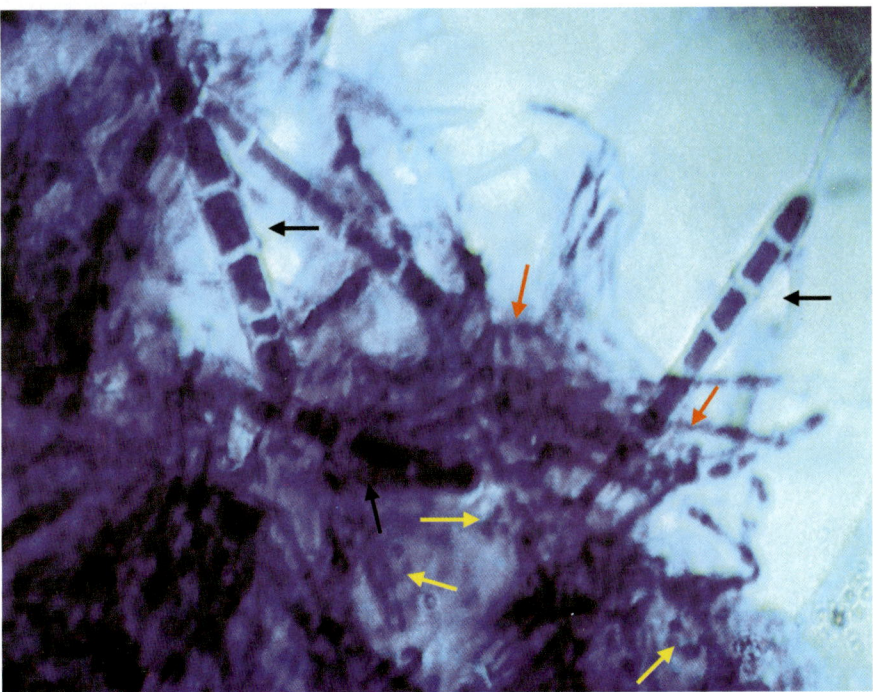

Fig. 1.162: *Microsporum fulvum.* The macroconidia (black arrow) are more clavate, cylindrical or bullet shaped but less often in clusters. Microconidia (yellow arrow) are indistinguishable from other species of *Microsporum.* Spiral hyphae are often seen (red arrow) [LPCB mount ×400].

becomes a bright cherry red or strawberrry red.

Microscopic morphology

The macroconidia are 6 to 8 × 15 to 50 μ in size and are often elongate with a blunt tip (spatulate or slipper-shaped). There are two to ten cells, and the walls are usually echinulate. The conidia are often attached to dentate, pectinate and leaf-like hyphae. Clavate and pyriform microconidia are also found (Figs 1.163–1.170). This is a zoophilic species associated with fowl and rarely involved in human infection.

Microsporum distortum

Colony morphology

Obverse: The growth is rapid, producing a wooly or cottony, velvety to fuzzy white to yellowish, flat or spreading grooved colony with radiating edges.

Reverse: The underside of the colony has less pigmentation and the colour is usually reddish brown.

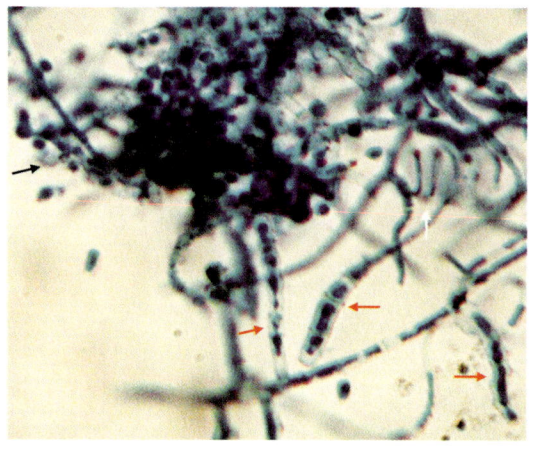

Fig. 1.163: *Microsporum gallinae*. Macroconidia are elongate with a blunt tip (red arrow); hence called 'spatulate' or 'slipper-shaped' and the walls of macroconidia are echinulate at the tip. Microconidia are clavate to pyriform (black arrow), spiral hyphae (white arrow) are also noticed [LPCB mount ×400].

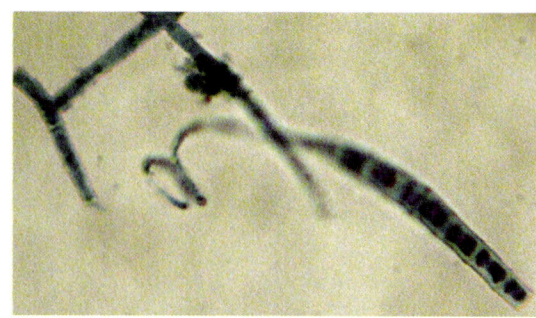

Fig. 1.164: An eight-celled long 'spatulate' macro-conidia of *Microsporum gallinae* [LPCB mount ×600].

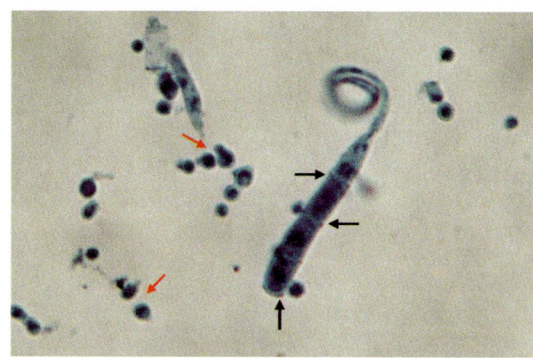

Fig. 1.165: 'Spatulate' macroconidia of *Microsporum gallinae*. Macroconidia are elongate, having two to ten cells and fine echinulations are present on the walls (black arrow). Microconidia are pyriform to clavate (red arrow) [LPCB mount ×400].

Microscopic morphology

The macroconidia (8 to 20 × 40 to 150 μ) are spindle shaped, similar to those of *M. canis* but grossly bent and distorted. They have thick walls, 5 to 10 septa and echinulate (Fig. 1.166). Sessile clavate microconidia are also produced. They are usually more abundant than isolants of *M. canis*.

Microsporum persicolor

Colony morphology

Obverse: A rapidly growing, flat to gently folded fluffy, yellowish buff to pale pink thallus is produced (Fig. 1.167).

Reverse: Pigmentation of the underside is variable. The colour ranges from peach or rose to deep shades of ochre. On sugar free media

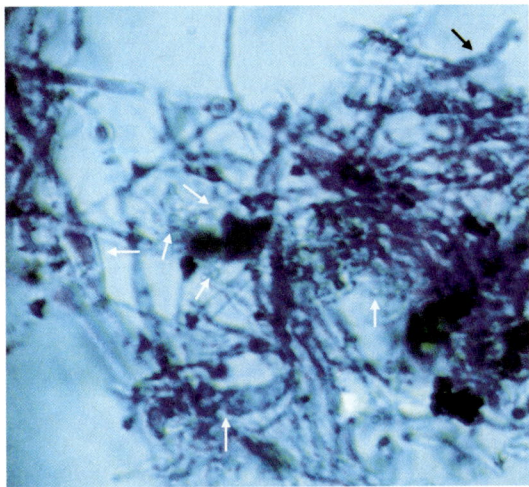

Fig. 1.166: *Microsporum distortum*. Macroconidia are similar to *M. canis* but grossly bent and distorted (black arrow). Spindle-shaped, echinulate macroconidia with curved or hooked ends are important characteristic feature. Sessile, clavate microconidia are abundant (white arrow) [LPCB mount ×400].

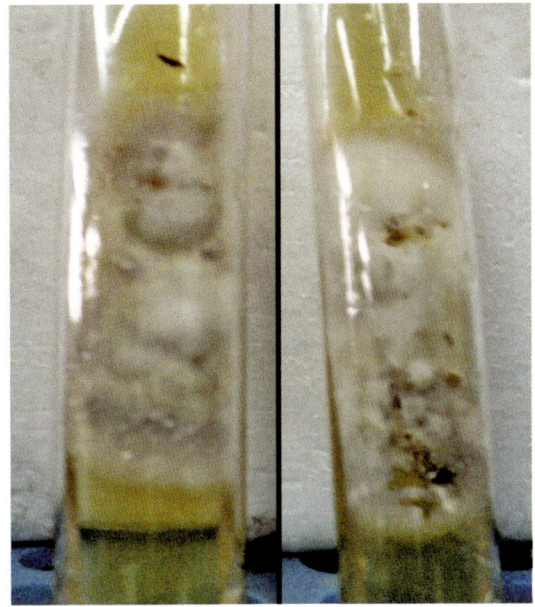

Fig. 1.167: Colony morphology of *Microsporum persicolor* grown on Sabouraud's dextrose agar. Flat, gently folded, fluffy, buff to pale pink colonies are produced. The reverse is deep peach to red in colour although deep wine tints are also sometimes noticed.

sectors of rose to red to deep wine tints are seen. This distinguishes it from *T. mentagrophytes,* which does not produce colour on these media. This red colour is produced on rice grain agar also.

Microscopic morphology
Microconidia are usually abundant. They are clavate or fusiform to globose, arranged in clusters resembling the microscopic morphology of *T. mentagrophytes,* but predominance of stalked, elongate clavate microconidia in *M. persicolor* is a distinguishing feature. Spiral hyphae are common. The macroconidia are sparsely produced. They are elongate, fusiform to clavate and usually six celled. The walls are thick with prominent echinulations (Figs 1.168 to 1.170). Hair perforation organs are produced.

This species is zoophilic and a rare pathogen for human. It is frequently found in bank voles and field voles. Human infections are noted for severity of the disease evoked.

Microsporum racemosum

Colony morphology
Obverse: The colony is flat, rapidly spreading, granular and white with a powdery cream central area.

Reverse: The underside of the colony is wine red in colour.

Microscopic morphology
The macroconidia are tapered and sparsely echinulate; have five to ten cells and may have a rat-tail terminal filament. Microconidia are noted for their arrangement in racemes (Figs 1.171 and 1.172).

It is a geophilic species and is cosmopolitan in distribution. These strains of this species have been isolated from three different cases of tinea corporis in our laboratory.

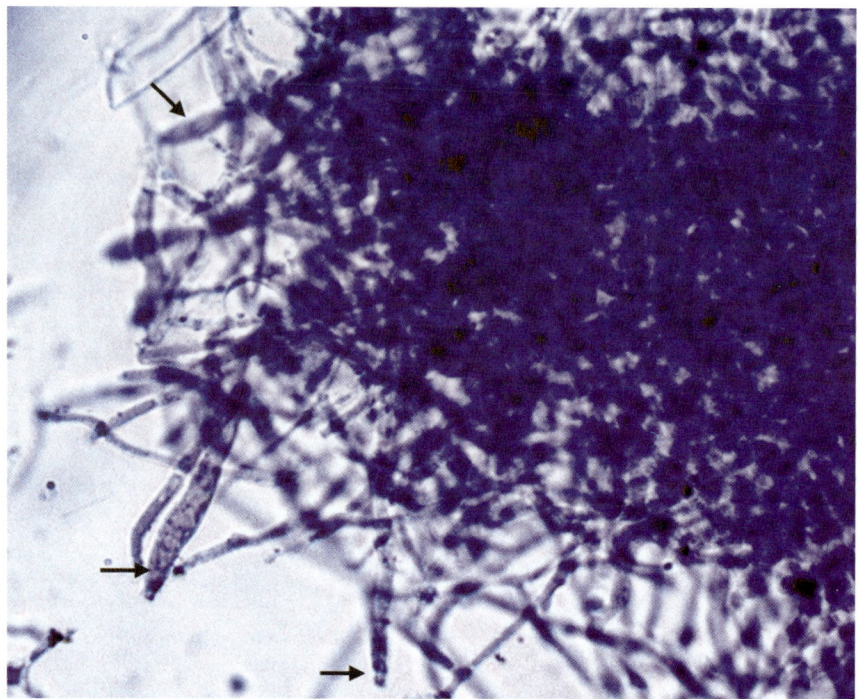

Fig. 1.168: *Microsporum persicolor.* Macroconidia (black arrow) are fusiform to clavate shaped and usually six celled. Fine echinulations are present on the walls [LPCB mount ×200].

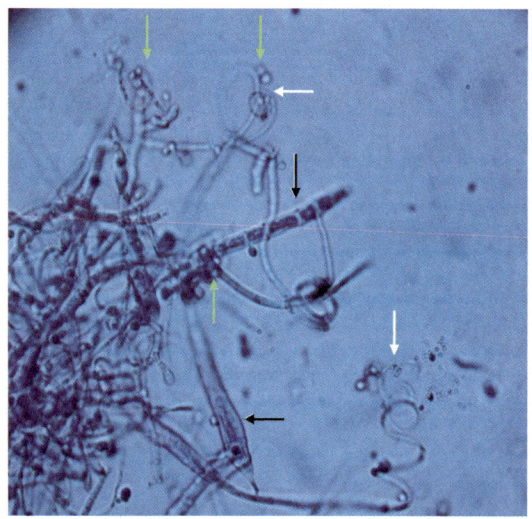

Fig. 1.169: *Microsporum persicolor.* Macroconidia elongate, fusiform to clavate (white arrow), microconidia, globose in clusters (black arrow) and spiral hyphae (red arrow) are seen (LPCB mount ×400).

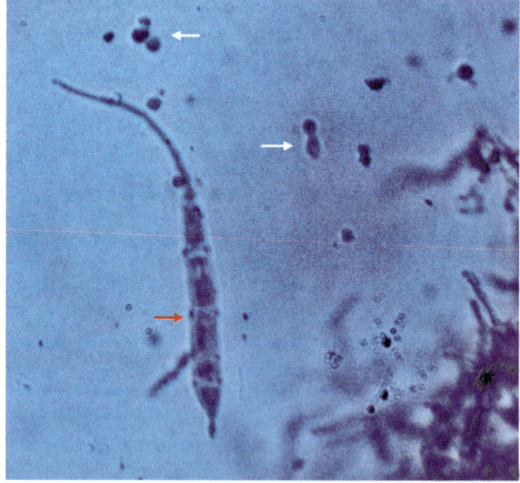

Fig. 1.170: *Microsporum persicolor.* Macroconidia are spindle shaped (red arrow) thin walled, with predominantly six cells. The finely echinulated walls may be more evident at the tip of the conidia and globose to clavate microconidia (white arrow) are seen in clusters [LPCB mount ×200].

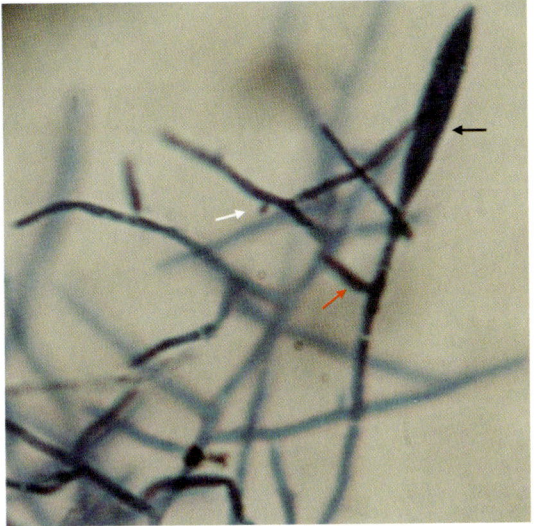

Fig. 1.171: *Microsporum racemosum*. Fusiform macroconidium (black arrow) are thin walled with sparse echinulations and a stalk (red arrow). Microconidia are pyrifom to wedge shaped, borne lateral to hyphae (white arrow) (×600).

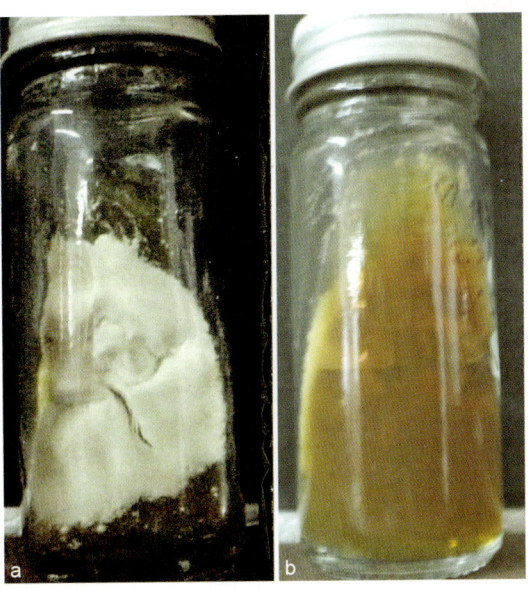

Fig. 1.173: Colony morphology of *Trichophyton yaoundei* grown on SDCA at 30°C after 3 weeks of incubation; (a) obverse, (b) reverse.

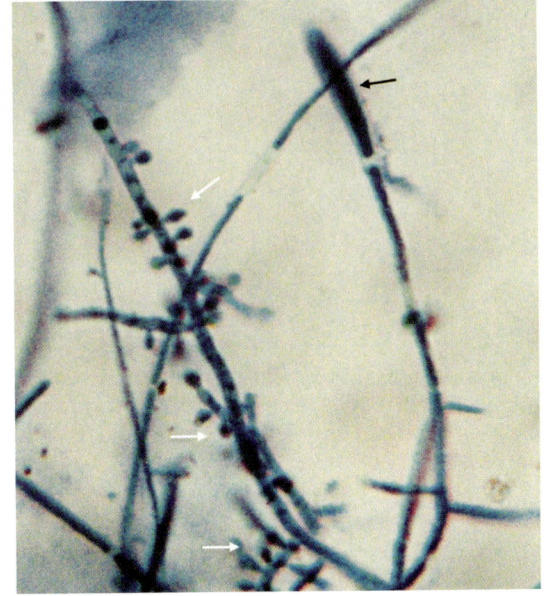

Fig. 1.172: *Microsporum racemosum*. Microconidia are arranged in racemes (white arrow). Tapered, fusiform macroconidium (black arrow) is also seen (×600).

Trichophyton ajelloi

Colony morphology

Obverse: A fast growing, flat, spreading colony is produced that is cottony and cream yellow to lavender pink (Fig. 1.173).

Reverse: The reverse is colourless to light yellow. The fungus rapidly becomes pleomorphic.

Microscopic morphology

Macroconidia are abundant, 59 to 62 × 11 μ in size, echinulate, thick walled (2–3 μ) and cylindro-fusiform in shape, with seven to ten cells. They are similar to those of *T. ajelloi* except that the latter has smooth walled conidia and a purple pigment. The microconidia are pyriform to obovate (Fig. 1.174).

This is a geophilic species rarely involved in ringworm of man. This species readily infects guinea pigs and produces hair perforation organs.

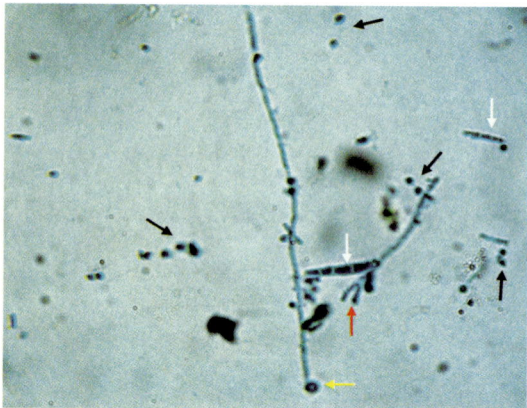

Fig. 1.174: *Trichophyton yaoundei.* Microconidia are pyriform in shape (black arrow) and produced abundant. Macroconidia (white arrow) are not *Trichophyton* type. Branched antler-like mycelial appendages (red arrow) and chlamydoconidia (yellow arrow) are formed [LPCB mount ×400].

SELF ASSESSMENT

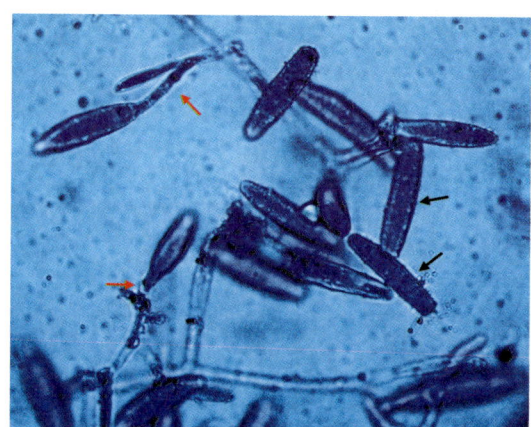

Fig. 1.175: Microscopic morphology of a fungus (dermatophyte) isolated from a eight years old boy presented with 'Kerion'. Spindle-shaped macroconidia, rough walled, having four to six septations (black arrow) and 'rat-tail' like appendages (red arrow) are noticed. Identify the fungus [LPCB mount ×400].

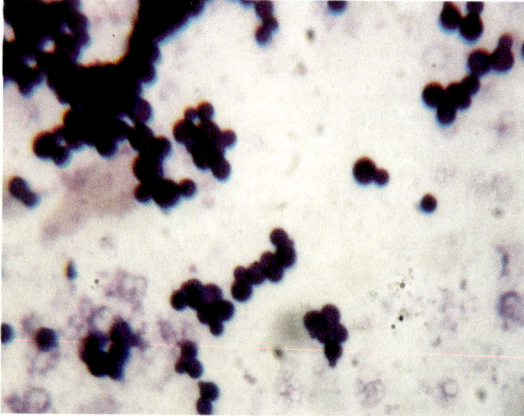

Fig. 1.176: Gram stained smear showing budding (unipolar and phialidic) yeast cells which are arranged in clusters and short chains but a few are lying singly. Multiple budding does not occur in this fungus. Identify the yeast [×1000].

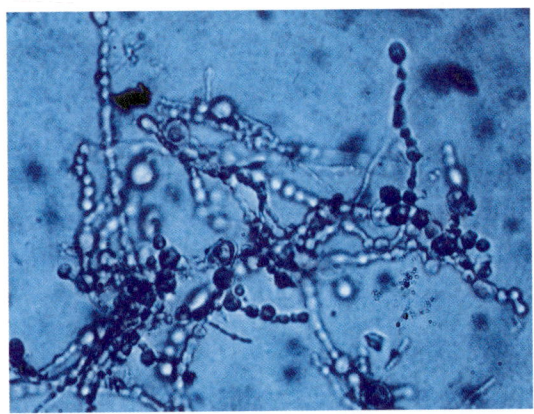

Fig. 1.177: Microscopic morphology of a dermatophyte isolated from a case of 'tinea capitis'. Identify the structures and the related fungi [LPCB mount ×400].

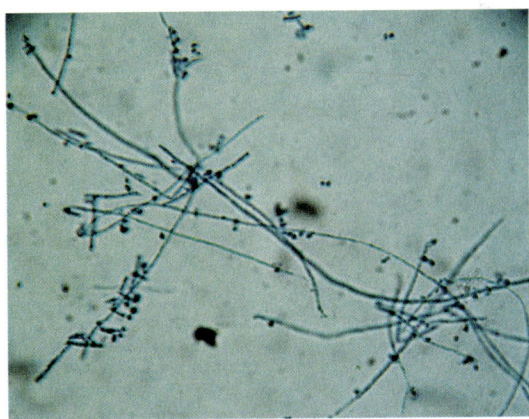

Fig. 1.179: Microscopic morphology of a clinical isolate of a dermatophyte from a case of 'tinea corporis'. Abundant microconidia are noticed. Macroconidia are rarely seen and are not specific for the particular genus. Identify the genus and species (if possible) of the isolate.

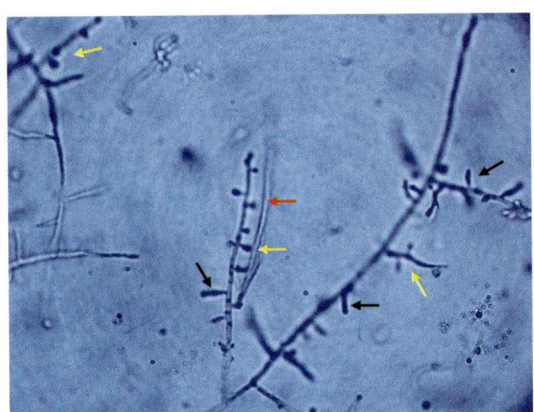

Fig. 1.178: Microscopic morphology of a clinical isolate of dermatophyte showing microconidia having different shapes. Identify them and the likely genus of the dermatophyte [LPCB mount ×400].

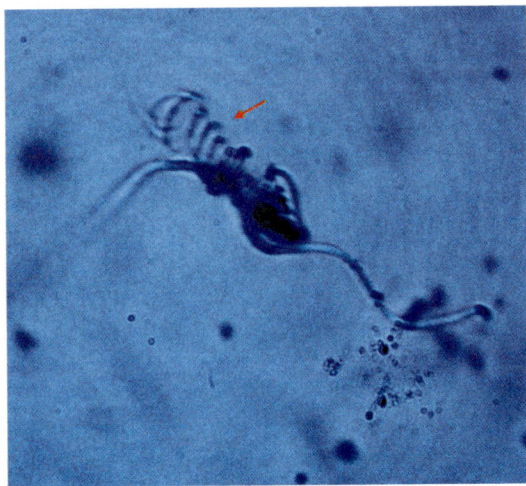

Fig. 1.180: Microscopic morphology of a dermatophyte showing hyphal modification of a vegetative hyphae (red arrow). Identify the structure and mention the genus where it is predominant [LPCB mount ×400].

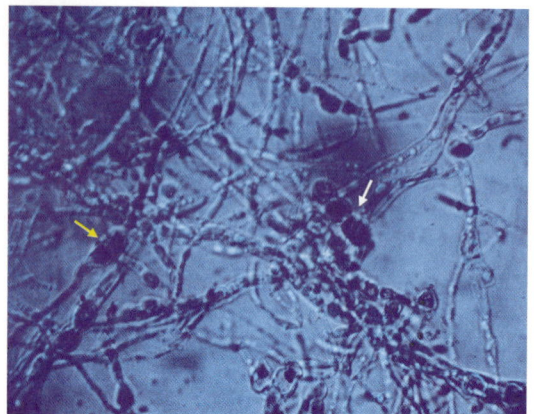

Fig. 1.181: Microscopic morphology of a dermatophyte isolated from a case of 'tinea corporis'. Identify the structures and the likely fungus.

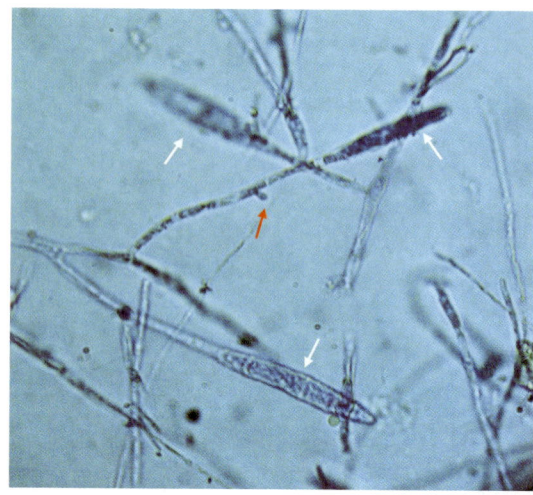

Fig. 1.183: Microscopic morphology of a clinical isolate of dermatophyte obtained from a case of 'tinea corporis' in a 48-year-old female. Identify the dermatophyte based on the morphological feature [LPCB mount ×400].

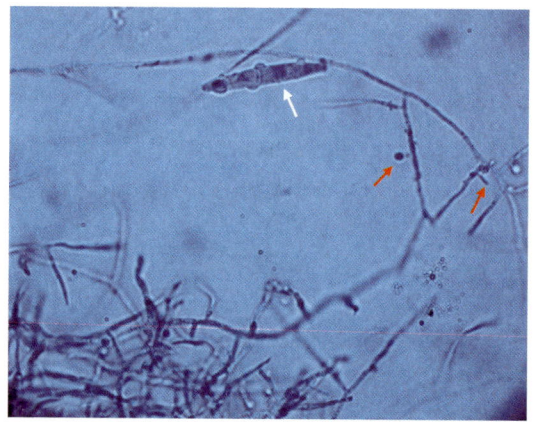

Fig. 1.182: Microscopic morphology of a dermatophyte causing both 'tinea cruris' and 'tinea capitis' in a eight-year-old boy. Identify the structures and the likely fungus responsible in this case [LPCB mount ×400].

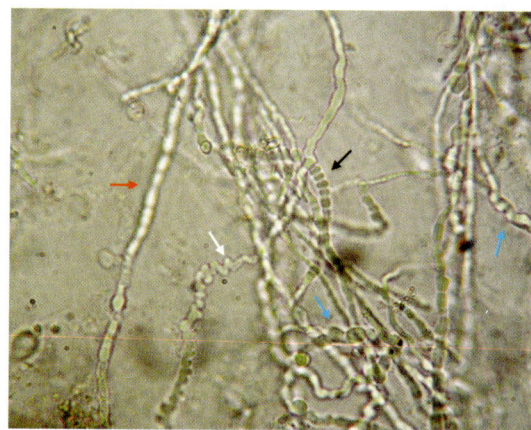

Fig. 1.184: Dermatophyte in nail sample of a child. Identify the structures that are in favour of dermatophytic etiology [KOH mount ×400].

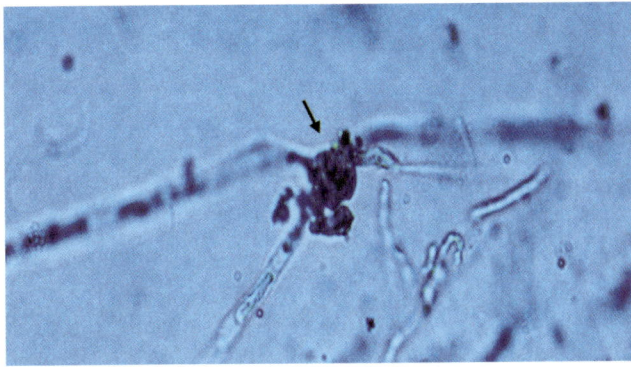

Fig. 1.185: Identify the structure (black arrow) which is found on vegetative hyphae (hyphal modification) and are predominant in Trichophyton species [LPCB mount ×600].

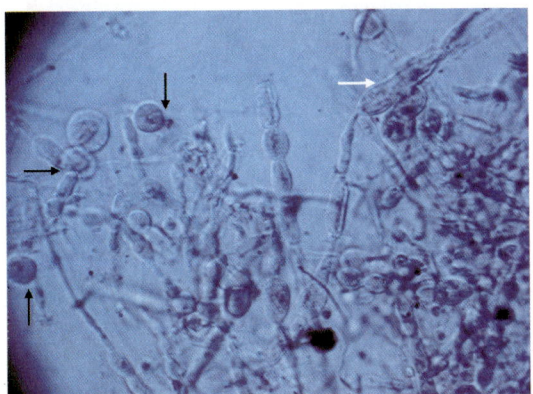

Fig. 1.186: Microscopic morphology of a dermatophyte isolated from a case of 'tinea corporis'. Identify the structures indicated and the relevant fungus [LPCB mount ×600].

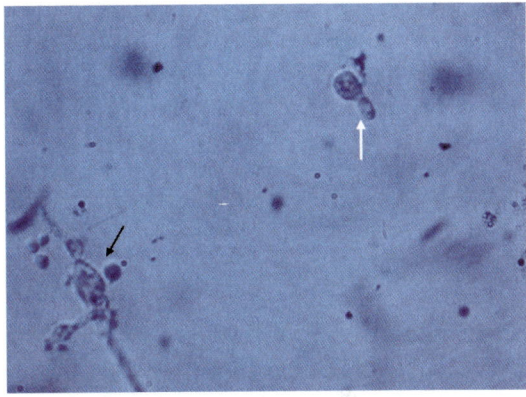

Fig. 1.187: Microscopic morphology of *Microsporum audouinii*. Identify the structures [LPCB mount ×400].

ANSWERS

- **Fig. 1.187:** Beaking of Chlamydoconidia (white arrow), bizarre looking macroconidia (black arrow) in *Microsporum audouinii*
- **Fig. 1.186:** Macroconidia (white arrow), Chlamydoconidia (black arrow); *Microsporum audouinii*
- **Fig. 1.185:** Nodular bodies
- **Fig. 1.184:** Chains of arthroconidia
- **Fig. 1.183:** *Microsporum gypseum*
- **Fig. 1.182:** Distorted macroconidia of *Microsporum canis*
- **Fig. 1.181:** *Epidermophyton floccosum*
- **Fig. 1.180:** Spiral hyphae; *Trichophyton* species
- **Fig. 1.179:** *Trichophyton yaoundei*
- **Fig. 1.178:** Pear shaped, clavate microconidia; *Trichophyton tonsurans*
- **Fig. 1.177:** *Microsporum audouinii*
- **Fig. 1.176:** *Malassezia*
- **Fig. 1.175:** *Microsporum gypseum*

Subcutaneous Mycoses

Subcutaneous mycoses include a hetero-geneous group of infections characterized by the development of a lesion at the site of inoculation. Unlike the systemic mycoses, these infections are the result of traumatic implantation of the fungus into the skin. The ensuing disease remains localized to this area or slowly spreads to surrounding tissue, a picture similar to that seen with the mycetoma. Diseases grouped under 'Subcutaneous mycoses' are as follows:

1. **Sporotrichosis:** Etiologic agent *S. schenckii* is a thermodimorphic fungus and slow extension via lymphatic channels is a frequent occurrence in this infection.
2. **Chromoblastomycosis:** Group of clinical entities caused by a variety of dematiaceous (pigmented) fungi where hematogenous and lymphatic dissemination is rarely recorded.
3. **Rhinosporidiosis:** Etiologic agent is *Rhinosporidium seeberi*, which has not yet been isolated *in vitro*. It is a chronic granulomatous disease involving the mucocutaneous tissue (Fig. 2.1).
4. **Entomophthoromycosis:** The disease is caused by a member of the 'zygomycetes' but it is completely different from diseases caused by other members of this family, i.e. mucormycosis. This disease has a little tendency to spread.
5. **Lobomycosis:** It is a chronic localized subepidermal infection caused by spheroidal

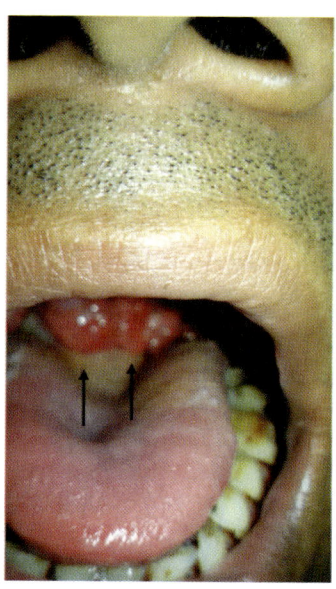

Fig. 2.1: Rhinosporidiosis. Lesion is on the hard palate.

yeast like organism known as *Loboa loboi*. The infection is characterized by presence of keloidal, verrucoid, nodular lesions or by vegetating crusty plaques and tumours. There is no systemic spread of the infection.

SPOROTRICHOSIS

Sporotrichosis is most commonly a chronic infection characterized by nodular lesions of the cutaneous and subcutaneous tissues and adjacent lymphatics that suppurate ulcerate and drain. The etiologic agent is *Sporothrix schenckii*. The fungus gain entrance by traumatic implantation into the skin or very rarely by inhalation into the lungs.

Clinical types
- Lymphocutaneous (Figs 2.3, 2.5 and 2.7)
- Fixed cutaneous (Figs 2.2 and 2.6)
- Mucocutaneous
- Extracutaneous and disseminated
- Primary pulmonary

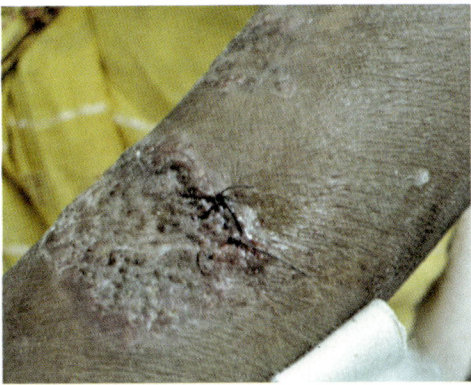

Fig. 2.4: Gummatous sporotrichosis. Necrotic and ulcerative lesion is on the forearm.

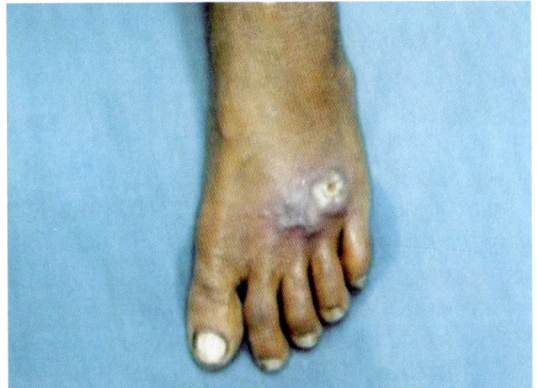

Fig. 2.2: Fixed cutaneous sporotrichosis. Verrucous ulcerative lesion is on the dorsum of the foot, near the base of third, fourth and fifth toes.

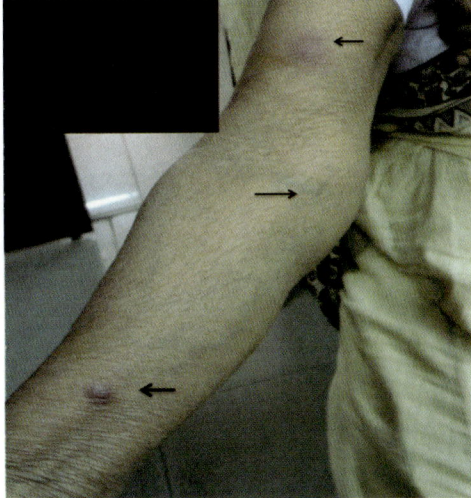

Fig. 2.5: Lymphocutaneous sporotrichosis. Subcutaneous nodules have appeared along the lymph channels (black arrow).

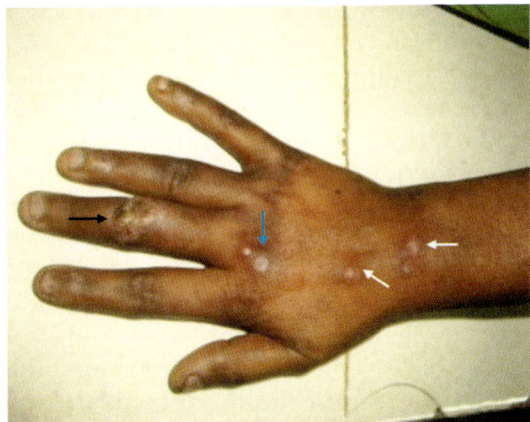

Fig. 2.3: Lymphocutaneous sporotrichosis. The initial lesion is discoloured, ulcerated and draining (black arrow); secondary lesions are deep, subcutaneous nodules (white arrow) except one which have ulcerated (blue arrow).

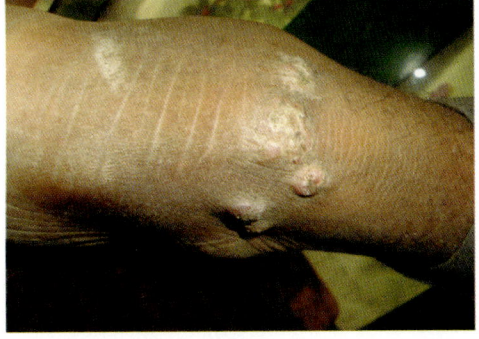

Fig. 2.6: Fixed cutaneous sporotrichosis. Nodular and ulcerative lesions are seen.

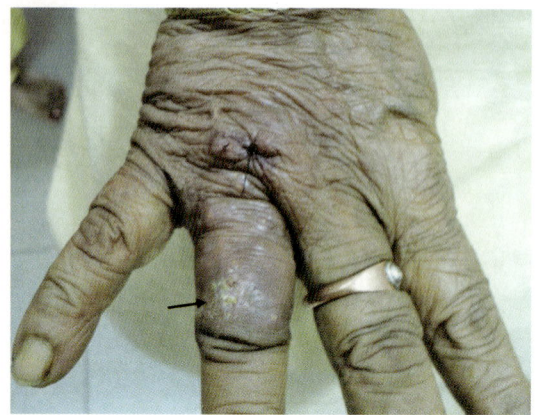

Fig. 2.7: Lymphocutaneous sporotrichosis. Note the primary ulcerative lesion (black arrow).

Laboratory Identification

Direct Examination

Samples like pus, exudates, aspirates and biopsy material are collected from different clinical types of sporotrichosis depending upon the availability of the sample. In general, direct examination with 10% potassium hydroxide preparation of such material is

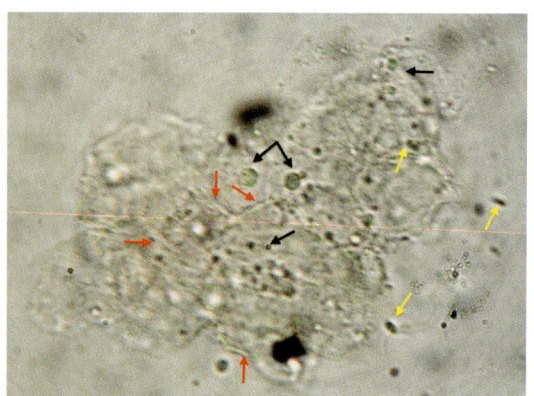

Fig. 2.8: Spherical to oval yeast cells with occasional budding (black arrow), a few cigar-shaped yeast cells (yellow arrow) are suggestive of yeasts of *Sporothrix schenckii*. A few thin hyphal strands (red arrow) are also noticed; might be due to colonization of saprophytic fungi. The sample is a postnasal discharge of a clinically diagnosed fungal sinusitis case who had undergone endoscopic sinus surgery 3 months back [KOH mount × 600].

unrewarding. An exception to this is the fluorescent antibody staining technique. Utilizing this procedure, material from lesions, histologic slide preparations and mycelia or conidia from cultures can be specifically stained.

Culture is the most reliable method for diagnosis as the percentage of culture positivity in cases of the disease is very high.

Colony Morphology

S. schenckii grows well on almost all culture media. Aspirates from cutaneous nodules, pus, exudate and material from curettage or swabbing from open lesions can be planted on Sabouraud's dextrose agar or blood agar and incubated at 25 to 27°C.

Surgical incision and biopsy are contra-indicated as methods for obtaining material for culture since this procedure may result in spread of the disease.

The initial colony of *S. schenckii* isolated from clinical material is moist, glabrous and yeast-like but becomes tough, wrinkled and folded in time. The colour is usually dirty white at first, although in some strains it is yellow, brown or quite black. Pigmentation is extremely variable. Unusually the whitish colony develops an overgrowth of fuzzy mycelium and turns darker in sectors (Fig. 2.9). Old laboratory strains often lose their pigmentation and are a dirty white colour. Primary isolates vary considerably in their colony morphology and may be creamy white, cottony white, various shades of brown and intense black (Fig. 2.10). Some white colonies may not show darkness for many months or never; however, most become dark-streaked in time.

At 37°C on SDCA, BHI blood or other media containing high concentration of glucose (10–20%), the organisms grow in the yeast phase. Colony morphology varies from pasty white and yeast-like to grayish yellow, sometimes glabrous bacteria like colony (Fig. 2.13).

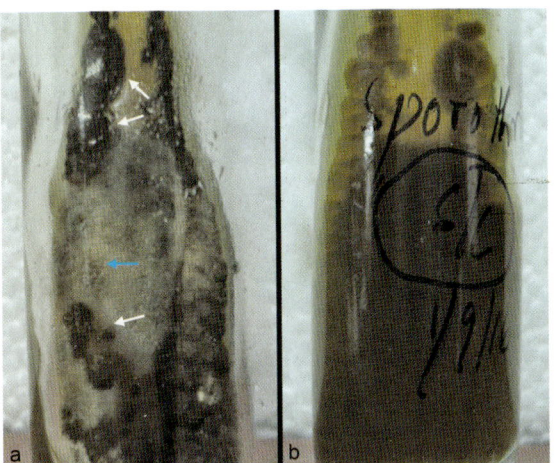

Fig. 2.9: Colony morphology of *Sporothrix schenckii* grown on Sabouraud's dextrose agar at 25°C for 3 weeks; (a) obverse, (b) reverse. Colonies are tough, wrinkled, dirty white and folded at first, gradually develops an overgrowth of fuzzy mycelium (blue arrow) and turns darker in sectors (white arrow). Reverse is dark brown to black in colour.

Fig. 2.10: Colony morphology of *Sporothrix schenckii* grown on Sabouraud's dextrose agar at 25°C for 3 weeks; (a) and (b) obverse, (c) reverse. Colonies are cottony white to light brown, tough, wrinkled and folded (yellow arrow). Reverse is dark brown to intense black at places (red arrow).

Microscopic Morphology

LPCB mount from colonies grown on SDCA at 25°C. Thin septate, branching hyphae, 1 to 2 m in diameter, are formed at room temperature. Frequently they will appear as twisted ropes containing several mycelial strands (Fig. 2.11).

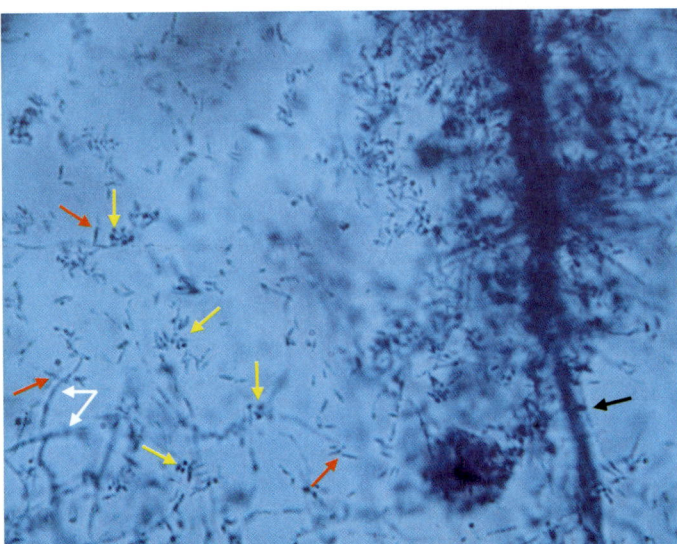

Fig. 2.11: *Sporothrix schenckii*. Several thin mycelial strands appear as twisted rope (black arrow) at 25°C and also at room temperature. The conidiophores are thin, delicate, of variable length, borne erect or recumbent (red arrow) on thin septate, branching hyphae of 1 to 2 μ in diameter (white arrow) [LPCB mount ×400].

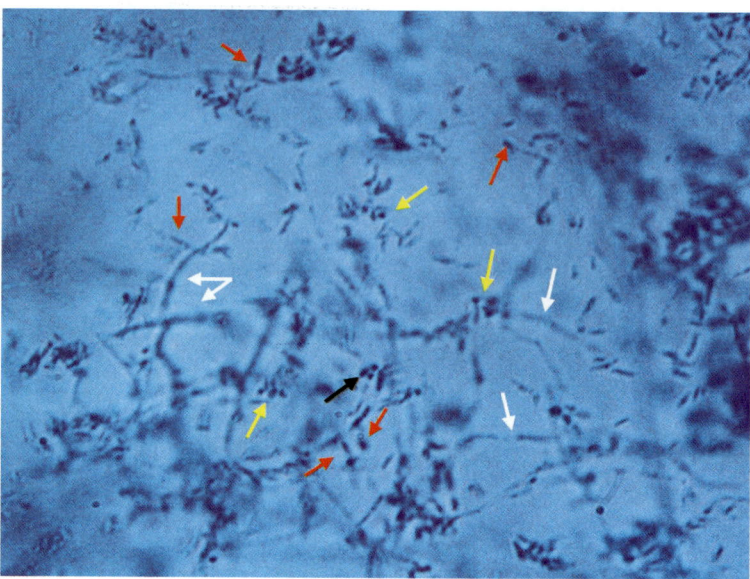

Fig. 2.12: *Sporothrix schenckii.* Several thin mycelial strands appear (white arrow) at 25°C and also at room temperature. The conidiophores are thin, elongate showing expanded denticulate vesicle at apex (red arrow) bearing conidia sympodially (yellow arrow) at 25°C [LPCB mount ×600].

At first conidiation is from long, slender, tapering conidiophores rising at right angles from the hyphae. The conidiophores are erect or recumbent, 1 to 2 m in diameter at the base, narrowing to 0.5 to 1 m at the tip. The length is quite variable. The apex of the conidiophores may expand to form a denticulate vesicle. Simple, ovate hyaline conidia 2 to 3 × 3 to 6 m are formed at first on the apex. Their arrangement suggests a palm tree or a flower head (Fig. 2.12). With age, conidiation increases, so that conidia are formed along the sides of the conidiophores and eventually along the undifferentiated hyphae as well. Dense sleeves of conidia are seen in old cultures.

A second conidial form produced by some strains consists of brown, thick-walled triangular one-celled macroconidia. These pigmented conidia may be more resistant to untoward environmental factors than are the thin-walled hyaline conidia. Malt extract rather than Sabouraud's dextrose agar favours macroconidia formation.

Mycelial to Yeast (M → Y) Conversion

Demonstration of dimorphism is important for specific identification of *S. schenckii.* To induce mycelial to yeast transformation, the fungus is inoculated on Sabouraud's dextrose agar, BHI blood agar or moist blood agar containing high concentration of glucose (10 to 20%) and incubated at 37°C. Conversion to the yeast form sometimes restricted to the outer edge of the colony (Fig. 2.13). The colony morphology varies from pasty, white and yeast like to a grayish yellow sometimes glabrous, like that of a bacterial colony (Figs 2.14 and 2.15). In the yeast form of growth at 37°C, the cells are spherical to ovate blastoconidia. The size is variable, but averages 1–3 μ × 3–10 μ. Several buds may appear on the yeast-like cells (Figs 2.18 and 2.19). Two morphologic transformations are actually found to occur in mycelial to yeast (M → Y) conversion. The first one is formation of club-shaped structures at the hyphal tips or on lateral branches which give rise to budding units, the blastoconidia (yeasts) (Fig. 2.20). The second type is formation of 'oidia' within the mycelium, followed by fragmentation. These free 'oidia' subsequently bud and blastoconidia are formed (Fig. 2.21). The yeast to mycelium (Y → M) transformation is effected by system elongation of the parent cell and rearrange-ment of the cytoplasmic membrane followed by septal formation. The elongation continues and several branching of mycelium occurs. **All dimorphic fungi convert from the yeast to the mycelial form in the similar manner.**

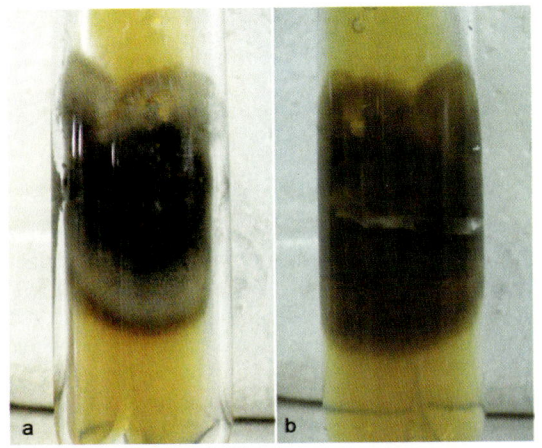

Fig. 2.13: Colonial form of *Sporothrix schenckii*. The dark area is dirty brown-black; the periphery is off-white to cream, may be an indication of yeast conversion. This colonial morphology is obtained after serial subculture on SDCA at 3 weeks interval during a period of four months.

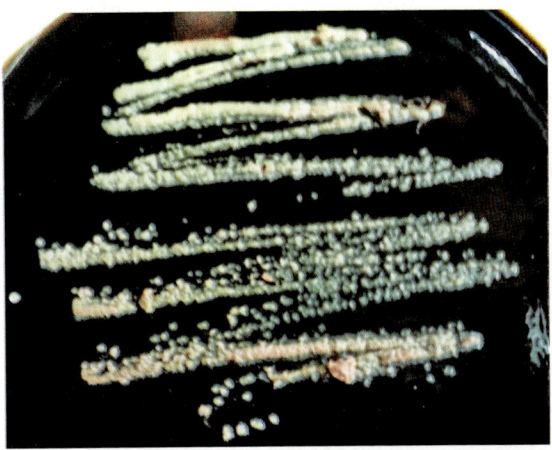

Fig. 2.15: *Sporothrix schenckii*. Colonies grown on blood agar containing 10% glucose at 37°C for 4–5 days. White to light pink glistening yeast like colonies are produced (M → Y conversion) and become more tough as the colony ages.

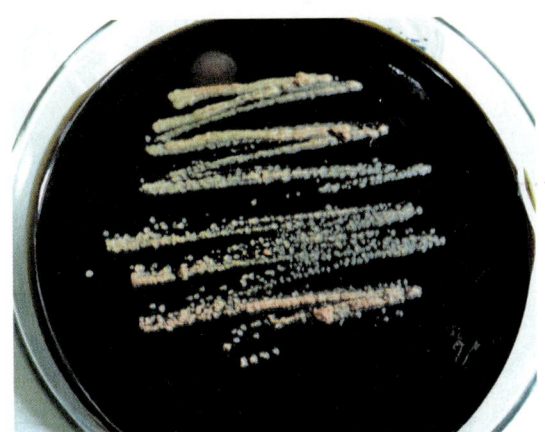

Fig. 2.14: *Sporothrix schenckii*. Transfer to blood agar containing 10% glucose at 37°C, the organism grow in the yeast phase. Pasty white glistening yeast like colonies are produced (M → Y conversion).

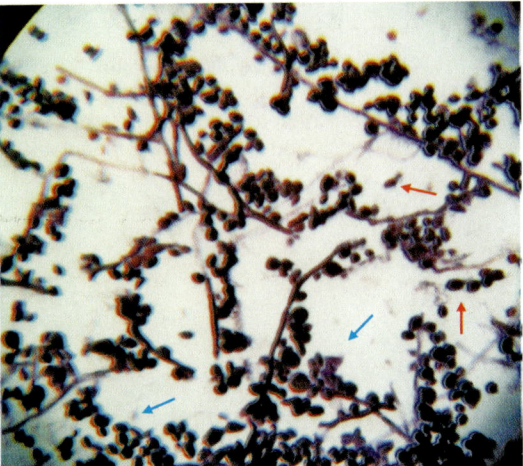

Fig. 2.16: Gram stained smear shows yeast cells of varied shapes and size. Yeast cells are spherical, ovate (blue arrow) or club shaped (red arrow). The smear is prepared from colonies appeared on blood agar (M→Y conversion. *Sporothrix schenckii* [×400].

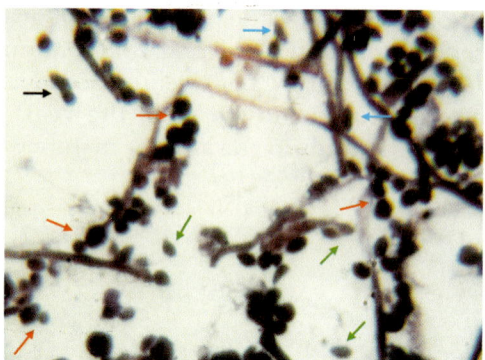

Fig. 2.17: Budding yeast cells of varying size and shapes are noticed. Some are spherical to oval in shape having prominent budding (red arrow); a few cigar shaped (blue arrow), some elliptical cells (green arrow) and one club shaped yeast cell with budding (black arrow) which is very much suggestive of yeasts of *Sporothrix schenckii* [Gram stained smear ×1000].

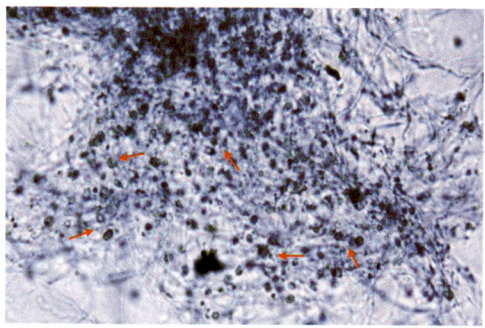

Fig. 2.18: *Sporothrix schenckii*. Mycelium to yeast conversion. Morphologic transformation of the mycelium occurs which then give rise to budding units of blastoconidia (yeasts, red arrow), [LPCB mount ×400].

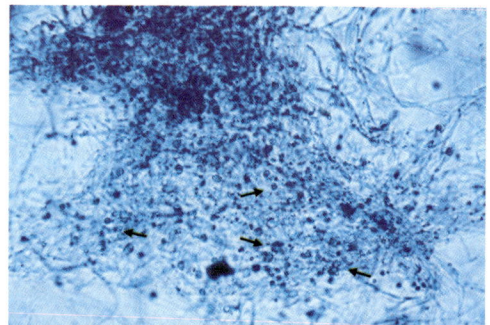

Fig. 2.19: Mycelium to yeast conversion in *Sporothrix schenckii*. Several budding units, spherical to oval, a few elongate blastoconidia (yeasts) are seen which indicates yeast conversion (black arrow) [LPCB mount ×400].

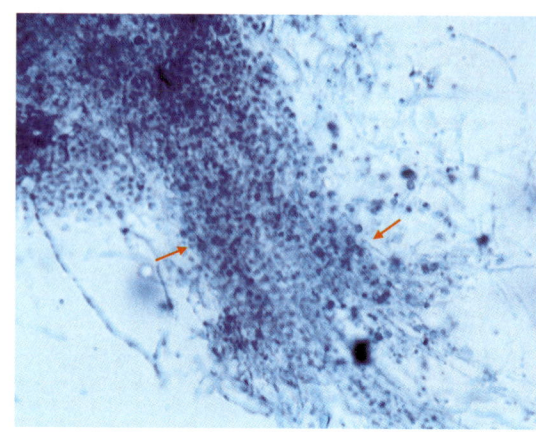

Fig. 2.20: *Sporothrix schenckii*. Mycelium to yeast (M→Y) conversion (initial stage). Plenty of dark coloured structures (red arrow) are seen against dense mass of thin, septate mycelia. These are actually club-shaped structures or 'oidia' formed within the mycelium which get fragmented and subsequently bud producing blastoconidia [LPCB mount ×400].

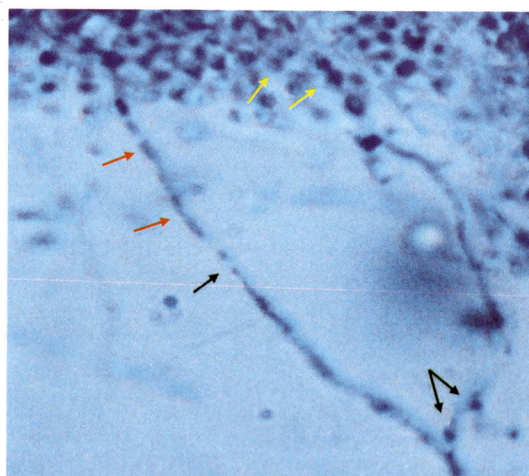

Fig. 2.21: *Sporothrix schenckii*. Mycelium to yeast conversion. Morphological transformation occurs by 'oidia' formation (black arrow) and also by formation of club-shaped structures within the mycelium (red arrow) followed by subsequent fragmentation. Several budding cells (blastoconidia, yellow arrow) arising from these structures are also seen [LPCB mount ×600].

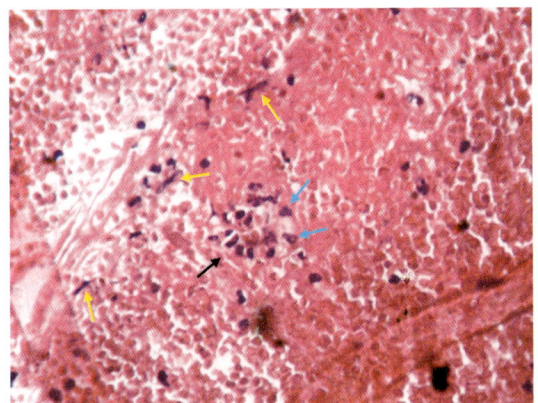

Fig. 2.22: Histopathology section of tissue material from maxillary sinus (obtained by FESS) shows presence of oval to round budding yeast cells (blue arrow), a few yeast cells of varied size and shapes (black arrow) and also cigar-shaped yeast cells (yellow arrow) suggestive of *Sporothrix schenckii* infection [H&E stain ×400].

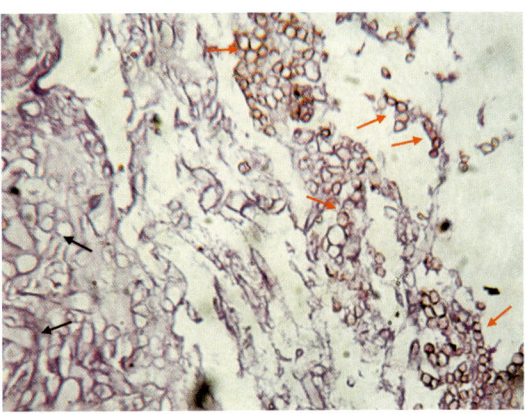

Fig. 2.24: Tissue section of paranasal sinus material shows plenty of dark coloured yeast cells of varied size and shapes (red arrow) and also clusters of thin walled, broad hyphae in wide angle branching and having regular septation (black arrow). These features are suggestive of infection caused by dual pathogenic fungi *Sporothrix schenckii* and *Conidiobolus incongruus* (after corroborating with culture finding) [PAS stained section ×400].

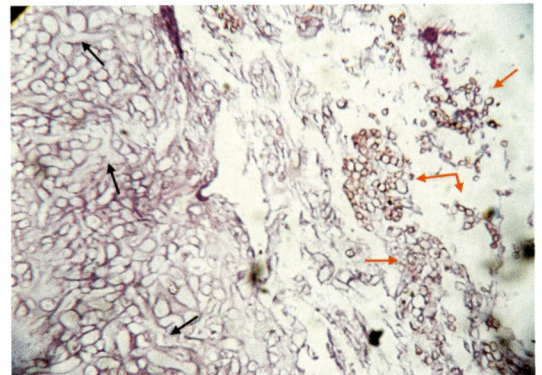

Fig. 2.23: Periodic acid–Schiff (PAS) stained section shows budding yeast cells of varied size and shapes (red arrow) along with cluster of weakly stained broad hyphae (both longitudinal and transverse section) in wide angle branching (black arrow) suggestive of dual infection sporotricosis and entomophthoromycosis conidiobolae [×400].

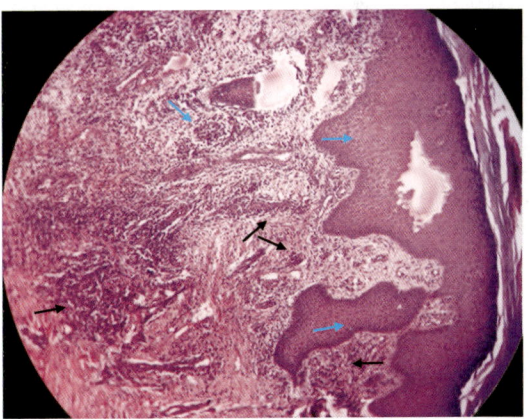

Fig. 2.25: H and E stained section shows pseudo-epitheliomatous hyperplasia (blue arrow), yeast cells in clumps and sheets with frequent budding (black arrow), microabscesses (red arrow) and inflammatory cell infiltration into the subcutaneous tissue; the histologic features suggestive of sporotrichosis [Punch biopsy material from subcutanuous nodule; low power view].

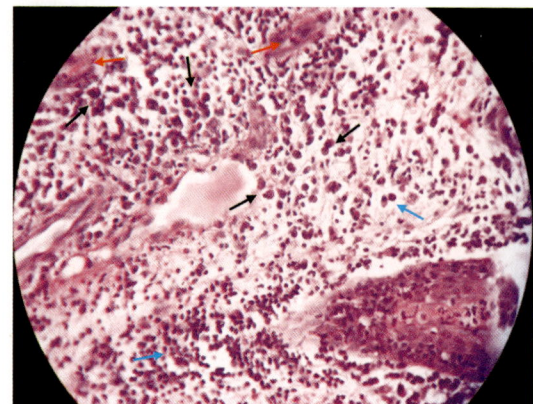

Fig. 2.26: Hematoxylin and eosin stained section shows numerous budding yeast cells (black arrow), infiltration of inflammatory cells of both acute and chronic (blue arrow), fibroblasts and a few giant cells (red arrow); the histologic features suggestive of sporotrichosis [A punch biopsy taken from an ulcerative lesion on the skin high power view].

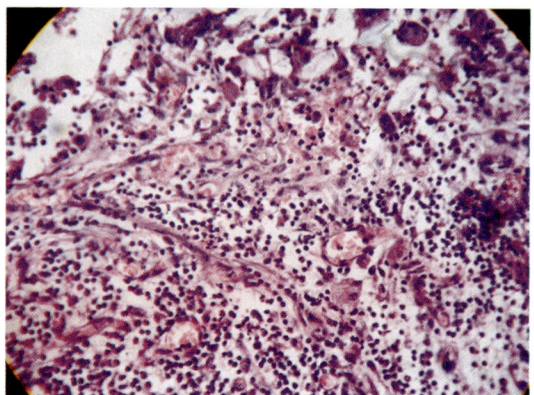

Fig. 2.28: Histopathology of sporotrichosis. Focal infiltration of polymorphonuclear neutrophils, epithelioid cells and giant cells in the surrounding area and presence of fibroblasts are suggestive of granulomatous inflammation [H&E stained section ×400].

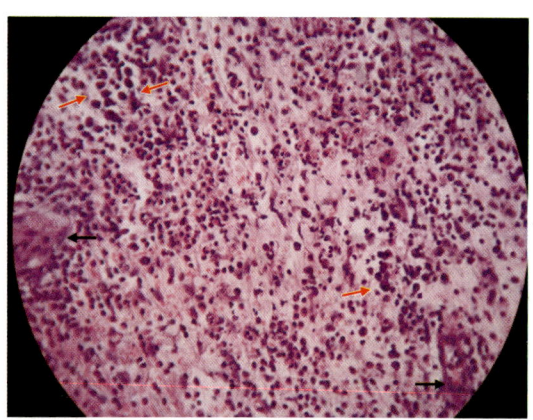

Fig. 2.27: Sporotrichosis. Inflammatory response with neutrophils predominating, epithelioid cells and giant cells (black arrow) in the surrounding area. Yeast cells are oval to cigar shaped, found in cluster (red arrow) [H&E stained section from skin infection, ×400].

RHINOSPORIDIOSIS

Rhinosporidiosis is an infection of the mucocutaneous tissue caused by *Rhinosporidium seeberi.* It is a chronic granulomatous disease characterized by the production of large polyps, tumours, papillomas or wart-like lesions that are hyperplastic, highly vascularized, friable, and sessile or pedunculated. The nose is most commonly affected with the conjunctiva, the second most frequently involved site. Areas of infection rarely involved include pharynx, larynx, ears, vagina and anus. The infection has also been described in a variety of wild and domestic animals.

Laboratory Identification

Direct Examination

Examination of the lesions often reveals macroscopically visible subsurface sporangia that can be seen with the naked eye as small white dots (Fig. 2.29). Dissected or excised tissue or nasal discharge can be slightly macerated and examined in a potassium hydroxide preparation. Mature sporangia up to 350 μ in diameter and spores 7 to 9 μ can be seen. Only spores are seen in nasal discharge, but a few sporangia may be present (Figs 2.31 and 2.32). The mucoid exudate on the surface of the lesion may show the presence of liberated spores from sporangia.

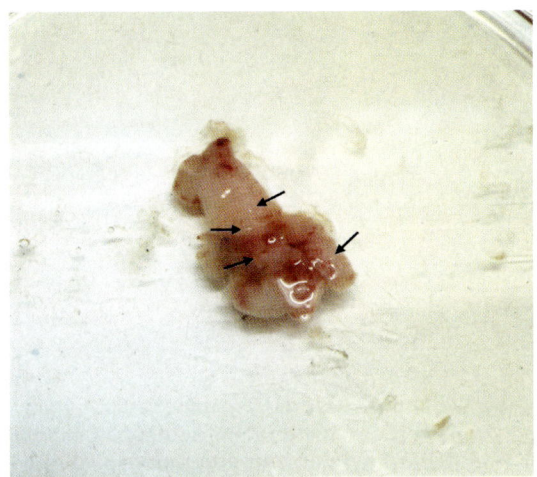

Fig. 2.29: Gross appearance of the specimen from a case of rhinosporidiosis. Polyp developed in nasal opening. The polypoidal mass is lobulated, soft, reddish pink to dark red and minute opaque spherules (white dots) are also readily visible.

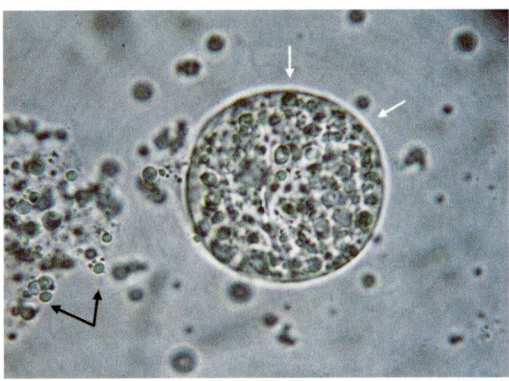

Fig. 2.31: Rhinosporidiosis. Mature spherules showing thick wall (white arrow) and endospores which are released through pores (black arrow). Nuclei can be seen within the endospores [KOH mount ×600].

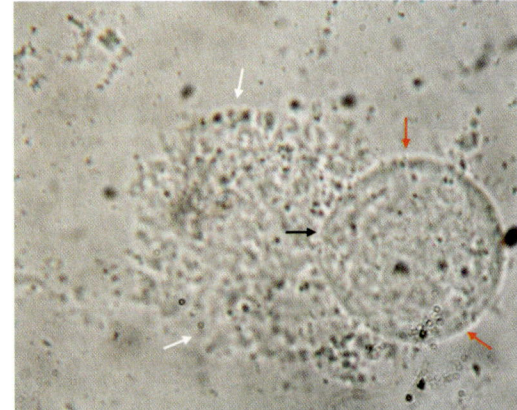

Fig. 2.32: Potassium hydroxide preparation of an excised polyp in a case of nasal rhinosporidiosis. Mature sporangium is filled up with endospores and the wall becomes thinner (red arrow). Subsequently pore is formed on the wall (black arrow) which ruptures and spores are released into the surrounding area (white arrow) [×400].

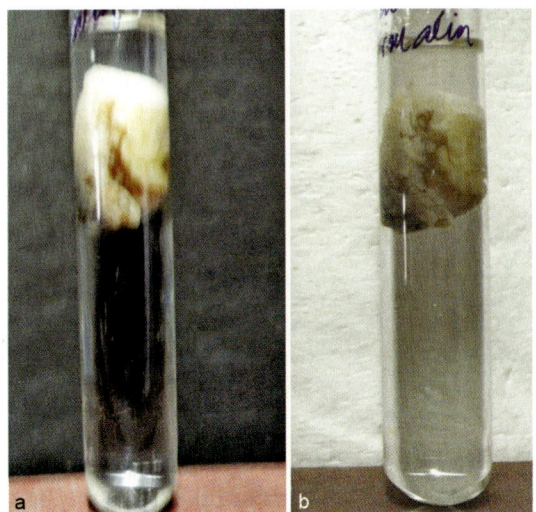

Fig. 2.30: Specimen of polyp from a case of rhino-sporidiosis. The lesion involved hard palate. Polyp of rhinosporidiosis are dense, opaque grayish white and granular material is apparent which represents the mature sporangia; (a) front and (b) back view of the same specimen.

The sporangia of **Rhinosporidium seeberi** should not be confused with spherules of **Coccidioides immitis.**

- The sporangium of **R. seeberi** is much larger and has thicker.
- The size and number of endospores in the sporangia of **R. seeberi** are greater.
- Sporangium of **R. seeberi** stains with mucicarmine unlike **C. immitis.**

Culture Methods

Rhinosporidium seeberi cannot be cultured on artificial media in the laboratory. Diagnosis of the disease can be made from histopathologic section (Figs 2.33 to 2.37) or by direct examination (both macroscopic and microscopic visualization in a KOH preparation).

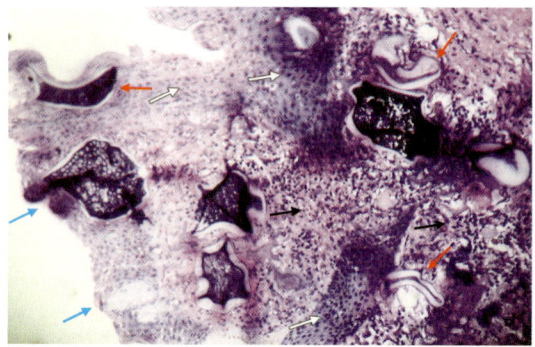

Fig. 2.35: *Rhinosporidiosis*. Histopathology section of the nasal polyp showing numerous sporangia in the submucosal, some of them are found collapsed or empty (red arrow). The submucosa contains variable number of inflammatory cells (black arrow), the linning mucosal epithelium is hyperplastic (white arrow) but may be quite thinned in some areas. The mature sporangia often lie just beneath the thinned areas (blue arrow) [H&E stained section ×400].

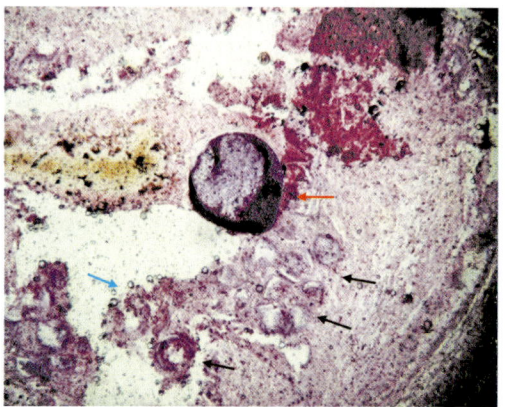

Fig. 2.33: Hematoxylin and eosin stained section shows a mature sporangium (red arrow), cysts in varying stages of development (black arrow) and numerous spores (blue arrow) are released into fibomyxomatous stroma. *Rhinosporidium seeberi* [×400].

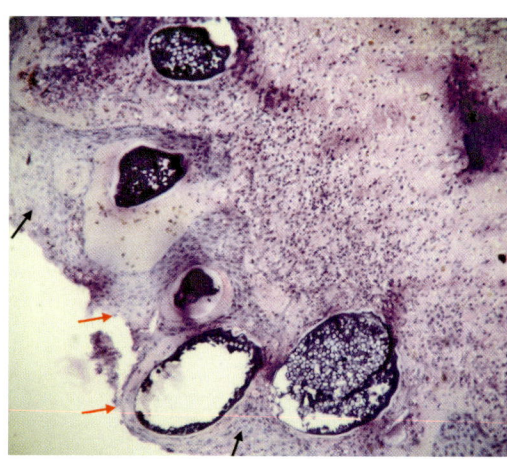

Fig. 2.36: Histopathology of nasal rhinosporidiosis. Mild degrees of pseudoepitheliomatous hyperplasia (black arrow) hyperkeratosis and thinning with areas of erosion (red arrow) are noticed. Various stages of sporangial development within the epithelium is seen [H&E stained section ×400].

Histopathological Examination

Microscopic examinations of the stained tissue sections confirm the diagnosis.

Hematoxylin and eosin stained section shows hyperplastic mucosal epithelium

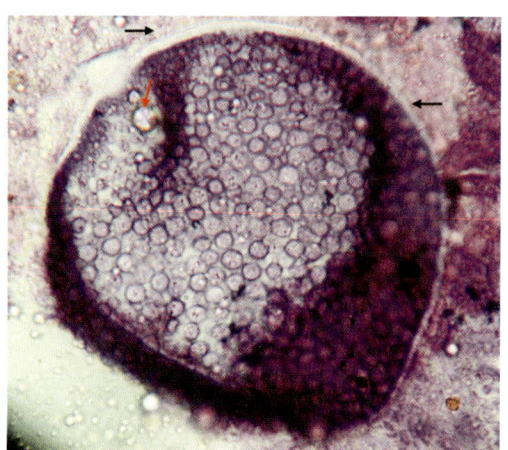

Fig. 2.34: *Rhinosporidium seeberi*. A matured sporangium (spherule) containing endospores. The sporangium has a thick covering made up of cellulose (black arrow) which becomes thinned out on verge of rupture. Mature spores contain globular bodies which are lipid globules, appear as small vacuoles (red arrow) in hematoxylin and eosin stain [H & E stain ×600].

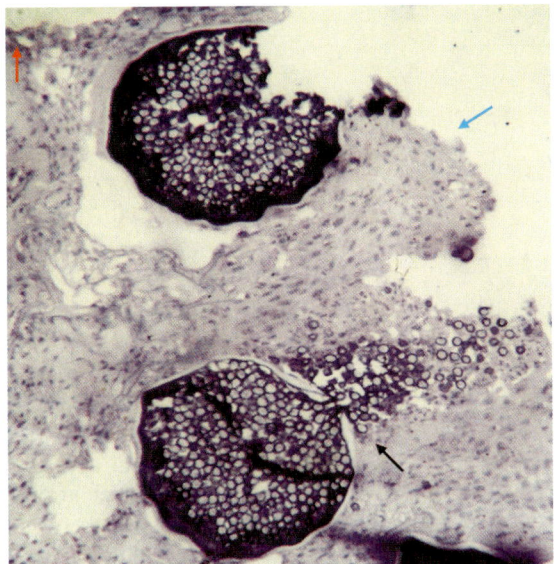

Fig. 2.37: *Rhinosporidium seeberi* infection of the nasal mucosa. Matured sporangia are found in fibromyxomatous connective tissue stroma. One sporangium (below) showing release of spores through a pore on the wall (black arrow) into the stroma. Thinning (red arrow) and ulceration (blue arrow) of the mucosal epithelium are also noticed [H&E stained section × 400].

though it may be quite thinned in some areas. Mature sporangia often lie just beneath the thinned mucosal epithelium (Figs 2.35 and 2.36). The major portion of the growth consists of very vascular fibromyxomatous connective tissue in which parasites are found in various stages of development (Fig. 2.36). The cellular infiltrate consists of plasma cells, lymphocytes, histiocytes and neutrophils. The mature sporangium enlarges to 250 to 350 µ, the wall becomes thinner, and the annulus begins to disappear. The mature spores migrate toward the periphery near the pore. Rupture of the pore occurs, possibly from internal pressure and the spores are released into the surrounding connective tissue (Figs 2.33 and 2.37). The spores at maturity are 7 to 9 µ. They contain nucleus, a basophilic karyosome-like body, and globular bodies in the cytoplasm. These bodies are lipid globules and usually appear reddish pink with H and E staining (Fig. 2.34).

CHROMOBLASTOMYCOSIS

Chromoblastomycosis, recently used term chromomycosis, included a group of clinical entities caused by a group of dematiaceous (pigmented) fungi. The lesion appears at the site of some trauma or punctured wound. Initially the lesion is a small, raised, erythematoid, non-prurigenous papule. Frequently these lesions become raised to 1 to 3 mm above the skin surface and are hypertrophic with a scaly, dull, and red to grayish surface (Fig. 2.38). Sometimes there is peripheral spread with healing in the centre as in cutaneous blastomycosis.

In mature lesions of chromoblastomycosis, the planate, yeast-like bodies (sclerotic cells) are found. These are referred to as "copper pennies" or "medlar bodies" (Fig. 2.45).

Etiologic agents of chromoblastomycosis and phaeomycotic cyst are:

- *Fonsecaea pedrosoi*
- *Fonsecaea compacta*
- *Wangiella dermatitidis*
- *Phialophora verrucosa*
- *Phialophora richardsiae*
- *Exophiala spinifera*
- *Cladophialophora carionii*
- *Cladophialophora bantianum*

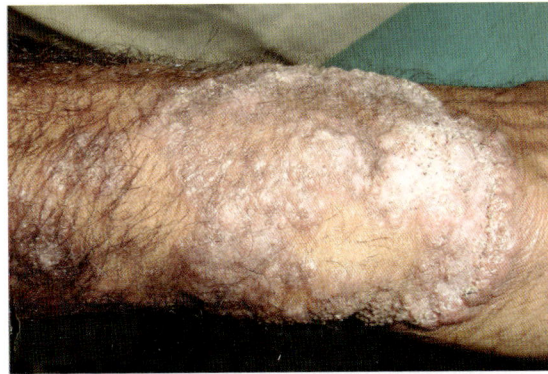

Fig. 2.38: Chromoblastomycosis. Pedunculated and verrucous lesions resembling florets of cauliflower.

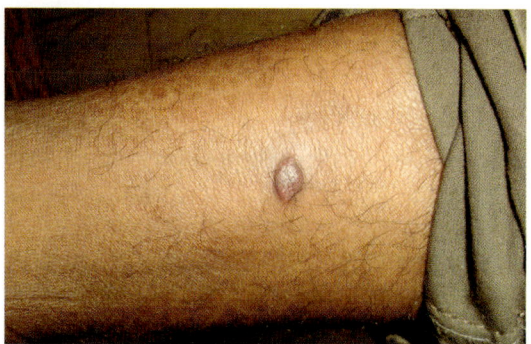

Fig. 2.39: Phaeomycotic cyst. Lesion is on the lateral aspect of leg. Subcutaneous involvement following nonpenetrating injury. Lesion is fluctuant, tender, blue-gray with no connection to surface.

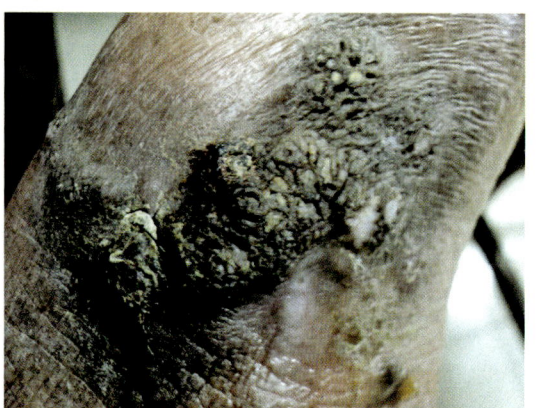

Fig. 2.40: verrucous chromoblastomycosis. The lesions are above the later malleolus of the left leg. *Fonsecaea pedrosoi* was cultured.

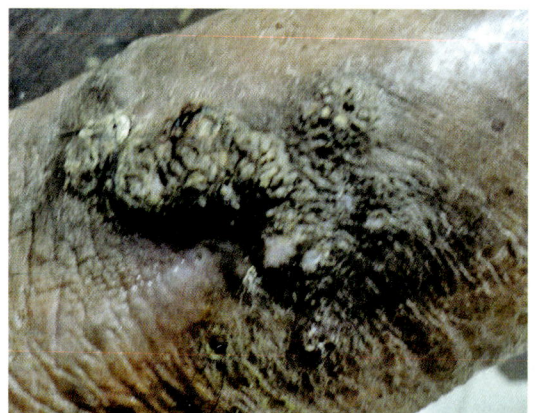

Fig. 2.41: Lesions of verrucous chromoblastomycosis resembles florets of a cauliflower.

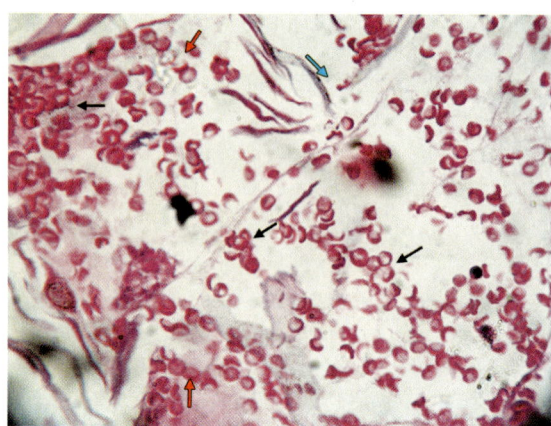

Fig. 2.42: Histopathology section of biopsy material from verrucous chromoblastomycosis. Predominance of 'sclerotic bodies' are noticed. These are thick walled, brown pigmented, rounded to pleomorphic cells that exhibit planate division (black arrow) or some are grouped in *chainlike* formation (red arrow) [H&E stain ×600].

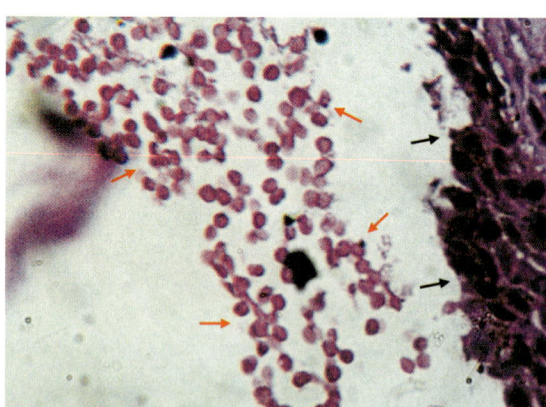

Fig. 2.43: Chromoblastomycosis. Brown coloured, thick walled, round to pleomorphic cells of varied size are 'sclerotic bodies' (red arrow) diagnostic of chromo-blastomycosis. Black arrow shows pseudoepithelio-matous hyperplasia of the surface epithelium [H&E stained section of punch biopsy from skin lesion ×400].

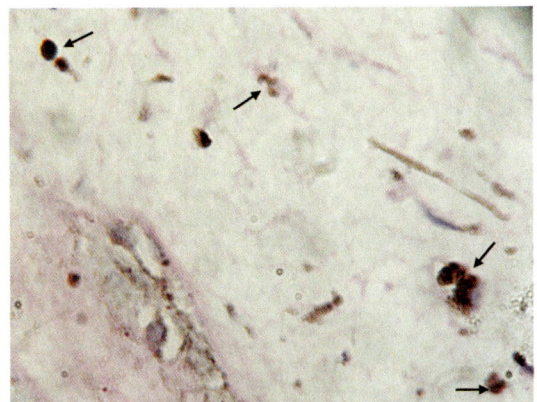

Fig. 2.44: Chromoblastomycosis. Histopathology section showing brown coloured 'sclerotic bodies' of varying size [H & E stain ×400].

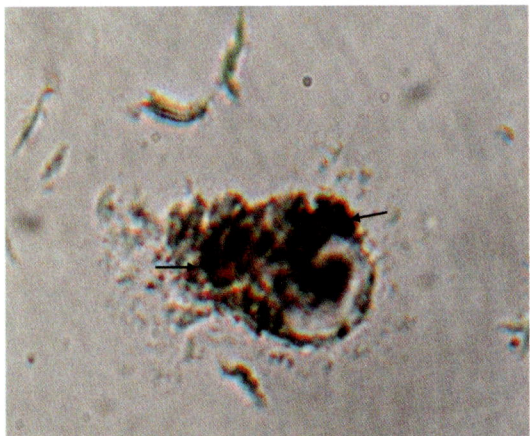

Fig. 2.45: 'Sclerotic bodies' in KOH preparation of punch biopsy material from verrucous chromoblastomycosis. These are thick walled, brown-pigmented cells and exhibits planate division (black arrow) [×600].

Laboratory Identification

Direct Examination

Laboratory diagnosis of chromoblastomycosis by direct examination of suspicious material is relatively easy, but it must always be confirmed by culture. Skin scrapings, crusts, aspirated debris, biopsy and excised material can be examined in a potassium hydroxide (KOH) mount. Brown-pigmented, branching, hyphal strands (2 to 6 µ) are easily seen in skin scrapings, crusts and aspirates. In pus from cysts, very distorted hyphae (3 to 8 µ wide) and pleomorphic brown bodies (up to 20 µ in diameter), which sometimes appear to bud, may be found. In granulation tissue obtained by curettage, excision, or biopsy from verrucous chromoblastomycosis, the sclerotic bodies predominate. They are thick walled, brown-pigmented, exhibit plantae division and may be grouped in a chainlike formation. The size varies from 4 to 12 µ (Fig. 2.46).

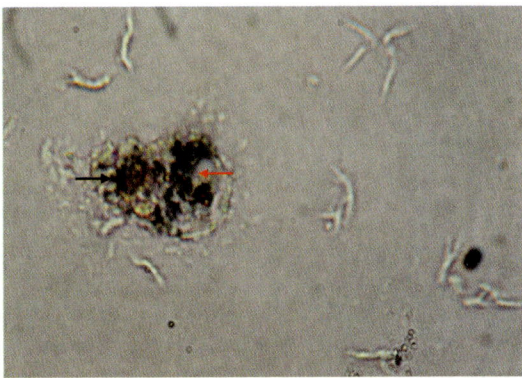

Fig. 2.46: Chromoblastomycosis. Plantae dividing rounded 'sclerotic bodies' (black arrow) of fungus in verrucoid chromoblastomycosis. Some sclerotic bodies may be grouped in a chainlike formation (red arrow) [KOH mount ×400].

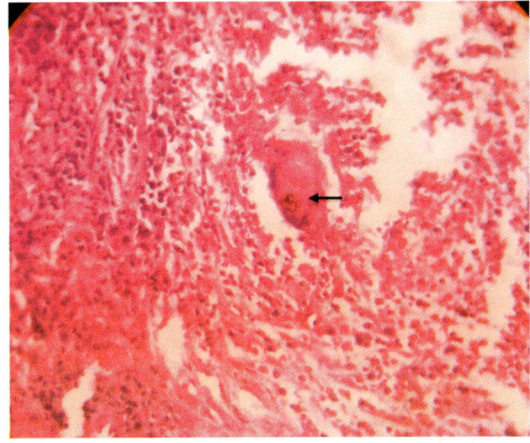

Fig. 2.47: Chromoblastomycoses. High power view of an abscess showing brown coloured sclerotic bodies (black arrow) of fungus within a giant cell [H&E stained section ×400].

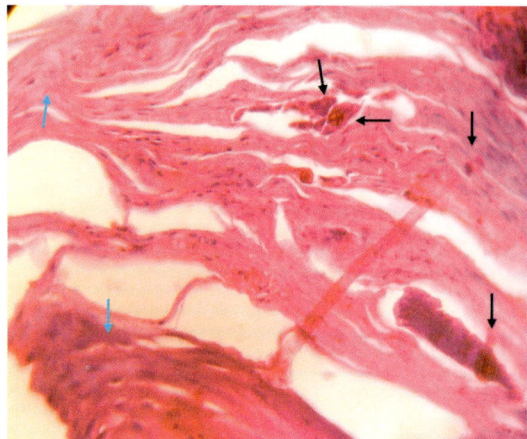

Fig. 2.48: Hematoxylin and eosin stained section of phaeomycotic cyst showing presence of sclerotic bodies (black arrow) and also pseudoepitheliomatous hyperplasia (blue arrow ×400).

Culture Methods

The agents of chromoblastomycosis are not inhibited by cyclohexamide (actidione) or chloramphenicol; hence selective media using these antibiotics may be used. Culture should be kept at 25 to 27°C for at least six weeks. The specific identification of the organism depends on conidia types, percentage of conidia types present, fine details of conidia production and perhaps the position of the planets. Three general types of conidiation are found in this group.

1. **Phialophora type**: Vase (flask) shaped phialides give rise to conidia which accumulate around the neck area giving a picture of "flowers in a vase". Conidia are oval, smooth walled, and hyaline and have no attachment scars.

2. **Rhinocladiella type**: The conidia are borne at the ends and sides of conidiophores and have one scar of attachment. Hyphae, conidia, and conidiophores are a pale greenish brown.

3. **Cladosporium type**: A simple stalk serves as a conidiophores, distal end of which is slightly enlarged and two or more conidia are formed at the tip. These in turn bud and form

secondary conidia at their distal poles. Conidiation continues with the formation of a long chain. The youngest conidium is the

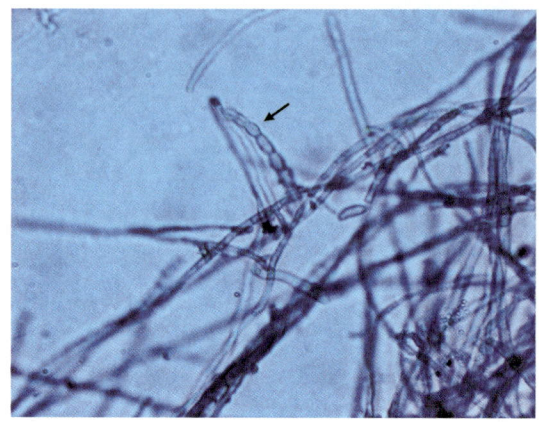

Fig. 2.49: *Cladophialophora carionii.* Conidial chains arise directly from the tip or side of the hyphae (black arrow). Conidia are pale brown, oblong to ellipsoidal with a truncate base. The width of the conidia in the same chain is remarkably uniform but the length varies depending on the position in the chain. This fungus is a frequent isolant from verrucous chromoblastomycosis [LPCB mount ×600].

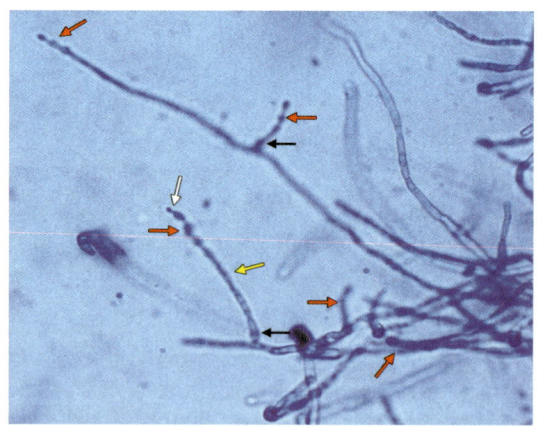

Fig. 2.50: Branched or unbranched acropetal (white arrow) chains of conidia (red arrow) are produced on poorly differentiated conidiophores (black arrow). The length of conidia in a chain varies depending on its position. The first few conidia (yellow arrow) proximal to conidiophore are longer than the conidia distal (red arrow) to conidiophore. *Cladophialophora carionii* [LPCB mount ×400].

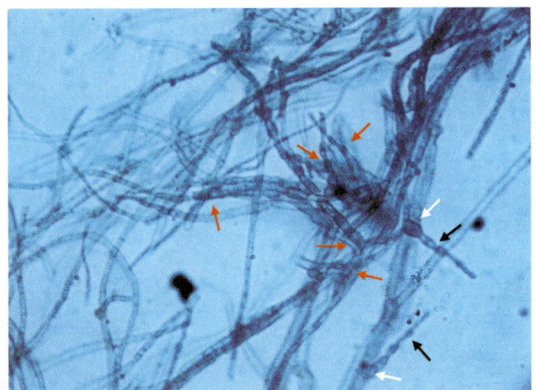

Fig. 2.51: *Cladophialophora carionii*. Conidial chains are branched (red arrow) or unbranched (black arrow) produced on poorly differentiated conidiophores or denticles (white arrow). Conidia are olivaceous brown, oblong to ellipsoidal with a truncate base [LPCB mount ×600].

one distal to the conidiophore. Detached conidia show a thickening or scar, called a disjuncture, where they were connected to the other conidia. A conidium having three disjunctures is described as "shield-shaped" cell.

Fonsecaea pedrosoi

Colony morphology

In culture *F. pedrosoi* grows very slowly, producing a black-brown, gray-black colony. The texture is velvety to fluffy and the surface varies from flat to heaped and folded (Fig. 2.52). The colony character may vary considerably between isolates and the organism is indistinguishable macroscopically from *P. verrucosa*.

Microscopic morphology

All three types of conidiation exist in this species, the population varying with the strain and the media used for growth. The *Cladosporium* type sometimes predominates with frequent admixture of the *Rhinocladiella* type and occasional phialophora type (Figs 2.55 and 2.56). A few conidia are produced on Sabouraud's dextrose agar but on deficient media, such as cornmeal agar, conidiation is enhanced. In *Fonsecaea pedrosoi* conidia are

borne in short chains (in *Cladosporium* type conidiation) rather than long chains, from distal end of conidiophores as it is found in

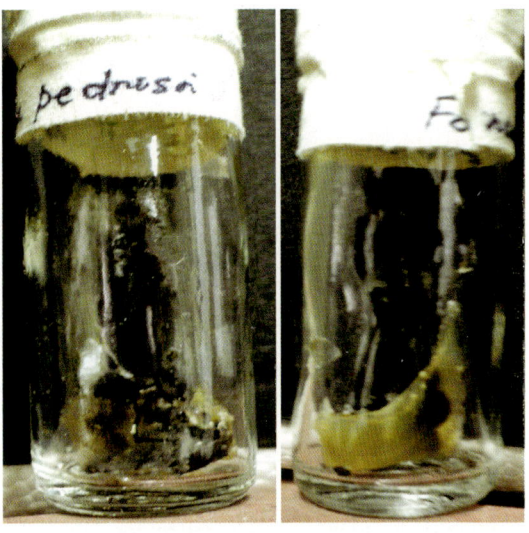

Fig. 2.52: Colony morphology of *Fonsacaea pedrosoi* grown on SDCA at 30°C for four weeks. Black brown, velvety, heaped and folded colonies are produced; (a) obverse, (b) reverse.

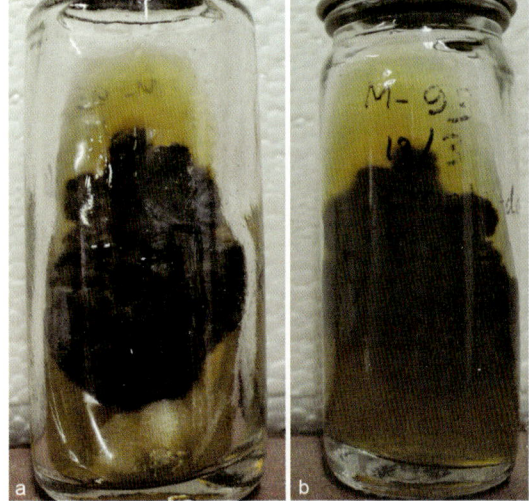

Fig. 2.53: *Exophiala jeanselmei*. Colonies on SDCA are olive to black, moist yeast-like at first but may remain as such or short mycelial element can overgrow on the surface of the colony; (a) obverse, (b) reverse.

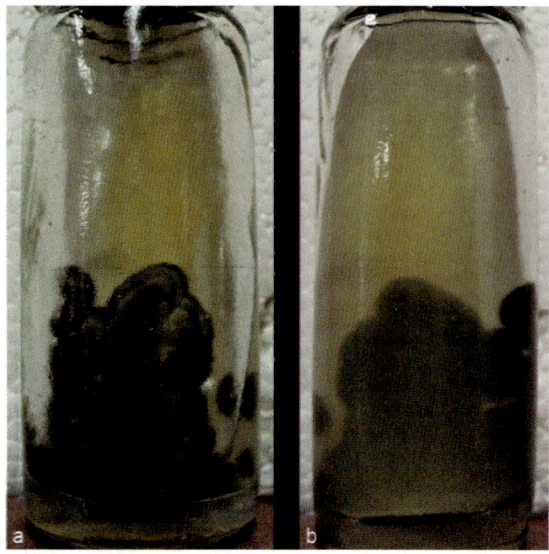

Fig. 2.54: Colony morphology of *Cladophialophora carionii* grown on Sabouraud's dextrose agar after 4 weeks of incubation at 30°C. Colonies are dark olive-gray to nearly black, compact and folded. The edges are entire and marginated by black submerged hyphae (white arrow). The reverse is black; (a) obverse, (b) reverse.

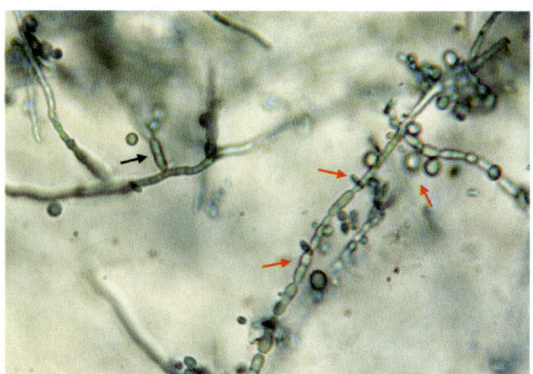

Fig. 2.56: *Fonsecaea pedrosoi*. Rhinocladiella type conidiation (red arrow) and Phialophora type of conidiation (black arrow) are shown here [LPCB mount ×400].

Cladosporium species (Figs 2.57 and 2.58). Conidiophores are of varying lengths. The conidia are elliptical, cylindrical to ovoid. They exhibit two dark thick scars (disjuncture) where they were attached in chains. 'Shield cells' with three scars may be found among conidia on the terminal end of conidiophores. The last cell of chain has only one scar.

Rhinocladiella type of conidiation is formed from bare hyphae or from knobby, denticulate conidiophores. The conidia are arranged at the tip and along the side of conidiophores (Fig. 2.58).

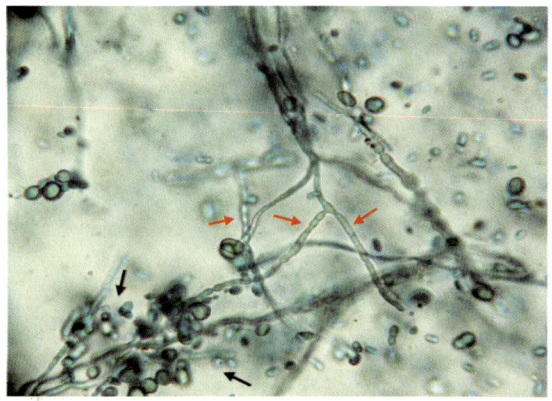

Fig. 2.55: Microscopic morphology of *Fonsecaea pedrosoi* showing predominantly 'Cladosporium' type of conidiation (red arrow). 'Rhinocladiella' type of conidiation (black arrow) is also noticed [LPCB mount ×400].

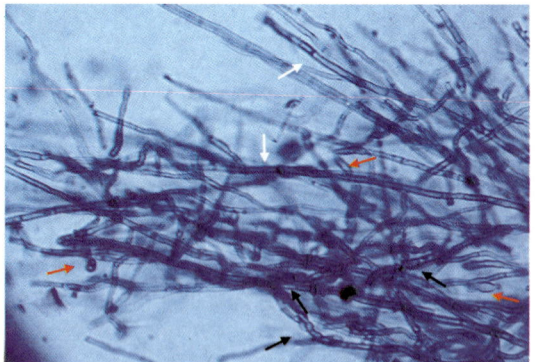

Fig. 2.57: *Fonsecaea pedrosoi*. Microscopic morphology showing pigmented (phaeoid) hyphae with regular septation (white arrow), Phialophora type of conidiation (red arrow) and also Cladosporium type of conidiation (black arrow) [LPCB mount ×400].

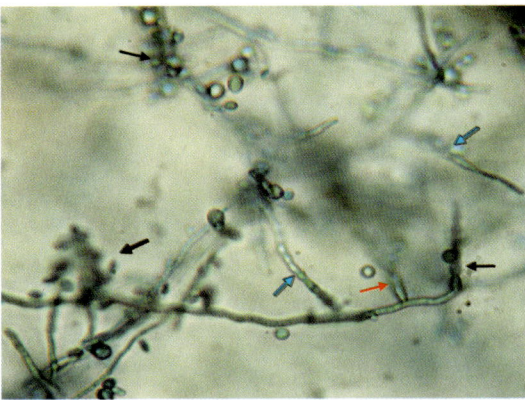

Fig. 2.58: All three types of conidiation are found in *Fonsecaea pedrosoi*. Cladosporium type (blue arrow), Rhinocladiella type (black arrow) and Phialophora type (red arrow) [LPCB mount ×400].

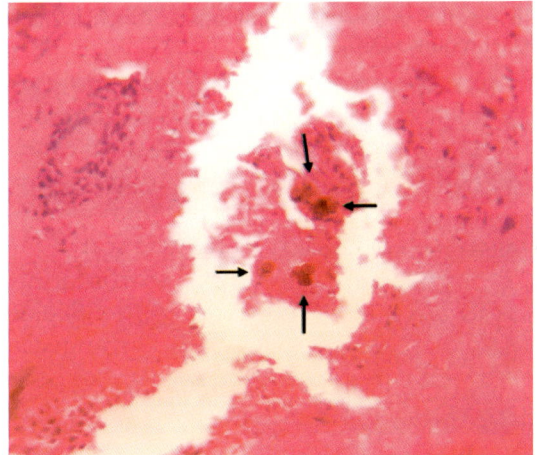

Fig. 2.59: Histopathology section in verrucous chromoblastomycosis showing planate dividing round sclerotic bodies (black arrow) of fungus [H&E stain ×400].

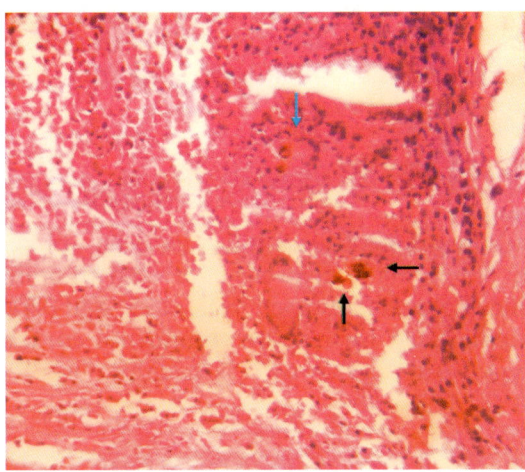

Fig. 2.60: Chromoblastomycosis. Hematoxylin and eosin stained histopathologic section showing planate dividing round sclerotic bodies within an abscess (black arrow). Sclerotic body within a giant cell (blue arrow) is also noticed [×400].

ENTOMOPHTHOROMYCOSIS

Entomophthoromycosis is a chronic inflammatory or granulomatous disease which is generally restricted to the subcutaneous tissue or the nasal submocosa. It includes clinically and mycological two distinct diseases caused by species of the order entomophthorales. These are referred to as:

1. **Entomophthoromycosis conidiobolae:** The etiologic agent is *Conidiobolus coronatus* and *Conidiobolus incongruous*. Nasal mucosa is usually involved and lesions are characterized by presence of polyps or extensive palpable subcutaneous masses which usually remain restricted to that area.

2. **Entomophthoromycosis basidiobolae:** The etiologic agent is *Basidiobolus ranarum*. The disease is characterized by massive, palpable, indurated, non-ulcerating, subcutaneous masses on the limbs, trunk, chest, back or buttock.

Entomophthoromycosis Conidiobolae

Primary infection, in most cases, appears to have originated in the nasal mucosa, and disease is usually restricted to the local subcutaneous tissue. Rarely, paranasal sinuses, facial muscles and pharynx may be involved due to local spread.

Laboratory Identification

Direct Examination

Materials for direct examination are scrapings of the affected nasal mucosa or tissue biopsy from the affected site. Potassium hydroxide mount of the specimens obtained reveals broad hyphae with occasional septation (Fig. 2.61). The hyphal walls are doubly refractile and granular inclusions are readily seen (Fig. 2.62).

Culture Methods

Samples collected from the affected site for culture are gently cut into pieces and plated on Sabouraud's dextrose agar with chloramphenicol and incubated both at 25° and 37°C. Media used for culture should not contain cyclohexamide. Growth is usually observed at 48 to 72 hours.

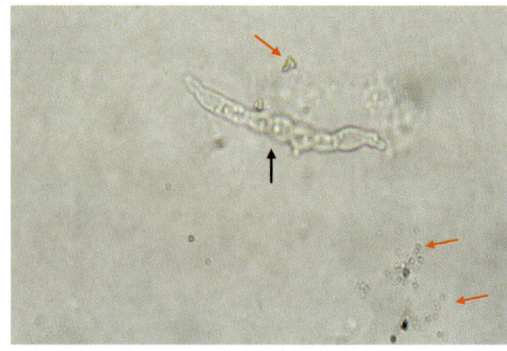

Fig. 2.62: Direct microscopy of nasal discharge (posterior) after potassium hydroxide digestion reveals broad hyphae with sparse septations. The hyphal walls are doubly refractile and granular inclusions are readily seen (black arrow). Yeast cells with occasional budding (red arrow) are also noticed indicating that the infection is due to dual pathogenic fungal invasion [KOH mount ×200].

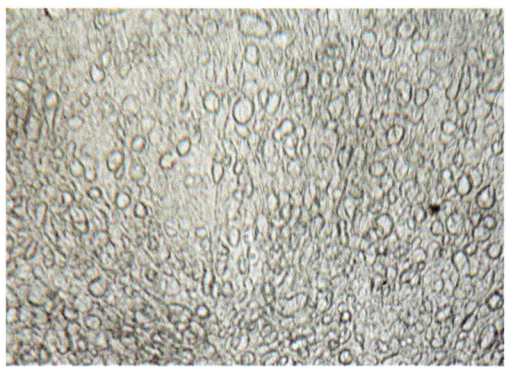

Fig. 2.63: Entomophthoromycosis conidiobolae. Direct examination of nasal discharge after 3 weeks of treatment with potassium iodide (SSKI) [KOH mount ×400].

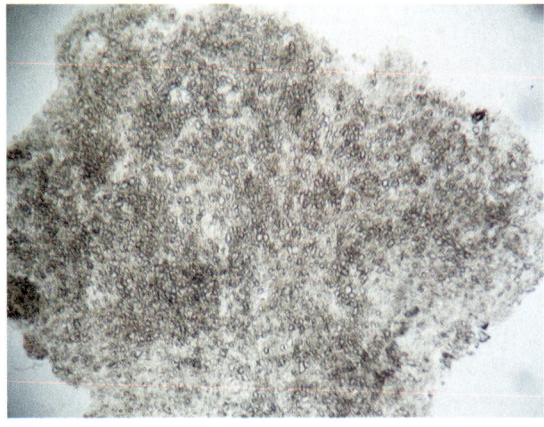

Fig. 2.61: Entomophthoromycosis conidiobolae. Potassium hydroxide mount of scraping from maxillary sinus mucosa [Low power view].

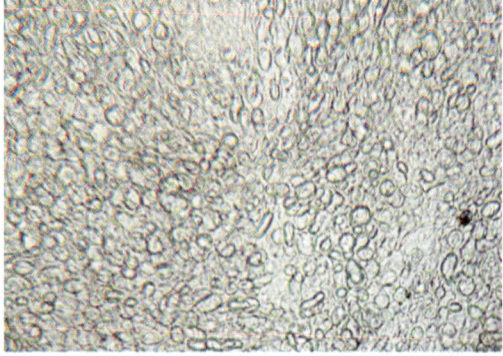

Fig. 2.64: Entomophthoromycosis conidiobolae. KOH preparation of paranasal sinus scrapings after six weeks of continued treatment with SSKI [×400].

Colony Morphology

The colony grows rapidly and is glabrous and adherent at first (Fig. 2.65). Soon the colony becomes covered with short, white, aerial mycelia and conidiophores (Fig. 2.66). Furrows

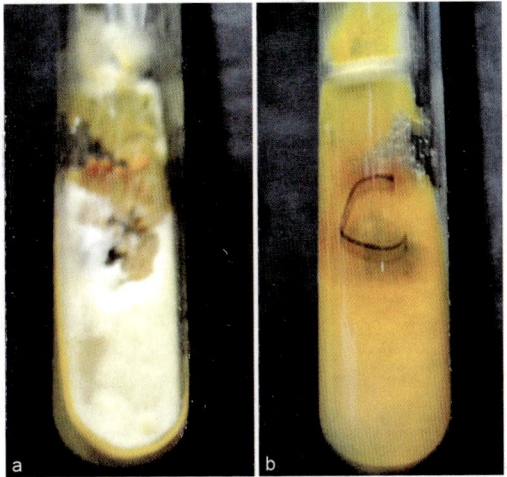

Fig. 2.65: Colony morphology of *Conidiobolus coronatus* grown on Sabouraud's dextrose agar at 25°C for 3 days. The colony grows rapidly and is glabrous and adherent at first (primary culture); (a) obverse, (b) reverse.

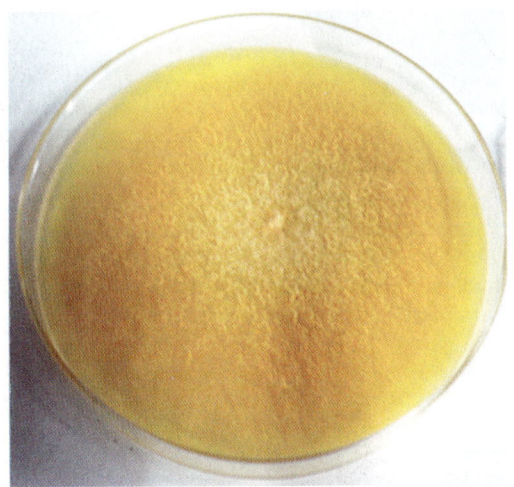

Fig. 2.66: A five-day-old culture of *Conidiobolus incongruus* grown on Sabouraud's dextrose agar at 30°C. The centre of the colony sometimes become covered with short, white aerial mycelia and conidiophore (obverse).

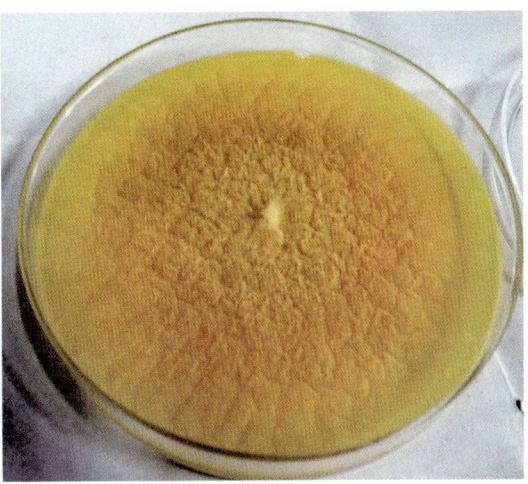

Fig. 2.67: *Conidiobolus incongruus*. Furrows and foldings occur particularly when the fungus is grown at 37°C. Colony morphology (obverse) on SDA for 7 days.

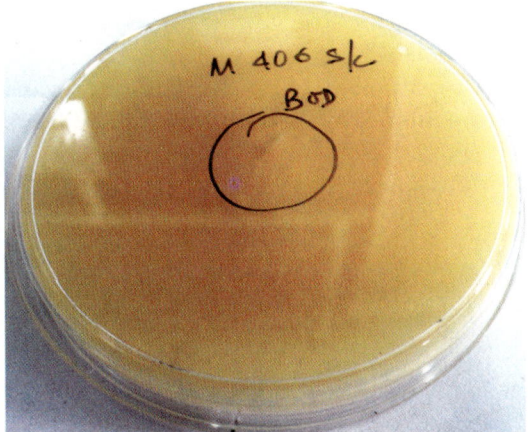

Fig. 2.68: Colony morphology (reverse) of *Conidiobolus incongruus* grown on Sabouraud's dextrose agar at 30°C for 5 days. Reverse is light yellowish brown.

and folding occur, particularly when the organism is grown at 37°C (Fig. 2.67). The colour of the colony becomes tan to yellowish brown and reverse is also light yellowish brown (Figs 2.66 and 2.68).

Microscopic Morphology

Sporangiola are formed and these are single celled and appear as large conidia (25–45 μ in diameter). They are produced on the end of short, erect, unbranched sporangiophores. The spores are ejected and travel distances up to 30 mm. The sides of the lid of the plates or tubes soon become covered with conidia which are forcibly discharged by the sporangiophores (conidiophores). The spores have prominent papillae on the wall that may give rise to secondary spores (Fig. 2.69). Several papillae and secondary spores may be produced on the wall of the primary (original) spore giving it an appearance of 'corona' of secondary spores. A spore may also produce multiple short hair-like appendages called 'villae'. Presence of this characterizes the species *Conidiobolus coronatus*. *Conidiobolus incongruus* also produces multiplicative spores with papillae, as similar to *C. coronatus* but the villose corona, characteristic of *C. coronatus* are not produced by *C. incongruus* (Fig. 2.70).

Histopathology of entomophthoromycosis is quite interesting and important. It is found that like all 'Zygomycetes' diseases, hyphal elements are readily stained in routine

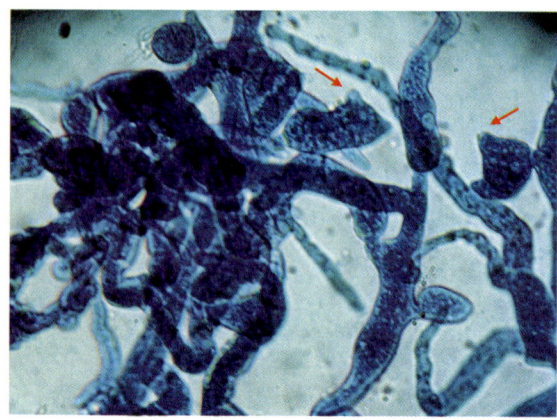

Fig. 2.70: *Conidiobolus incongruus*. Microscopic morphology shows large conidia with prominent papillae (red arrow) but villose corona (hair like appendages on the surface of conidia) characteristic of *Conidiobolus coronatus* is not produced [LPCB mount ×400].

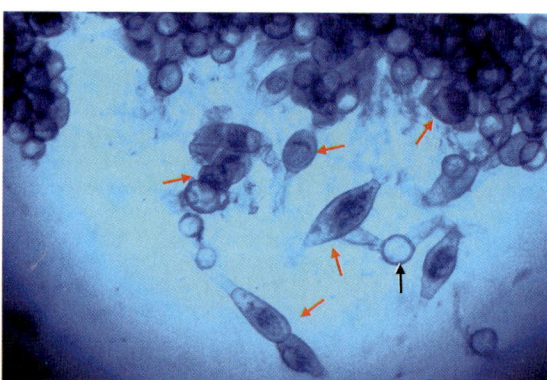

Fig. 2.71: Microscopic morphology of *Basidiobolus ranarum* showing large unicellular sporangium (red arrow) at the apical part of sporangiophore. Sometimes chlamydospores are also noticed in old culture (black arrow) [LPCB mount ×400].

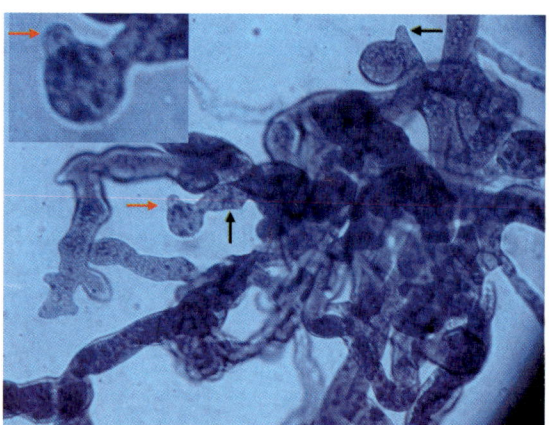

Fig. 2.69: Microscopic morphology of *Conidiobolus incongruus*. Large conidia (single celled sporangiola) are produced on the end of short erect, unbranched sporangiophore (black arrow). Primary conidia have a prominent conical papillae (inset, red arrow) on the wall that may give rise to secondary conidia [LPCB mount ×400].

hematoxylin-eosin preparation but in contrast, with special fungal stain like PAS, Gridley or GMS (stain fungi weakly), these are not well stained. The hyphae of *Conidiobolae* are broad, ribbon-like, with variations in diameter between 4 µ to 10 µ (mean diameter 8 µ) and sometimes up to 22 µ. They are regularly septate and fewer in number. In tissue, hyphae

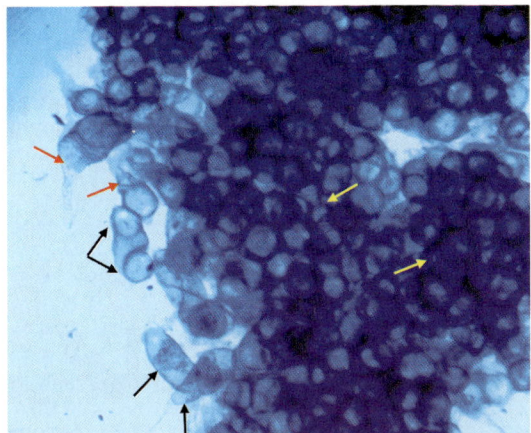

Fig. 2.72: Microscopic morphology showing numerous zygospores and chlamydospores (round structures; yellow arrow). Sporangium (black arrow) are borne at the enlarged apical portion (sporangiola; red arrow) of sporangiophore. *Basidiobolus ranarum* [LPCB mount ×400].

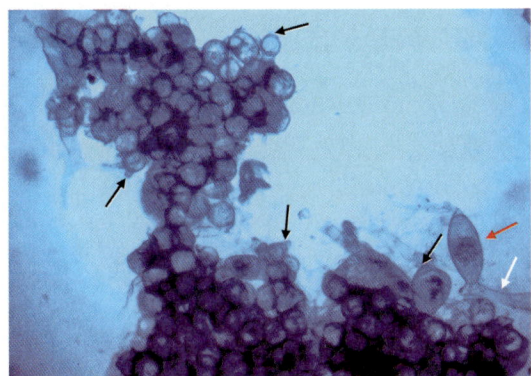

Fig. 2.73: Microscopic morphology of *Basidiobolus ranarum* showing zygospores. The zygospores of Basidiobolus species have a prominent 'beak' (black arrow) attached to one side, representing the copulatory tubes. The sporangium and sporangio-phore are indicated by red and white arrow respectively [LPCB mount ×400].

may lie singly or in clusters (Figs 2.74 and 2.75). The walls are thin but easily defined and surrounded by bright, radiating, granular eosinophilic material (Splendore-Hoeppli phenomenon). The hyphae do not infiltrate the walls of blood vessels, are not seen within the

lumen of the vessels and there is no vascular thrombosis, in contrast to mucormycosis.

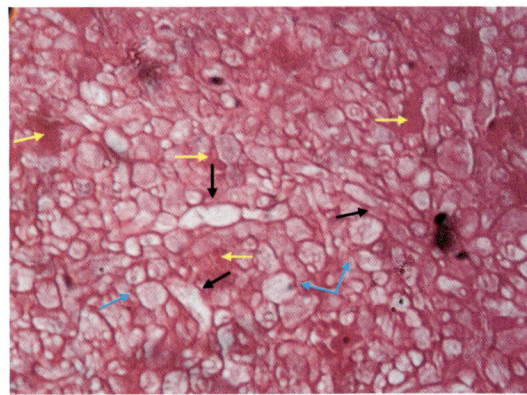

Fig. 2.74: Histopathology section shows broad, thin walled and regularly septate hyphae (oblique section, black arrow) which are surrounded by bright, granular eosinophilic sleeves (yellow arrow) and is called Splendore-Hoeppli phenomenon. Blue arrow indicates cross sections of hyphae; features suggestive of entomophthoromycosis conidiobolae [Tissue obtained from para nasal sinus by FESS; H&E stained section ×400].

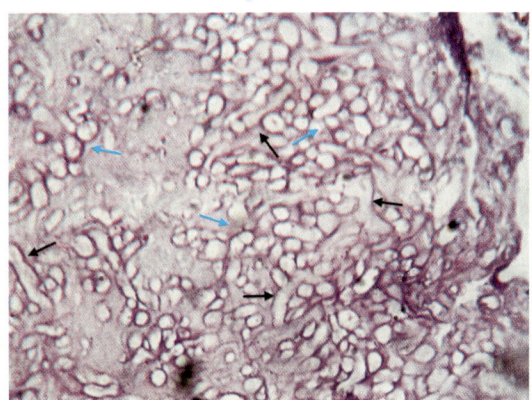

Fig. 2.75: Entomophthoromycosis conidiobolae. Section shows clusters of broad thin walled regularly septate hyphae where some are found in oblique section view (black arrow) and others are in cross section view (blue arrow). The most striking feature is that the hyphal elements are not well stained in periodic acid–Schiff (PAS). Tissue obtained from left maxillary sinus mass in a case of fungal sinusitis [PAS stained section ×400].

The histological features of entomophthoromycosis (both conidiobolae and basidiobolae) contrast sharply to that of mucormycosis. **The three major points of difference between entomophthoromycosis and mucormycosis are:**

1. The eosinophilic sheath (Splendore-Hoeppli phenomenon) around the hyphae is a characteristic feature in entomophthoromycosis but it is not found in mucormycosis.

2. Vascular invasion is a characteristic histopathologic feature found in mucormycosis which is lacking in entomophthoromycosis.

3. Hyphal elements of fungi causing mucormycosis are sparsely septate in tissue, whereas frequent septation is found in entomophthoromycosis.

BASIDIOMYCOSIS

Basidiomycota are very common in nature but rarely associated with human infection. Among all fungi belonging to 'Basidiomycota' *Schizophyllum commune* is the only pathogenic species responsible for human disease. Frequently it has been documented in the literature as a causative agent of fungal sinusitis from eastern India and a few discrete foci in North-East India. We have recovered *Schizophyllum commune* from clinically diagnosed six cases of chronic fungal sinusitis who were not responding to conventional treatment. These patients were undergone FESS (functional endoscopic sinus surgery) and from the biopsy material, this fungi were isolated. We had also recovered *S. commune* from sputum sample of a case with a fungal ball in the left lung on radiology. Repeated isolation of the fungus confirmed the diagnosis. Another fungi which is in the 'Basidiomycota' is teleomorphic stage of *Cryptococcus*, that is genus *Filobasidiella.*

Schizophyllum commune

Colony morphology

Colonies grown on Sabouraud's dextrose agar are white to pale grayish, wooly (Fig. 2.76). As the colony ages, fruit bodies (basidiocarp) are formed on the surface of the colony in concentric zones which are visible macroscopically. The colony reverse is yellowish brown.

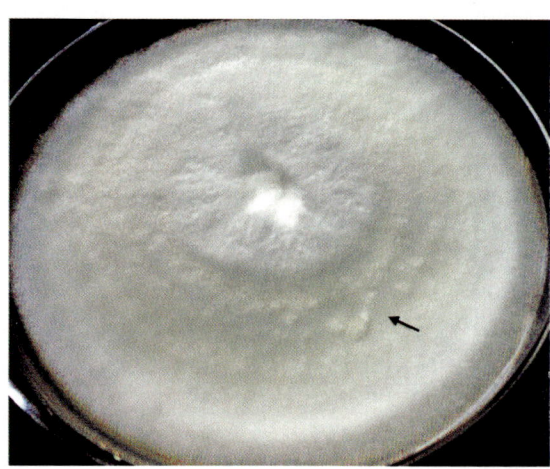

Fig. 2.76: Colony morphology of *Schizophyllum commune* grown on Sabouraud's dextrose agar at 25°C for 3 weeks. White wooly colony and appearance of basidiocarps (black arrow) are characteristic features.

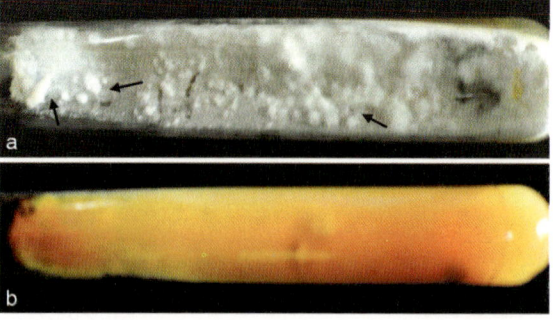

Fig. 2.77: Colony morphology of *Schizophyllum commune* on potato dextrose agar (PDA). Mycelia are beginning to organize into a basidiocarp (black arrow); (a) obverse, (b) reverse.

observed here although other species of *Aspegillus,* namely *A. fumigates, A. terreus* and *A. parasiticus,* are not uncommon agents in FRS. It is worth mentioning that *A. parasiticus* have been isolated from several patients of FRS in our institution.

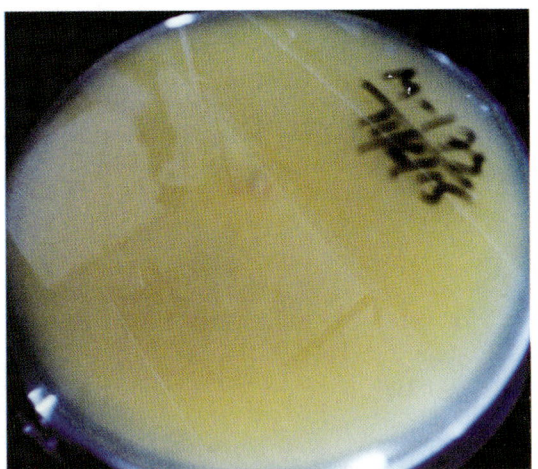

Fig. 2.78: Colony morphology (reverse) of *Schizophyllum commune* grown on Sabouraud's dextrose agar 25°C for 3 weeks. Reverse is tan to light yellowish brown in colour.

Other common agents of fungal rhinosinusitis (FRS)

Aspergillus species is the most common etiology of fungal rhinosinusitis (FRS) in Kolkata and its surrounding region and *Aspergillus flavus* is the predominant species

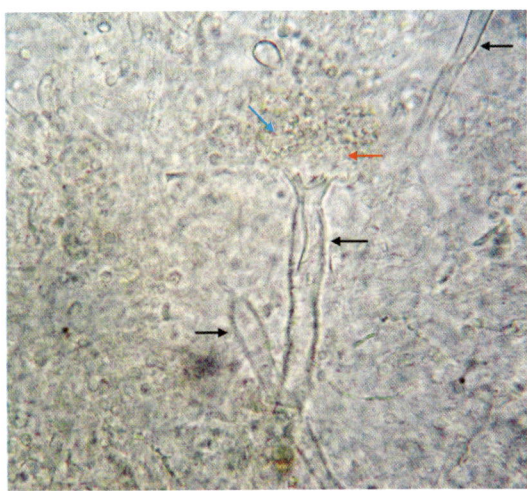

Fig. 2.80: Direct examination of nasal polyp (obtained by FESS) after potassium hydroxide digestion showing rough erect slightly pigmented conidiophore (black arrow), at the tip it enlarges into a hemispherical vesicle (red arrow). Series of sterigmata and conidia are seen surrounding the vesicle (blue arrow) [× 400].

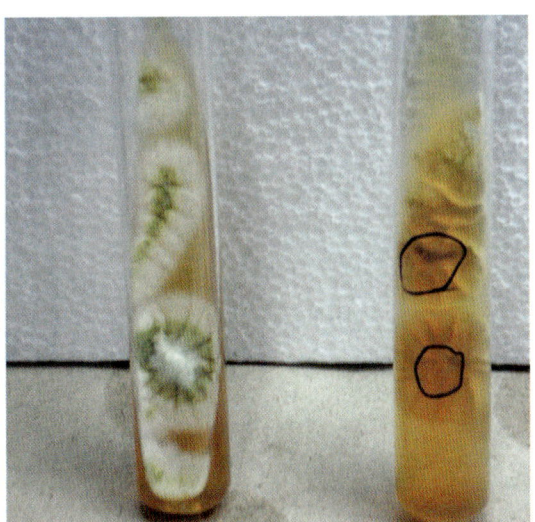

Fig. 2.79: *Aspergillus flavus* grew in culture of the same sample of nasal polyp (Fig. 2.80) when inoculated onto SDCA and incubated at 28°C in BOD incubator for 5 days.

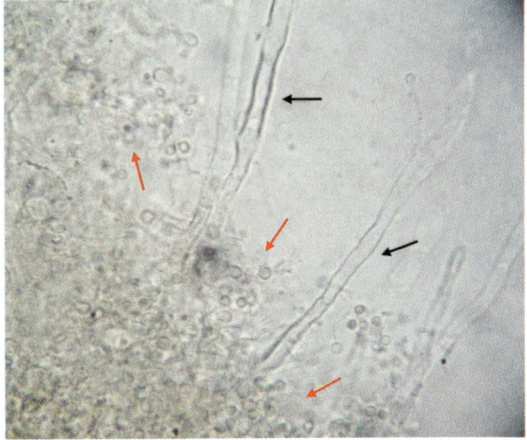

Fig. 2.81: Potassium hydroxide preparation of nasal scraping sample shows rough, dark coloured conidiophore (black arrow) and dense sheets of conidia (red arrow) [×400].

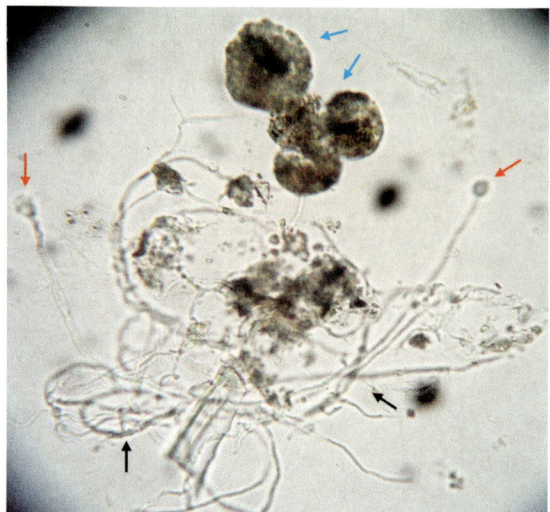

Fig. 2.82: Direct microscopy after potassium hydroxide digestion of a sample (scraping and swab) from a grayish-white patch at the poster pharyngeal wall of 3 months duration. Entangled mycelia (black arrow) which are hyaline, septate, branched in mostly acute angle are noticed along with aleuroconidia (red arrow) and grayish-brown cleistothecia, suggestive of *Aspergillus* colonization. *Aspergillus glaucus* was cultured from the lesion [KOH mount ×400].

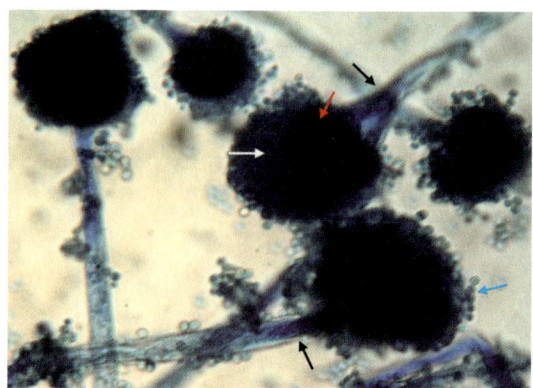

Fig. 2.84: Microscopic morphology of *Aspergillus flavus*. Conidiophores are hyaline, thick-walled and rough (black arrow). Vesicles are subglobose, globose or elliptical (red arrow). They produce sterigmata that cover either the entire or three-fourths of the vesicle surface (white arrow). Sterigmata may be uniseriate or biseriate and produce chains of conidia (blue arrow). Conidia are globose or subglobose to elliptical, yellowish green colour, echinulate [LPCB mount ×400].

Microscopic morphology

Mycelium is hyaline often with clamp connections and series of spicules which are characteristic of **Schizophyllum.** Gradually mycelium organize to form basidiocarp as the colony ages (Figs 2.85 and 2.86).

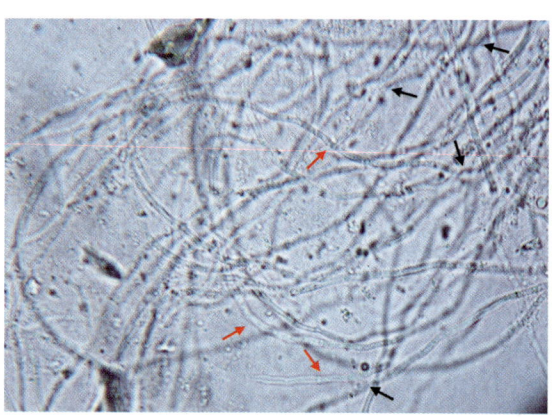

Fig. 2.83: KOH mount of an excised white patchy mass at the palatal region. The mycelia are hyaline, thick to moderate width and have regular septation with acute angle branching suggestive of colonization of *Aspergillus* species. *Aspergillus flavus* was isolated in pure culture.

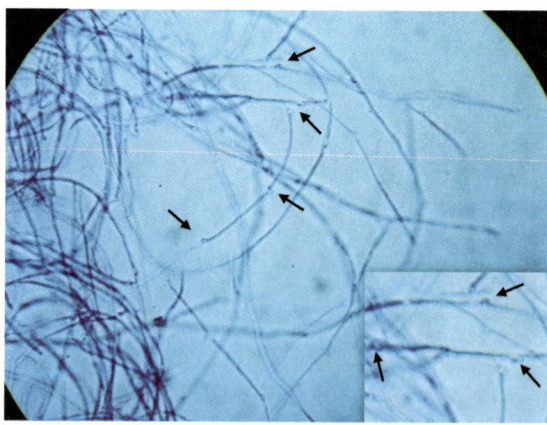

Fig. 2.85: Morphology of *Schizophyllum commune* in culture. Mycelium in culture showing clamp connections (black arrow) which indicate this to be a Basidiomycota [LPCB mount ×400].

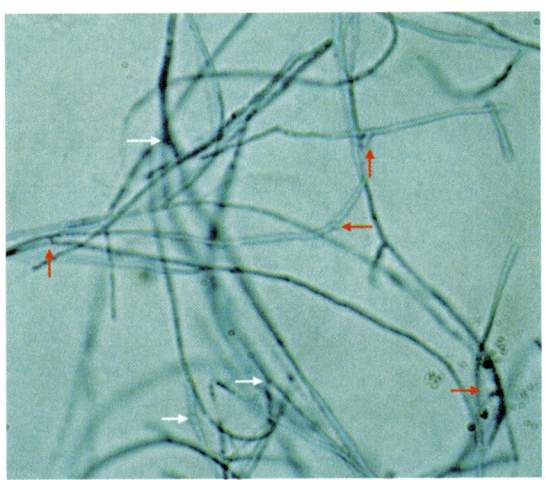

Fig. 2.86: Microscopic morphology of *Schizophyllum commune* reveals presence of 'clamp connections' (white arrow) and spicules (red arrow); the latter are characteristic of Schizophyllum [LPCB mount ×400].

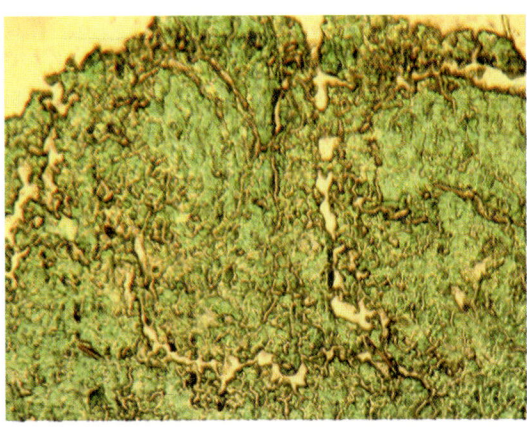

Fig. 2.88: Histopathology section of tissues obtained by endoscopic sinus surgery (FESS) from maxillary sinus showing extensive network of black colour thin septate fungal hyphae. *Schizophyllum commune* was cultured from the lesion [Gomori's methenamine silver stain ×400].

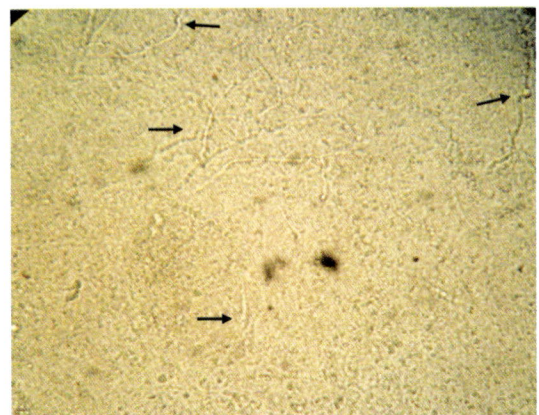

Fig. 2.87: Scraping from paranasal sinus in KOH preparation. Thin hyaline mycelia are observed and clamp connections are also evident (black arrow) [×400].

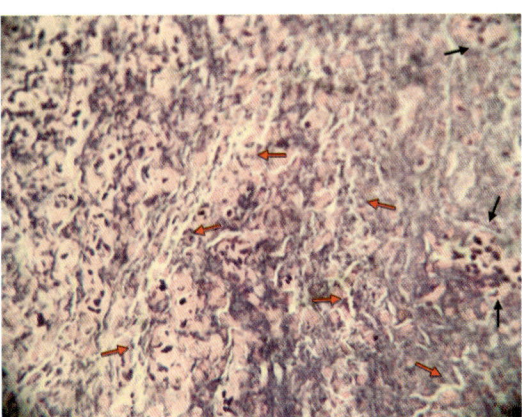

Fig. 2.89: Hematoxylin and eosin stained section of paranasal sinus tissue in fungal sinusitis caused by *Schizophyllum commune*. Numerous thin septate branching hyphae are noticed (red arrow). Plenty of giant cells (black arrow), histiocytes and chronic inflammatory cells seen, suggestive of granulomatous reaction [×400].

SELF ASSESSMENT

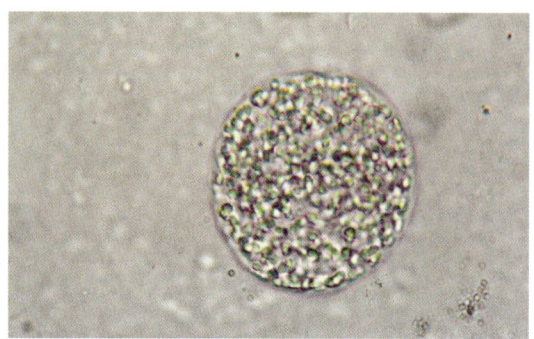

Fig. 2.90: Identify the structure and the likely fungus [KOH mount of nasal polyp ×400].

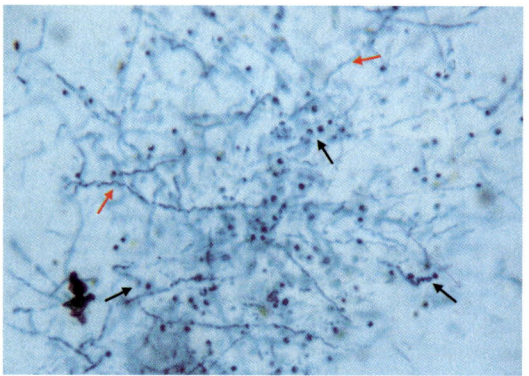

Fig. 2.91: A dimorphic fungi which causes subcutaneous mycoses. Identify the state of the fungus in this picture.

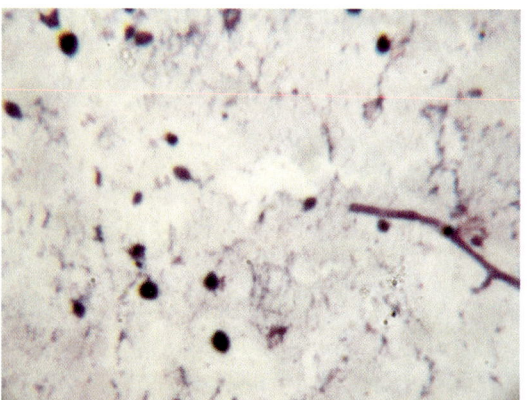

Fig. 2.92: Smear shows a few yeast cells, some fragmented mycelia and a viable mycelium. Identify the fungus with proper justification [Gram stained smear ×1000].

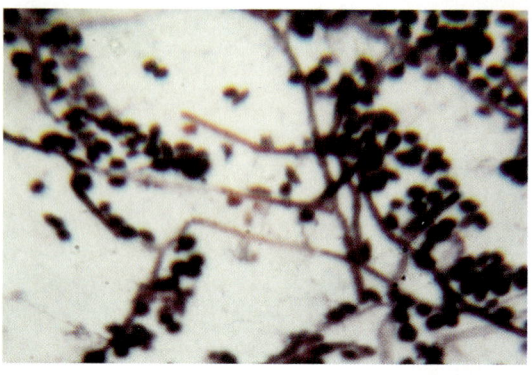

Fig. 2.93: Identify the yeast. [Gram stained smear ×1000].

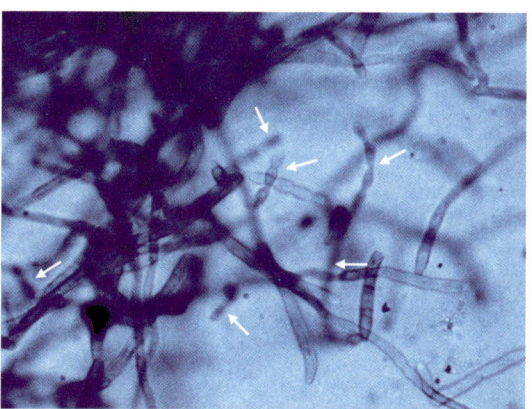

Fig. 2.94: Microscopic morphology of a fungal isolate recovered from a 45-year-old female having a verrucoid black pigmented lesion at the lateral aspect of the right leg. Identify the structure (white arrow) and the likely fungus.

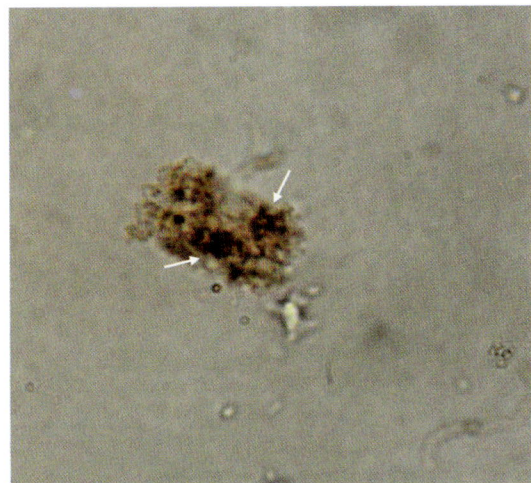

Fig. 2.95: Potassium hydroxide preparation of a tissue biopsy taken from a verrucous, lobulated, black pigmented lesion on the lateral aspect of the left leg of a 62-year-old female. The clinical diagnosis was verrucous chromoblastomycosis. Identify the structures indicated.

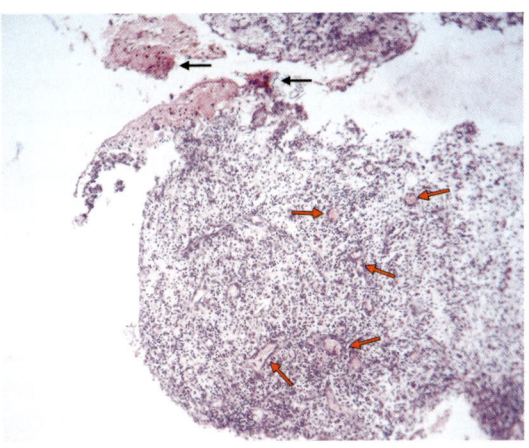

Fig. 2.97: Histopathology section of a punch biopsy from a verrucoid, ulcerated skin lesion. The clinical diagnosis is chromoblastomycosis. Identify the structures indicated and justify the reason to confirm the diagnosis. The lower part of the section shows newly formed capillaries (red arrow), fibroblasts and inflammatory cell infiltration (white arrow) suggestive of granulation tissue formation [H&E stained section ×200].

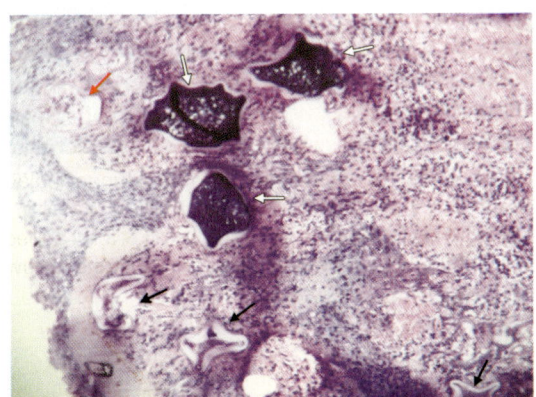

Fig. 2.96: H&E stained tissue section of a nasal mass excised from a 18-year-old male with a history of nasal obstruction for last six months. Identify the structures and the likely fungus.

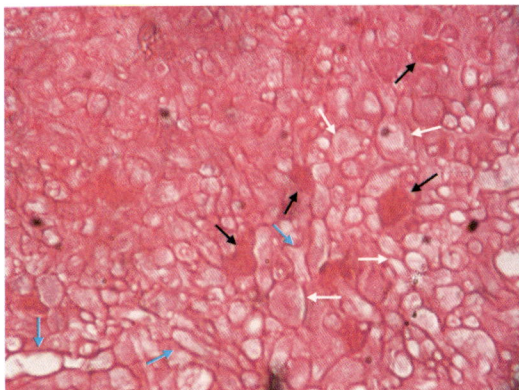

Fig. 2.98: H&E stained section of a biopsy material obtained by FESS from a clinically diagnosed case of fungal sinusitis. Identify the structures indicated and mention the clinical condition suggestive of this histopathology features [×400].

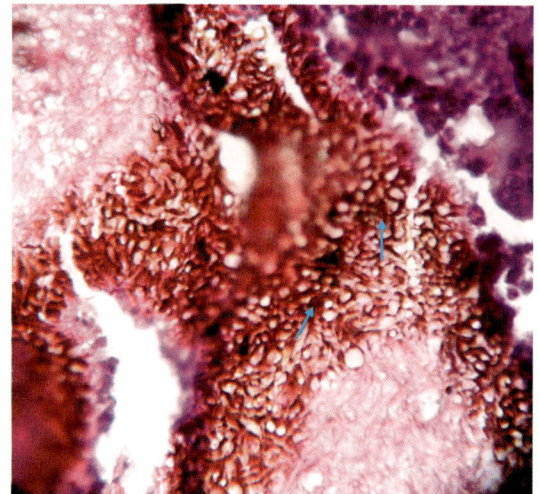

Fig. 2.99: Histopathology section of an excised blackish cauliflower growth appeared on right leg above medial malleolus of a 68 years old female. Identify the structures indicated (blue arrow) and the diagnosis [H&E stained section ×400].

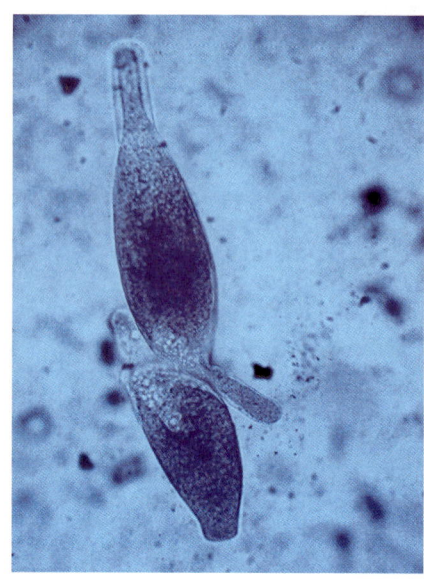

Fig. 2.100: Identify the structure and the relevant fungi [LPCB mount ×600].

ANSWERS

- **Fig. 2.100:** Sporangia of *Basidibolus ranarum*.
- **Fig. 2.99:** Blue arrow—sclerotic bodies; Chromoblastomycosis.
- **Fig. 2.98:** Longitudinal section (blue arrow) and transverse section (white arrow) of broad aseptate hyphae of *Zygomycetes*; Splendore-Hoeppli phenomenon (black arrow); *Entamophthoromycosis conidiobolae*.
- **Fig. 2.97:** Planate dividing cells; Sclerotic bodies
- **Fig. 2.96:** Ruptured sporangium of *Rhinosporidium seeberi*
- **Fig. 2.95:** Sclerotic bodies/medlar bodies/copper penny bodies
- **Fig. 2.94:** Cladosporium type of conidiation; *Cladophialophora carionii*
- **Fig. 2.93:** Yeasts of *Sporothrix schenckii*
- **Fig. 2.92:** M → Y conversion of *Sporothrix schenckii*
- **Fig. 2.91:** M → Y conversion of *Sporothrix schenckii*
- **Fig. 2.90:** Sporangium; *Rhinosporidium* species

Mycetoma

Mycetoma is a clinical syndrome of localize, indolent, deforming lesions and sinuses, involving cutaneous and subcutaneous tissues, fascia and bone. It usually occurs on a foot or hand. The disease results from the traumatic implantation of soil organisms into the tissues. The etiological agents are wide variety of bacteria (actinomycotic mycetoma) and fungi (eumycotic mycetoma) from plant debris and soil. The criteria for the diagnosis of mycetoma are:

1. Tumefaction
2. Multiple draining sinuses
3. Presence of grains which are characteristic granules of the etiologic agents.

The above three criteria are called 'triad of mycetoma' which confirms the clinical diagnosis of the condition. Otherwise these

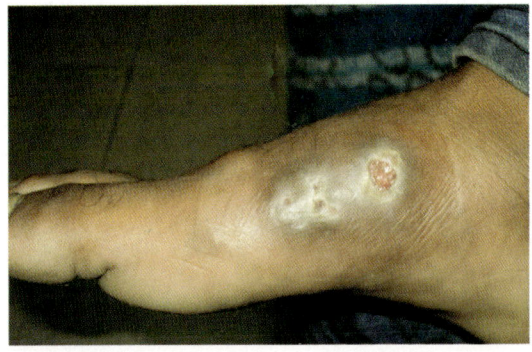

Fig. 3.2: Eumycotic mycetoma. Swollen and distorted foot. Few draining sinus tracts are seen but there is no invasion of muscle or bone. *Fusarium solani*

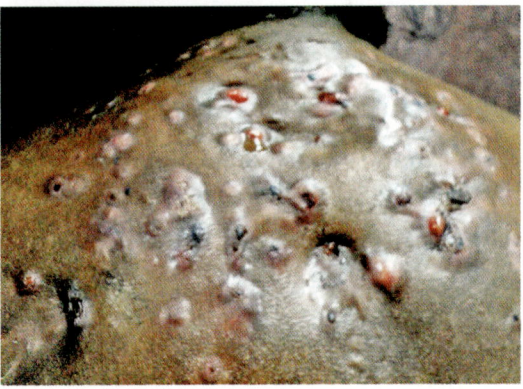

Fig. 3.3: Actinomycotic mycetoma. Multiple sinus tracts and there is hyperplasia at the openings of the sinus tracts which indicate an actinomycotic cause of disease. *Nocardia brazilliensis*

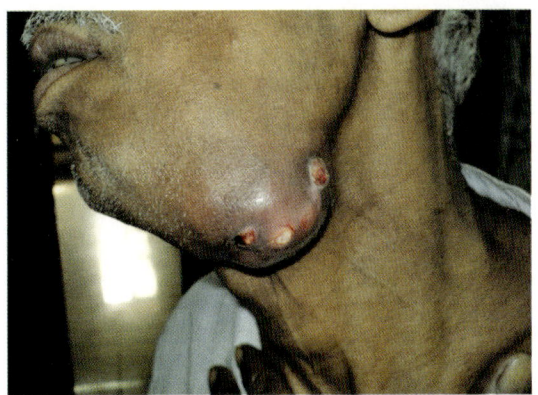

Fig. 3.1: Actinomycotic mycetoma. Multiple sinus tract opening over the ramus of mandible.

organisms cause other clinical diseases, such as actinomycosis, phaeohyphomycosis, mycotic granuloma, etc.

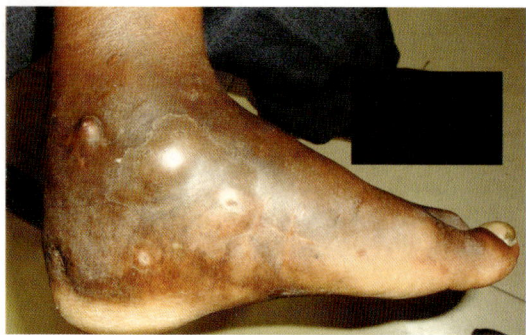

Fig. 3.4: Actinomycotic mycetoma. Swollen and distorted foot. Few draining sinus tracts with the characteristic hyperplasia at the openings of the sinus tracts are seen but there is no invasion of muscle or bone.

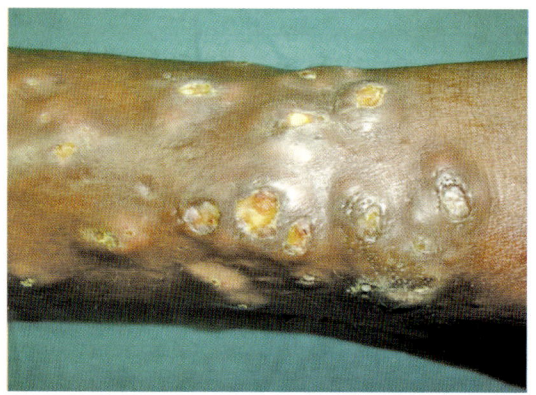

Fig. 3.5: Actinomycotic mycetoma. Multiple sinus openings in an infection caused by *Nocardia* species.

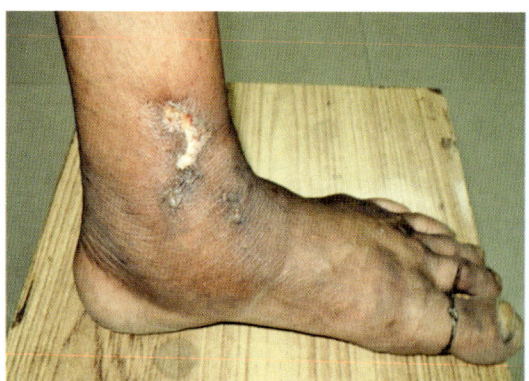

Fig. 3.6: Eumycotic mycetoma. Tumifaction and multiple sinus openings in an infection caused by *Curvularia geniculata*.

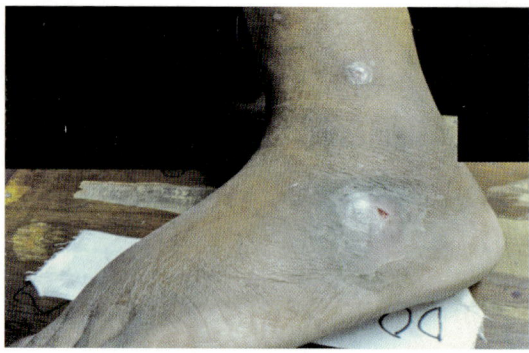

Fig. 3.7: Eumycotic mycetoma. Swollen distorted foot, few draining sinuses are present. In this case, there is no invasion of muscle or bone. The infection is caused by *Acremonium kiliense*.

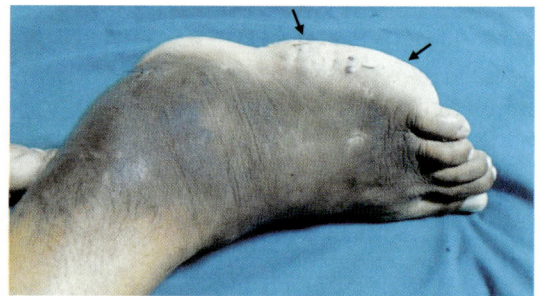

Fig. 3.8: Eumycotic mycetoma. Convex sole of the foot due to tumour like growth in a patient with advanced disease. Muscle involvement is noticed without any bone involvement.

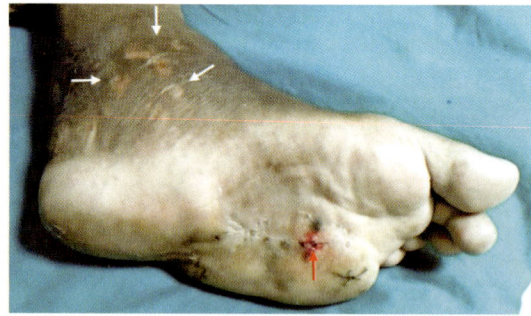

Fig. 3.9: Eumycotic mycetoma. Tumour like growth with a few discharging sinus tracts are present over the lateral aspect of the sole of the foot (red arrow). Multiple sinus tract openings are seen over the medial aspect of the ankle (white arrow). *Madurella mycetomatis* was isolated in pure culture in several occasions from the lesion before and after surgery in this patient.

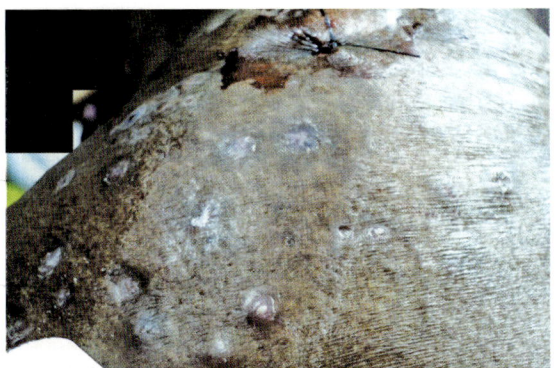

Fig. 3.10: Actinomycotic mycetoma. Punch biopsy taken from the hyperplastic sinus tract opening. *Actinomadura madurae* was cultured from lesions.

Common etiologic agents of mycetoma are:
1. Actinomycotic mycetoma (thin, branching intertwined filaments)
   - *Actinomyces israelii*
   - *Nocardia asteroides*
   - *Nocardia brasiliensis*
   - *Nocardia caviae*
   - *Actinomadura madurae*
   - *Actinomadura pelletieri*
   - *Streptomyces somaliensis*

2. Eumycotic mycetoma (wide, branching, intertwined hyphae and cyst like cells)
   - *Madurella mycetomatis*
   - *Madurella grisea*
   - *Acremonium falciforme*
   - *Acremonium kiliense*
   - *Curvularia geniculata*
   - *Curvularia lunata*
   - *Exophiala jeanselmei*
   - *Fusarium spp.*
   - *Aspergillus nidulans*
   - *Pseudoallescheria boydii*

In this section, only the eumycotic mycetoma will be discussed and actinomycotic mycetoma is beyond the scope of this book *"Atlas of Medical Mycology"*.

Laboratory Identification

Direct examination

Clinical specimens which are collected from the patient are usually pus, exudates or biopsy material. These are examined for the presence of grains. Although grains are macroscopically visible, their morphology, texture, colour and shape may help in identifying the causative agent. Eumycotic grains show intertwined, broad (2 to 5 μ) mycelia strands which may have larger cells at the periphery.

Gram stain is of limited value for observing true fungi. Giemsa stain is recommended and can give better result in staining the smear prepared from collected grains.

Culture method

Specimens suspected to have eumycotic agents may be washed in antibiotic containing saline and plated on Sabouraud's dextrose agar containing 0.5% yeast extract media without cyclohexamide. Plates should be incubated at 25°C.

Several plates should be planted as the number of single species obtained in different plates indicate true etiology.

As the growth of eumycotic agents is usually slow, plates should be kept for six to eight weeks. Identification depends on colony morphology, conidia types and assimilation patterns. Sometimes conidia production is enhanced by growth on nutritionally deficient media like cornmeal agar or potato-carrot agar.

Madurella mycetomatis

It is one of the most important causative agents of mycetoma in India. The infection remains localized and encapsulated at first but in the later stages tend to invade the anatomic barrier and spread along the fascial planes. In advanced stages osteolysis is marked without osteogenesis.

Grains of ***M. mycetomatis*** are black, 0.5 to 1 mm in size, round or lobed, hard or brittle. These are composed of hyphae. Hyphal fragments vary in content of pigment. Two types of grains are produced.

a. Compact form filled with dark brown granular cement between the hyphal elements. In hematoxylin and eosin stains, it appears as an uniform rust brown colour.

b. Vesicular type of grain in which the cement in the periphery is brown and filled with vesicle 6 to 14 µ in diameter. The center is light coloured (Figs 3.11 and 3.12).

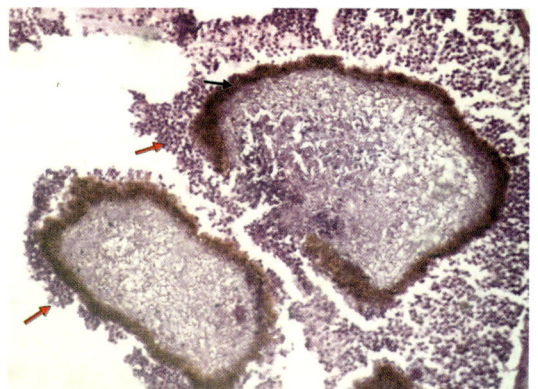

Fig. 3.11: Eumycotic mycetoma. Black grain mycetoma caused by Madurella species. There is heavy pigmentation at the periphery (white arrow) and neutrophils are attached to the periphery of the grain (red arrow). [Hematoxylin and eosin stained section ×600]

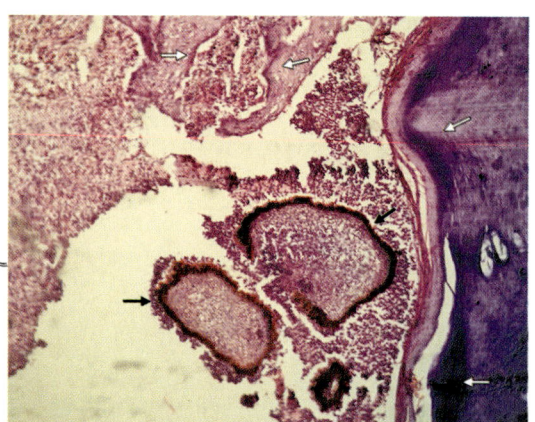

Fig. 3.12: Eumycotic mycetoma. Detail of grain showing thin active edge (black arrow) and soft amorphous interior. Pseudoepitheliomatous hyperplasia (white arrow) of the epidermis is also noticed [Hematoxylin and eosin stained section ×200].

Colony morphology

The colony is at first leathery, folded and heaped, white to yellow or ochreceous brown in colour (Fig. 3.13). As the colony ages, there is an overall growth of brownish aerial mycelia and diffusible pigment (Figs 3.14 and 3.15). In old culture (>2 months), black sclerotia (1 mm dia.) may be formed composed of rounded polygon-shaped mycelia element. Old colonies take on reddish-brown hue. Optimum growth occurs at 37°C.

Microscopic morphology

The mycelia average 1 to 5 µ with moniliform hyphae from 2 to 6 µ. Enlarged vesicle like cells

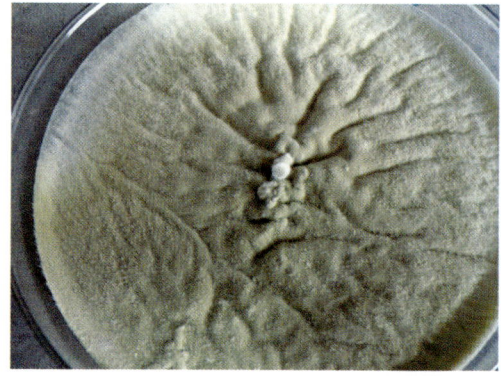

Fig. 3.13: *Madurella mycetomatis.* Colonies grown on SDCA at optimum temperature of 37°C is white to light yellowish to ochreceous brown, leathery, heaped and folded at first; obverse.

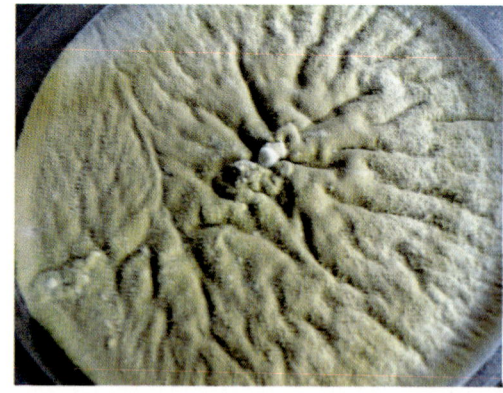

Fig. 3.14: *Madurella mycetomatis.* Brownish aerial mycelial overgrow on the surface of the colony in old culture.

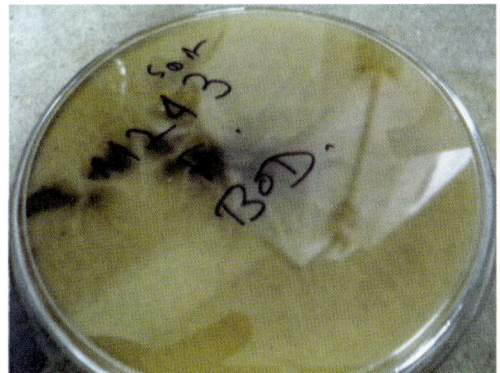

Fig. 3.15: Colony reverse of *Madurella mycetomatis*. Diffusible brown pigment production is characteristic in this species.

are formed. When grown on cornmeal agar, two types of conidiation are seen. Pyriform conidia (2–5 µ), with a truncate base, borne on the tip of simple conidiophores, and small, flask-shaped phialides producing spores (3 µ in diameter) (Figs 3.16 and 3.17).

Exophiala jeanselmei

Clinical disease produced by this organism is eumycotic mycetoma, subcutaneous abscesses, phaeohyphomycosis with sclerotic round

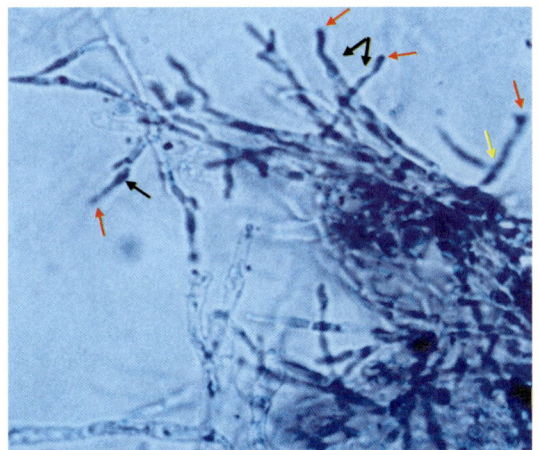

Fig. 3.16: Microscopic morphology of *Madurella mycetomatis*. Colony grown on Sabouraud's dextrose agar at 37°C for 6 days. Note the phialidic conidiation is more (red arrow—conidia; black arrow—flask shaped phialides). Yellow arrow shows conidiation on branched conidiophore. [LPCB mount ×400]

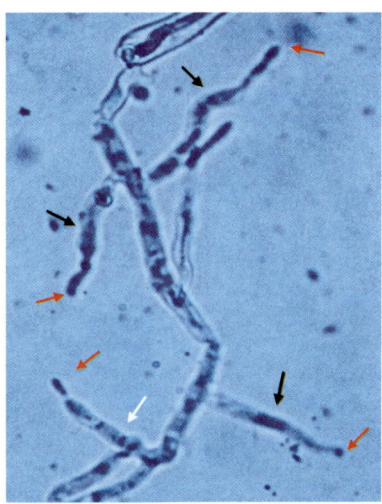

Fig. 3.17: Conidial structure of *Madurella mycetomatis*. Simple or branched conidiophore (white arrow) with pear-shaped conidia having a truncate base. Tapering phialides (black arrow) with small ovoid to globose conidia (red arrow ×600) or pear-shaped conidia having a truncate base (red arrow) or tapering phialides (black arrow) with small ovoid to globose conidia (red arrow) are characteristic features [LPCB mount ×600].

bodies in lesions and hypertrophied verrucous skin lesions.

In mycetoma grains produced by this fungus are characteristically soft, black, of variable size vermiform or serpiginous. It is composed of mainly swollen cells (5–10 µ in size); brown hyphal elements are also seen.

Colony morphology

Colonies of *E. jeanselmei*, when grown on Sabouraud's dextrose agar are perplexing. The initial slow growing colony is mucoid, dark, yeast-like or glabrous. Yeast cells predominate in this stage but in time, a grayish-black velvety aerial mycelium develops with black pigment on the reverse side giving a dematiaceous appearance (Fig. 3.18). The optimum temperature for their growth is 30°C but the fungus grows extremely slowly or not at all at 37°C.

Microscopic morphology

In yeast-like cultures, budding cells predominate in these primary culture and most of

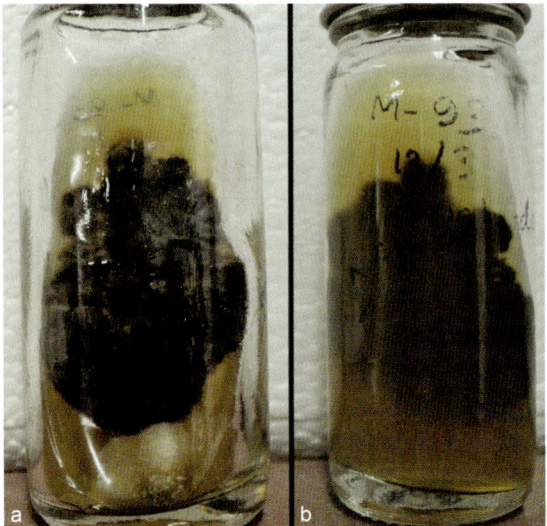

Fig. 3.18: *Exophiala jeanselmei.* Colonies on SDCA are olive to black, moist yeast-like at first but may remain as such or short mycelial element can overgrow on the surface of the colony; (a) obversel (b) reverse.

the conidiogenous cells are short with inconspicuous annellations and are produced laterally on the hyphae (Fig. 3.19). On repeated transfer of the cultures, more characteristic elongated conidiogenous cells (simple or branched) with a series of annellations are produced. Hyphae are moniliform and tube-like annelids are formed with narrow tapered tips. Conidia are quite variable in size and shape among the isolates but they are mostly elliptical measuring 5 to 6 μ × 1 to 2 μ (Fig. 3.20). The conidia are produced successively from the tip of the tapered annellides (phialides). They may be seen clustered above the tip of annelid and there is no attachment scar (Fig. 3.21). Primary isolates also produce a few phialides that are unstable and disappear in the subcultures.

Acrmonium kiliense

It is a common agent of eumycetoma and characteristically produces white grain. The grains are whitish to yellow, soft, irregular and about 1.5 mm in diameter.

Colony morphology

Colonies on SDA grow slowly producing a tufted and down colony is white to buff gradually the center changes to pinkish to brownish.

A diffusible red current pigment is produced at the underside (Fig. 3.22).

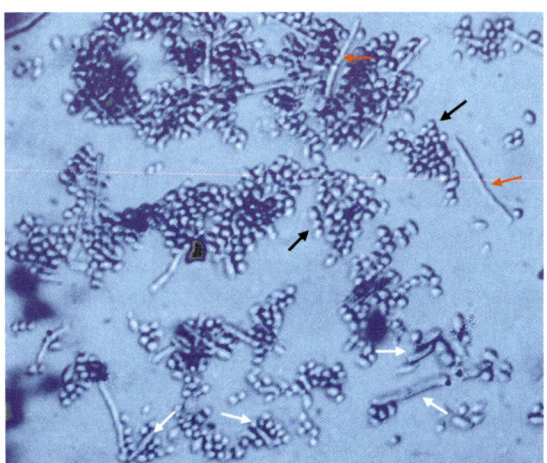

Fig. 3.19: *Exophiala jeanselmei.* In primary culture, yeast-like budding cells predominate (black arrow), conidiogenous cells are short with inconspicuous annellations (white arrow) and produced laterally on the hyphae (red arrow) [LPCB mount ×200].

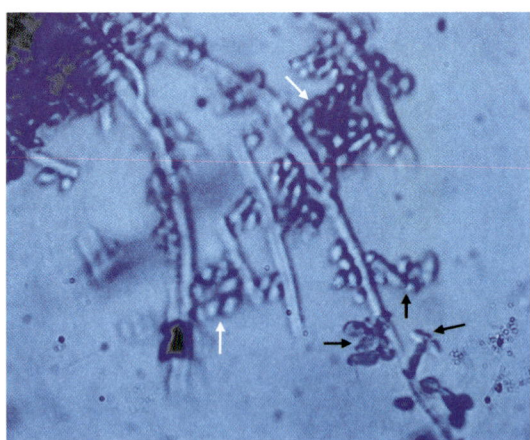

Fig. 3.20: *Exophiala jeanselmei.* In yeast like colony, conidial balls (white arrow) are produced laterally on the hyphae. Annelidic conidiogenous cells with pointed tip (black arrow) also produce conidia [LPCB mount ×600].

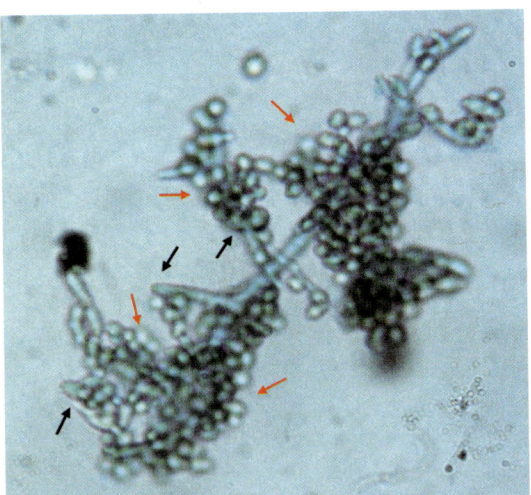

Fig. 3.21: *Exophiala jeanselmei*. Elongate, tubelike annelides (annelophores) are produced which has a narrow tappered tips (black arrow). Conidia (red arrow) are variable in size with no attachment scars and are clustered at the tip of annelide [LPCB mount ×600].

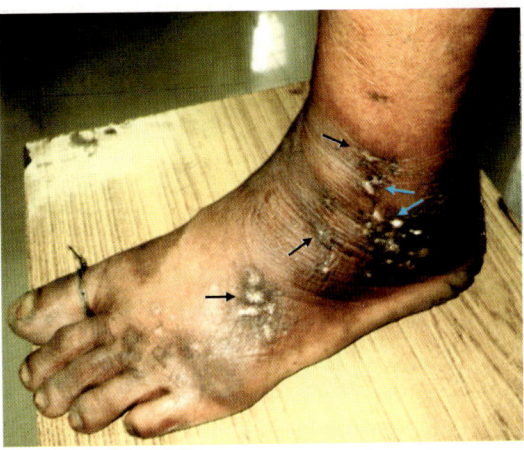

Fig. 3.23: Multiple sinus tract openings. Few are in the process of healing (black arrow) but some are with active discharge (blue arrow). The surfaces of the lesion are flat and somewhat discoloured which indicates an eumycotic cause of disease.

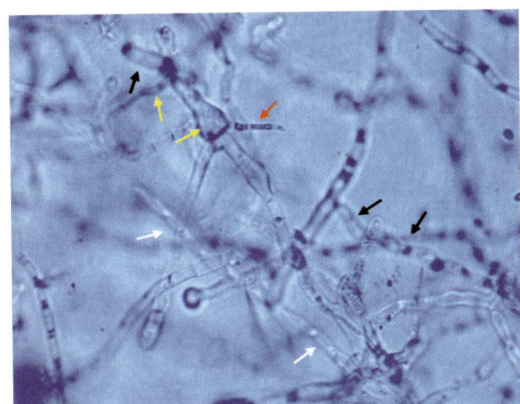

Fig. 3.24: *Madurella mycetomatis*. Moniliform hyphae (white arrow), chains of arthrospores (black arrow), polygon-shaped dark brownish mycelial element (yellow arrow), simple unbranched conidiophore (red arrow) arising from the hyphae near the septum and flask-shaped phialides (brown arrow) which produces round conidia are important features of this species [LPCB mount ×400].

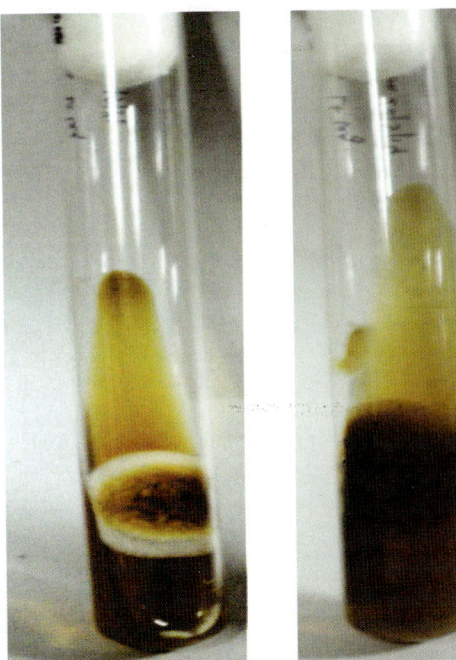

Fig. 3.22: *Acremonium kiliense*. Colonies grown on SDA at 30°C are white at the original colony which gradually changes to buff or reddish brown colour. A diffusible red current pigment is produced on the reverse side.

Microscopic morphology

Hyphae are hyaline, 2 to 4 μ in diameter, conidiophores are thin, delicate. Conidia are single celled, elliptical and are borne successively from the tips of conidiophores (phialides) and held there as a cephalic (head-

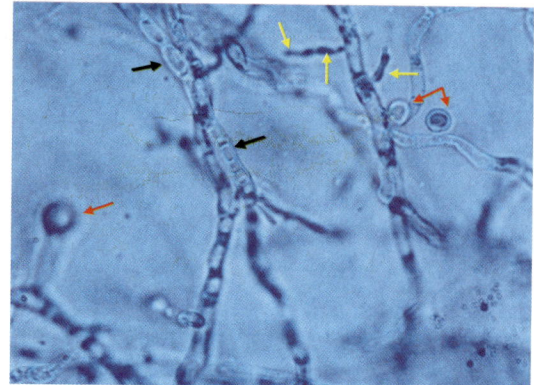

Fig. 3.25: Microscopic morphology of *Madurella mycetomatis* in aged culture. Colony grown on Sabouraud's dextrose agar at 37°C for 2 weeks. Presence of arthroconidia (black arrow), chlamydospores (red arrow), tapering phialides (yellow arrow) bearing small ovoid to globose conidia are diagnostic [LPCB mount ×600].

like) or 'ball-like' clusters by mucilaginous exudates (Fig. 3.24).

Aspergillus nidulans

Colony morphology
On Sabouraud's dextrose agar, the colonies grow rapidly at 25°C. Among the strains of

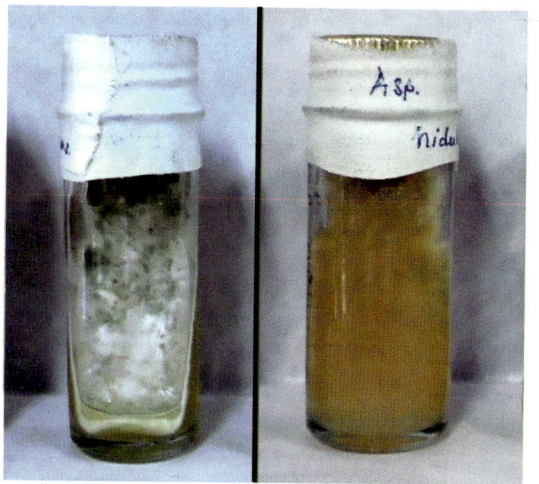

Fig. 3.26: Colony morphology of *Aspergillus nidulans* grown on Sabouraud's dextrose agar at 25°C for one week. Colonies appear white, cottony at first, grows rapidly and turns into deep green. Reverse is colourless to light yellow; (a) obverse, (b) reverse.

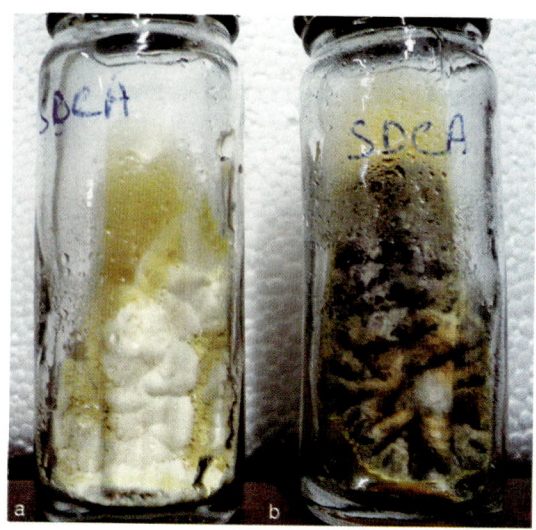

Fig. 3.27: Colony morphology of *Aspergillus nidulans* grown on SDCA at 30°C after 10 days of incubation. Colonies are white to cream to buff (a) at first but gradually changes to honey brown colour (b).

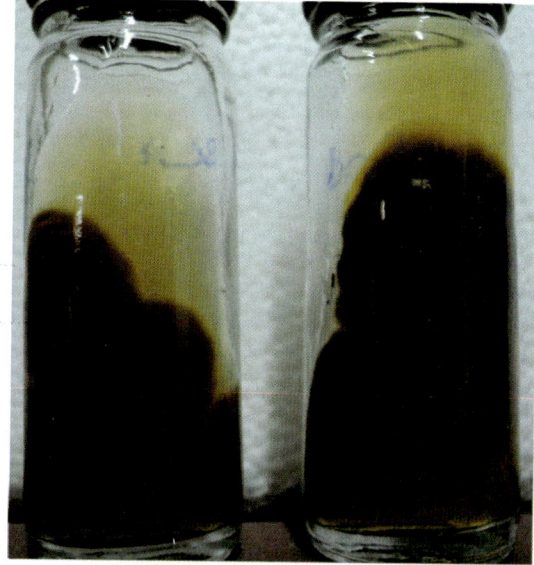

Fig. 3.28: *Aspergillus nidulans.* The reverse of colonies grown on Sabouraud's dextrose agar at 30°C; (a) young culture, (b) old culture.

this species, majority are almost cleistothecial and appear as dark olive buff with relatively few dark green, short, columnar conidial heads. The strains which produce abundant

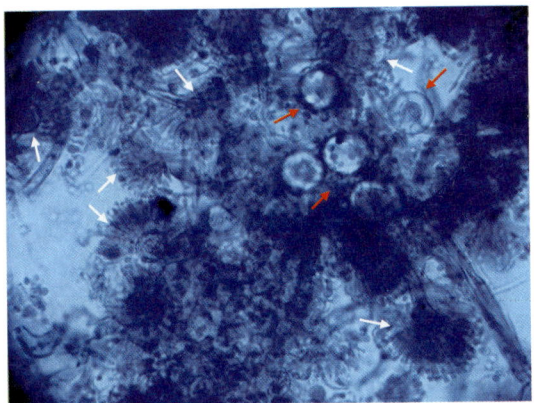

Fig. 3.29: *Aspergillus nidulans*. Globose to subglobose 'hulle cells' (red arrow) produced on Sabouraud's dextrose agar. Plenty of conidial structures (includes conidiophore, vesicle, sterigmata and conidia; white arrow) are noticed. The morphology of conidial structures and hulle cells are diagnostic of this species [LPCB mount ×400].

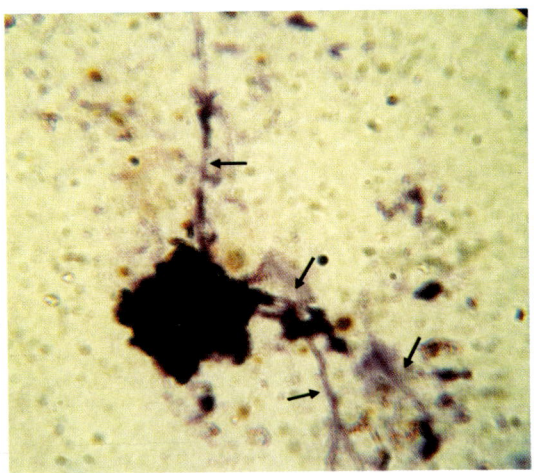

Fig. 3.31: Gram stained smear of discharge material collected from sinus opening shows presence of Gram positive mycelial structures (black arrow ×1000).

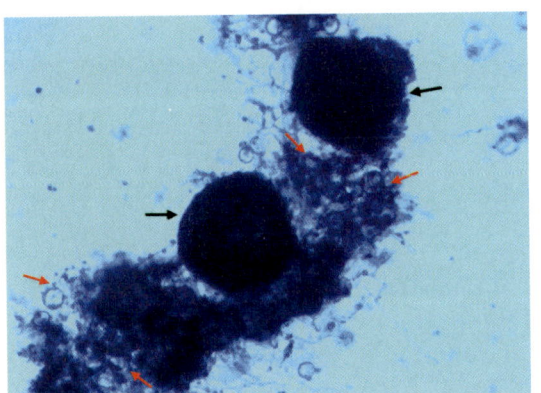

Fig. 3.30: 'Cieistotheicia' (black arrow) of *Aspergillus nidulans*. These are globose to subglobose, reddish brown sac like structures that are surrounded by a yellowish cinnamon-coloured layer of hyphae that bear globose 'hulle cells' (red arrow) [LPCB mount ×400].

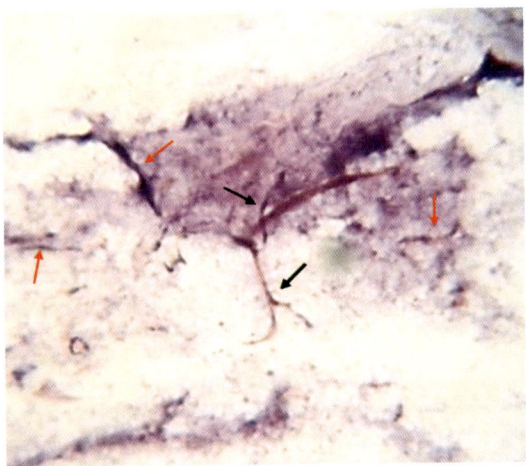

Fig. 3.32: Gram-positive hyphae with acute angle branching (black arrow) along with a few small fragments of hyphae (red arrow) are noticed in a smear of exudate collected from a sinus tract opening [Gram stain ×600].

conidia are deep green in colour (Fig. 3.26), and a few cleistothecia are produced within and upon the conidial layer.

Microscopic morphology

Hyphae are hyaline, regularly septate and have dichotomous branching. Conidiophores are frequently sinuous with smooth, brown, thick walls and end in hemispherical vesicles.

The sterigmata develops in double series, the primaries are longer and wider than the secondaries. The conidia are globose, rough and green (Fig. 3.36).

Actinomadura madurae

The grains produced by *Actinomadura madurae* in tissue are the largest (1 to 5 mm)

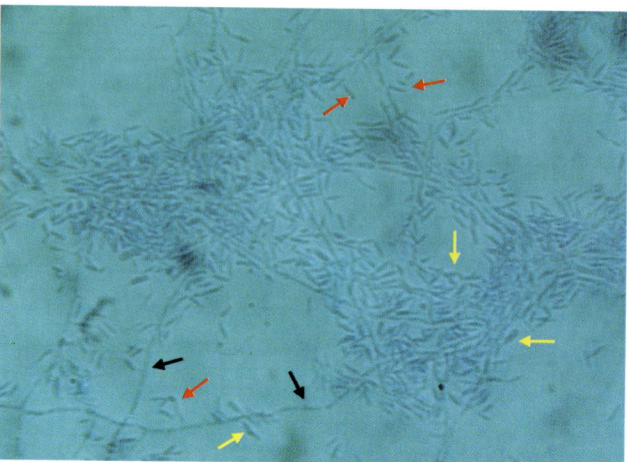

Fig. 3.33: *Acremonium kiliense*. Narrow, delicate, fragile hyphae (black arrow) and tapered thin walled conidiogenous cell (phialide; red arrow) giving rise to elliptical or short cylindrical single celled conidia (yellow arrow) are characteristic morphologic features [LPCB mount ×400].

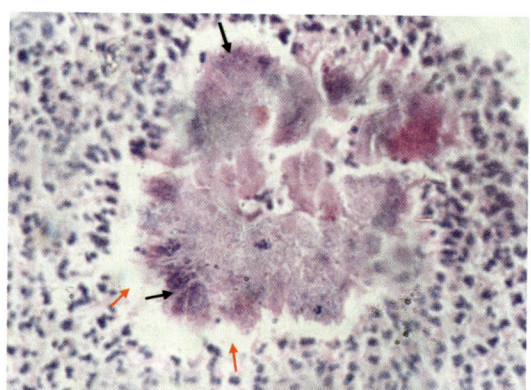

Fig. 3.34: Actinomycotic mycetoma. The centre of actinomycotic grain is light coloured and unorganized. There is a strong basophilia (black arrow) surrounding the periphery of the grains and a white fringed (red arrow) eosinophilic border [Hematoxylin & eosin stained section ×400].

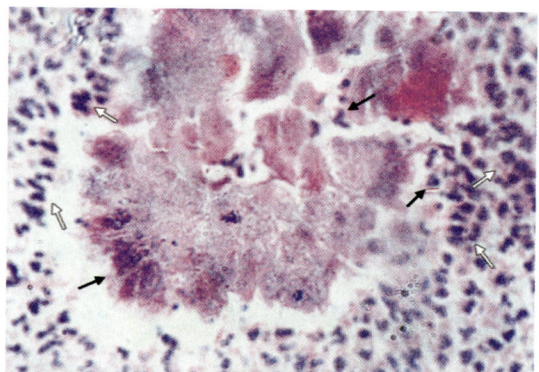

Fig. 3.35: Actinomycotic grain. Sulfur granule showing eosinophilic 'clubs' with attached neutrophils (black arrow). The centre of the granule is light coloured and unorganized. Surrounding the granule, plenty of inflammatory cells (both acute and chronic inflammation) along with a few giant cells are noticed (white arrow) [Hematoxylin & eosin stained section ×600].

in mycetoma. They are oval, spherical or angular with a lobulated (mulberry-like) surface. The colour of the grain is white to yellow. The margin of the grain is made up of fringe like hyphae.

Colony morphology

The colonies develop rapidly on Lowenstein-Jensen medium and blood agar but more slowly on Sabouraud's agar. Colonies are waxy, cerebriform at the center and have a flat peripheral zone (Figs 3.37 and 3.38). They are so tough and membranous that it may peel off the medium when a portion of it is attempted to be removed for microscopic examination or subculture.

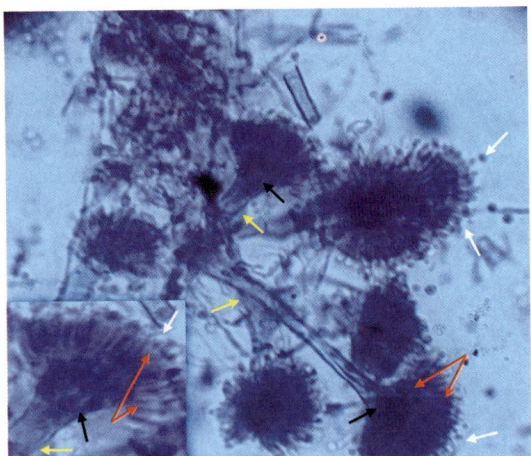

Fig. 3.36: *Aspergillus nidulans.* Conidiophores (yellow arrow) are frequently sinuous; smooth, brown, thick walls and produce hemispherical vesicle (black arrow). The sterigmata develop in double series (red arrow). The secondaries may be slightly narrower than the primaries. Conidia are globose, rough, green (white arrow) [LPCB mount ×600].

Microscopic morphology

Smear prepared from colony are Gram-positive (Figs 3.39 and 3.40) but non acid-fast (Fig. 3.41). The optimum growth temperature is 37°C. Acids are produced from arabinose, cellobiose, mannitol, rhamnose and xylose.

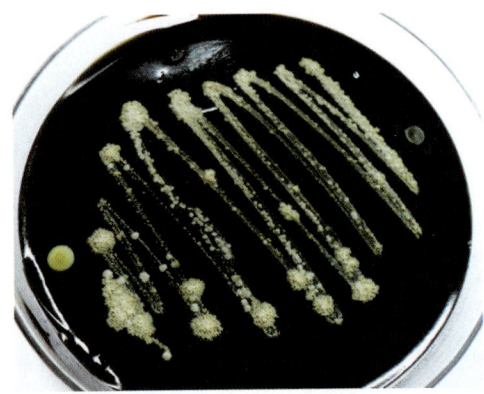

Fig. 3.38: *Actinomadura madurae.* Colony morphology on blood agar at 37°C after 5 days of aerobic incubation (subculture). Colonies are waxy, buff to light yellowish, cerebriform at the centre but have a flat peripheral zone. They are tough membranous and densely adherent onto the surface of the media.

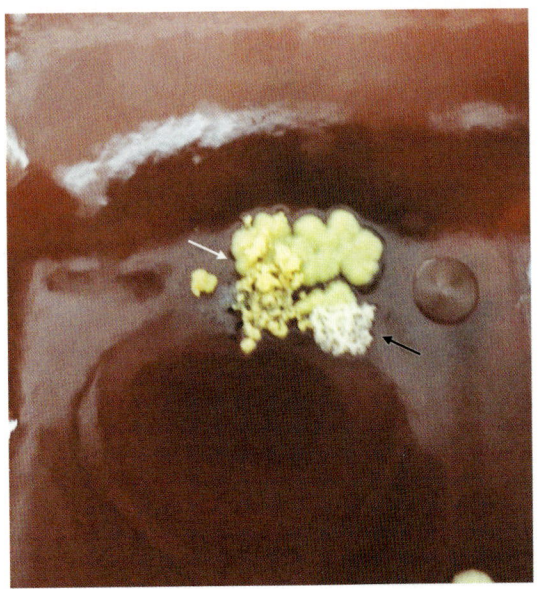

Fig. 3.37: Colonial morphology of *Actinomadura madurae* grown on blood agar at 37°C after 12 days of aerobic incubation (primary culture). The colony is moist, folded, dull white (black arrow) to yellow colour in some areas (white arrow).

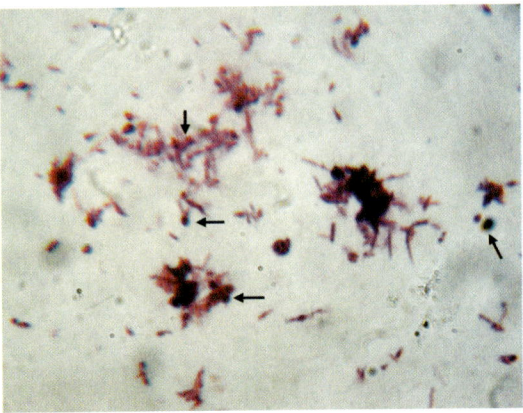

Fig. 3.39: Gram-positive filaments of *Actinomyces.* Presence of clubs are also appreciated (black arrow).

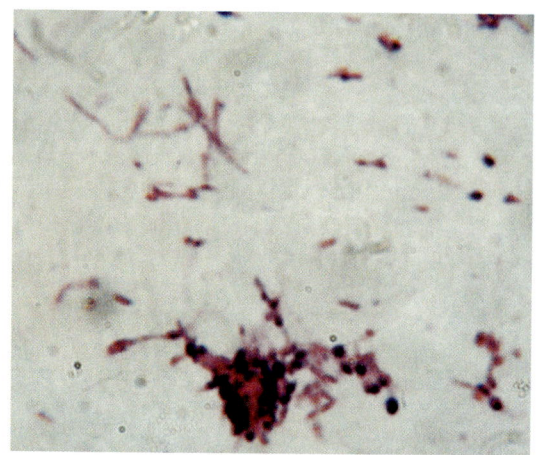

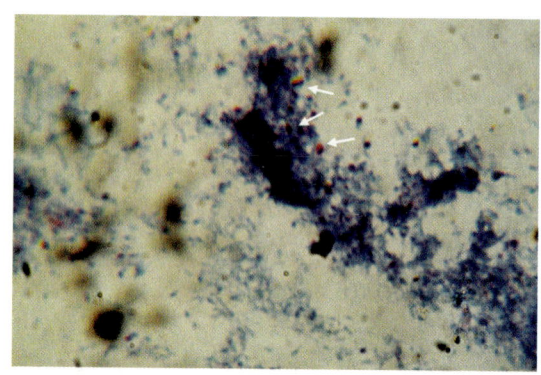

Fig. 3.41: Acid-fast 'clubs' (white arrow) of *Actinomyces* [Z-N stained smear with 1% sulfuric acid used as decolouriser ×1000].

Fig. 3.40: Smear shows Gram-positive branching filaments of *Actinomyces*. Darkly stained round to oval 'clubs' of actinomyces are also noticed [×1000].

EUMYCOTIC MYCETOMA

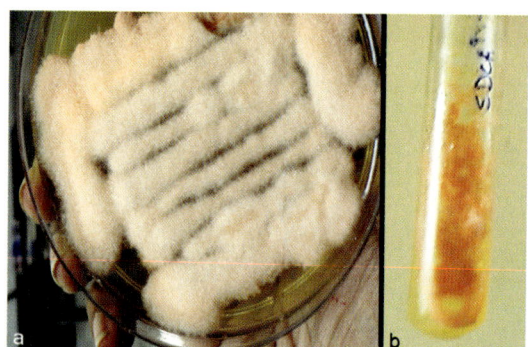

Fig. 3.42: Colony morphology of *Fusarium soiani* grown on Sabouraud's dextrose agar at 28–30°C for 1 week. Colony is rapidly growing, appears within 3–5 days as white, fluffy gradually develops a light pinkish orange colour. Orange brown pigment is obvious at the reverse side of the colony; (a) obverse, (b) reverse.

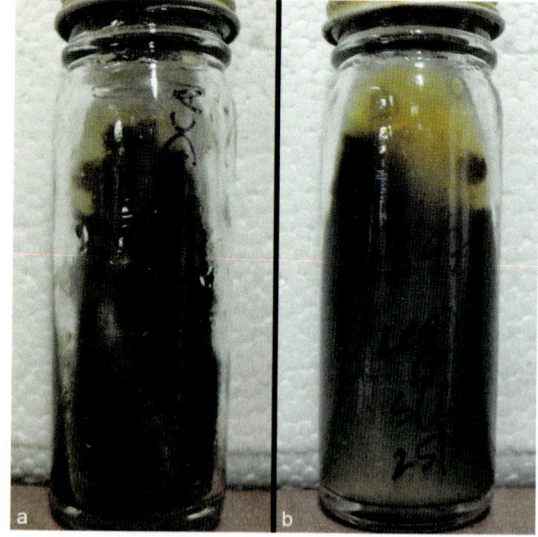

Fig. 3.43: *Curvularia* species. Colonies grown on SDCA are floccose to velvety, fast growing, at first appearing as grayish white but soon turns into dark brown to black. Reverse is black; (a) obverse, (b) reverse.

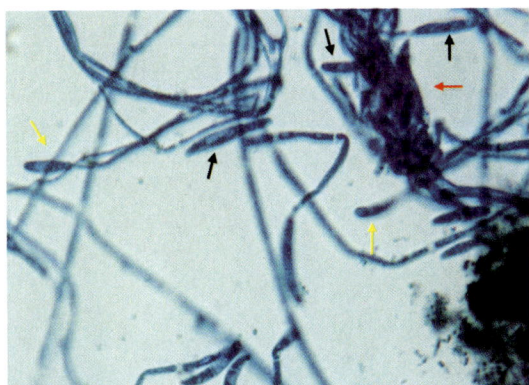

Fig. 3.44: Microscopic morphology of *Fusarium solani*. Macroconidia are fusiform, thick walled, widest in upper half (black arrow); macroconidia are borne on short, branched conidiophore which forms 'sporodochia' (red arrow); Microconidia are single celled, fusoid, atop an elongate microconidiophore (brown arrow) (Slide culture; LPCB mount ×400).

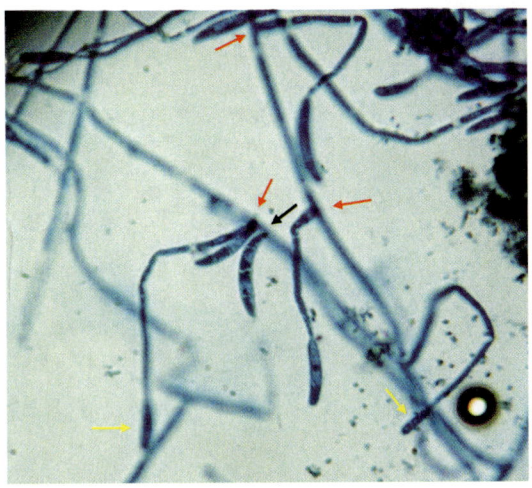

Fig. 3.46: *Fusarium solani*. Microscopic morphology shows conidiophores arising lateral to the hyphae from foot cells (red arrow); microconidia are fusoid, produced on elongate conidiophores (yellow arrow); macroconidia are slightly curved, fusiform and a short conidiophore (black arrow) [LPCB mount ×400].

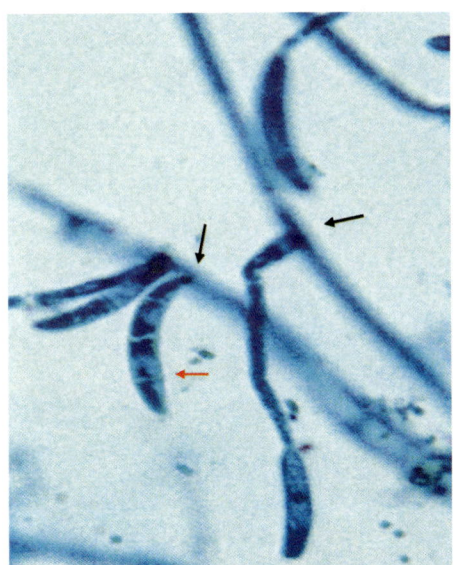

Fig. 3.45: Macroconidia of *Fusarium solani*. Macroconidia are fusiform, curved, widest at the upper part (red arrow) and have 'foot cells' with some type of 'heel' (black arrow) are definitive characteristics of genus *Fusarium* [LPCB mount ×600].

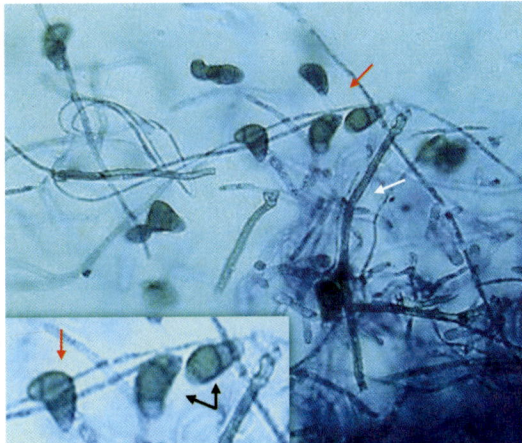

Fig. 3.47: *Curvularia geniculata*. Dematiaceous hyphae. Conidia (poroconidia) arise from a pore in the sympodially elongating conidiophore (white arrow). Conidia are slightly curved, fusiform (red arrow) with one of the central cells being darker and larger (Inset: Black arrow) [LPCB mount ×400].

SELF ASSESSMENT

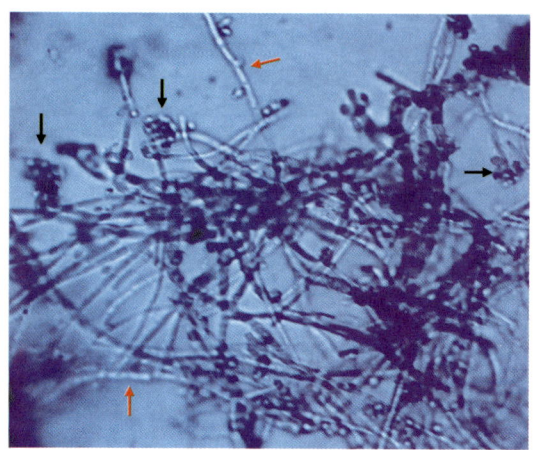

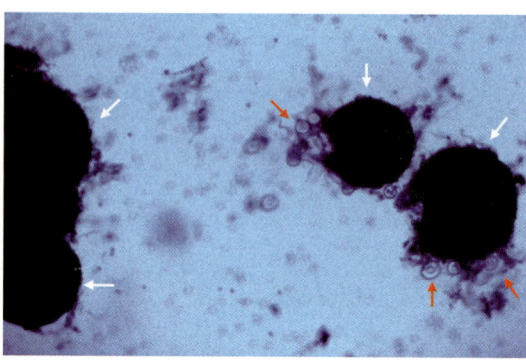

Fig. 3.50: Microscopic morphology of an *Aspergillus* species. Identify the structure and the likely species producing it [LPCB mount ×400].

Fig. 3.48: Microscopic morphology of a phaeoid fungi which causes both mycotic mycetoma and mycotic keratitis. Identify the structures and the likely fungus.

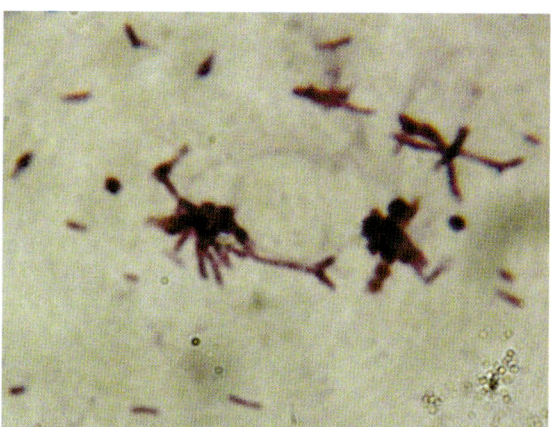

Fig. 3.51: Gram stained smear showing branching Gram-positive filaments and a few dark stained round to oval structures. Identify these structures [×1000].

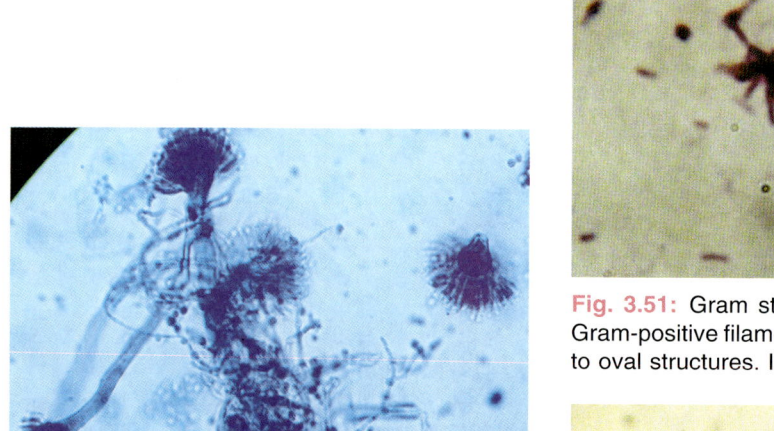

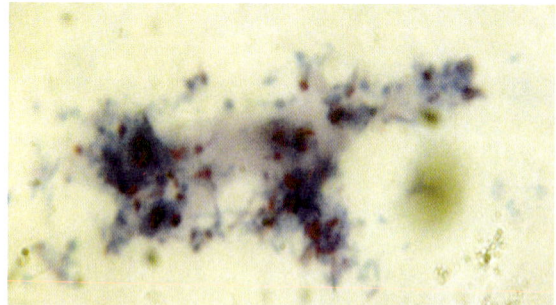

Fig. 3.49: Identify the *Aspergillus* species isolated from a case of mycetoma. Colony produced on SDA was white to olive green at first and gradually became buff to honey brown. LPCB mount showing microscopic morphology of the isolated fungus. Identify different parts of the conidial structures which might help in species identification [×400].

Fig. 3.52: Smear prepared from the grains of a case of actinomycotic mycetoma. Identify the red and blue structures [Z-N staining ×1000].

ANSWERS

- **Fig. 3.52:** Clubs of actinomycetes (red arrow); Filamentous actinomycetes (blue arrow)
- **Fig. 3.51:** Gram-positive filaments of actinomycetes
- **Fig. 3.50:** Cleistothecia of *Aspergillus nidulans*
- **Fig. 3.49:** *Aspergillus nidulans*
- **Fig. 3.48:** Conidial clusters; *Exophiala werneckii*

Systemic Mycosis

The systemic diseases caused by fungi fall into two very distinct categories. These categories are delineated by the interaction of two factors: Inherent virulence of the fungus and constitution adequacy of the host. These are:

1. True pathogenic fungus infections
2. Opportunistic fungus infections

The True Pathogenic Fungus Infections

The true pathogenic fungi are those species that have the ability to elicit a disease process in the normal human host when the inoculum is of sufficient size. Pathogenicity in fungi is an accidental phenomenon and is not essential to the survival or dissemination of the species involved. Vast majority of such infections, usually more than 90% are either completely asymptomatic or of very short duration and quickly resolved. Resolution imparts strong immunity.

Other characteristics of true pathogenic fungi includes:

- Restricted geographic distribution
- Age, sex and race are important in the statistics of pathogenic fungus infection
- Thermal dimorphism is exhibited by all of the major organisms that produce systemic infection and one agent that produces subcutaneous infection (sporotrichosis)

The true pathogenic fungi includes:

- *Histoplasma capsulatum*
- *Blastomyces dermatitidis*

- *Coccidioides immitis*
- *Paracoccidioides brasiliensis*
- *Penicillium marnefii*

The above five fungi are grouped under "systemic thermal dimorphic fungi"

- *Sporothrix schenckii*—subcutaneous thermal dimorphic fungus.

The Opportunistic Fungus Infections

The organisms involved are inherently low virulence, and disease production depends on diminished host resistance to infection. The common etiologic agents of opportunistic infections are *Aspergillus, Candida, Cryptococcus* and *Rhizopus*.

CANDIDIASIS

Candidiasis is a primary or secondary infection caused by a member of the genus *Candida*. Although *Candida albicans* is the most prevalent species in both mucocutaneous and disseminated infectious, the incidence of candidiasis due to *non-albicans Candida* (NAC) is increasing in recent years. The emergence of NAC species as a predominant cause of various infections are important to know as several NAC species are inherently resistant or acquire resistance to commonly used antifungal drugs.

A diversity of clinical pictures are encountered with various candidiasis. All of the tissue and organ systems are subject to invasion and the pathology evoked is as variable as are the clinical syndromes. The various manifestations are described according to the primary organ system involved.

1. *Infectious diseases*
   A. *Mucocutaneous involvement*:
      - Oral thrush, glossitis, stomatitis, cheilitis (Fig. 4.1)
      - Bronchial and pulmonary
      - Vaginitis, balanitis
      - Esophagitis, enteric and perianal disease
      - Chronic mucocutaneous candidiasis (Fig. 4.2)
   B. *Cutaneous involvement*:
      - Intertriginous and generalized candidiasis
      - Paronychia and onychomycosis
      - Diaper rash (napkin candidiasis)
      - Candidal granuloma
   C. *Systemic involvement*:
      - Urinary tract
      - Endocarditis
      - Meningitis

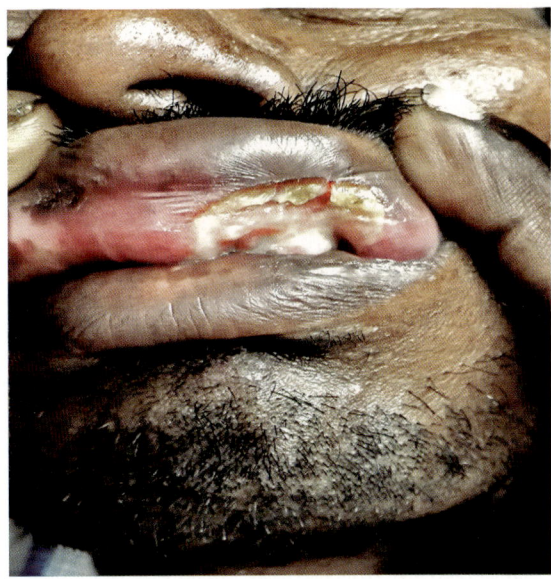

Fig. 4.2: Mucocutaneous candidiasis in HIV reactive patient.

   - Septicemia
   - Iatrogenic candidemia (barrier break candidemia)

2. *Allergic disease*
   - Eczema
   - Asthma
   - Gastritis, etc.

Laboratory Identification

Direct examination

Scrapings from cutaneous and mucocutaneous lesions can be examined directly either in potassium hydroxide slide mounts (KOH mount) or by Gram stain. The characteristic mixture of yeast and mycelial phase organisms permits a rapid diagnosis of such infections. Sputum, vaginal discharge, urine specimens, stool samples present more difficulty. **The mere finding of yeast in such material is of no diagnostic importance; however, mycelial form organisms usually connote an established colonization of the involved area.**

Direct culture

Freshly obtained, multiple specimens should be examined for maximum isolation of fungi.

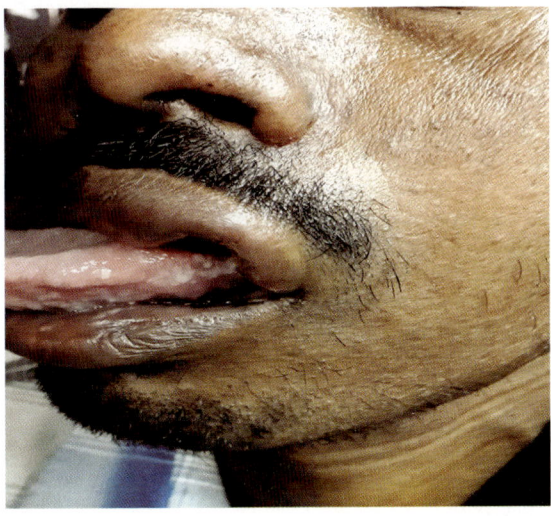

Fig. 4.1: Oral candidiasis—'thrush'. Cream white, cardy patches of pseudomembrane cover the front and lateral portion of the tongue in HIV reactive patient.

Sabouraud's dextrose agar with antibacterial antibiotics is recommended. Most species of *Candida* are unaffected by the cyclohexamide used in selective media for pathogenic fungi except *C. krusei* and *C. parapsilosis* which are sensitive to it. Optimal growth of all species occurs at room temperature. A pasty, yeast-like colony appears by 24 to 48 hours.

Many procedures have been proposed for rapid identification of unknown yeasts. These are as follows:

1. Germ tube production (Reynolds-Braude phenomenon)
2. Chlamydospore production in Cornmeal-Tween agar
3. Microscopic morphology (mycelial morphology) on Cornmeal-Tween plate
4. Carbohydrate fermentation
5. Carbohydrate assimilation

1. Reynolds-Braude Phenomenon

Unknown yeast is mixed with serum and incubated at 37°C for two hours. After such incubation *C. albicans* and *C. dubliniensis* shows sprout mycelium which are called 'germ tube'. This test is considered positive if more than 30% yeast cells produce sprout mycelium (germ tube). Essentially all strains of *C. albicans* and *C. dubliniensis* are positive in this test, and no other commonly encountered species demonstrates this reaction. Occasionally less than 5% sprout mycelium (Germ tube) production are noticed in a few strains of *C. tropicalis* (Fig. 4.3).

2. Microscopic Morphology on Cornmeal-Tween Agar

Candida albicans

Candida albicans is the most common species causing human infection.

Colony morphology

Colonies grown on Sabouraud's dextrose agar for three days at 25°C are white to cream coloured, smooth and glistening (Fig. 4.4). After 1 month they are cream coloured, waxy

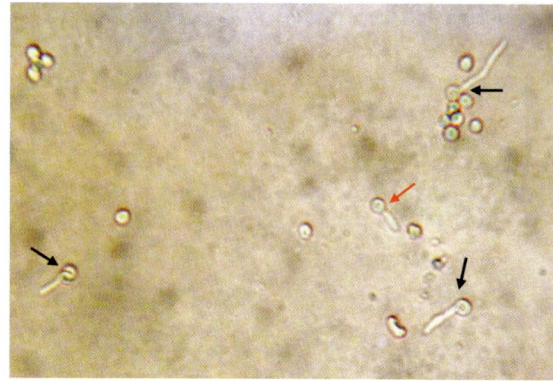

Fig. 4.3: 'Germ tube' formation (black arrow) in *Candida albicans* (Reynolds-Braude phenomenon) which differs from pseudohyphae formation (red arrow) [×400].

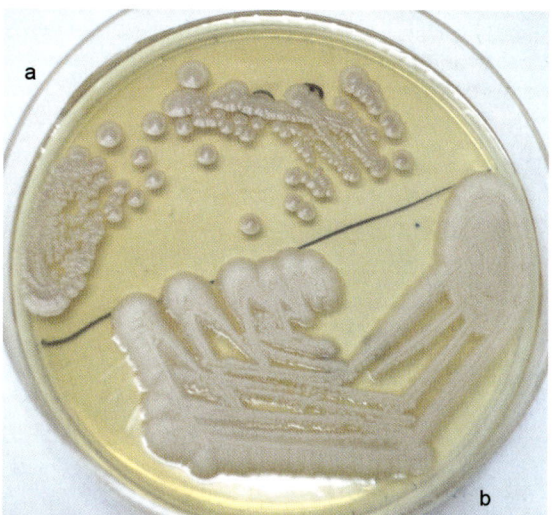

Fig. 4.4: Colony morphology on Sabouraud's dextrose agar; (a) *Candida albicans*; (b) *Candida tropicalis*.

or soft, smooth to somewhat reticulated or wrinkled and with or without mycelial fringes.

Microscopic morphology

On SDCA at 25°–30°C for three days, the colony is composed of globose to oval to elongate yeast cells of various sizes (Figs 4.5 and 4.7). Some isolates frequently produce large globose cells with small uniform sized multiple polar buds (Figs 4.6 and 4.8). The yeast cells can undergo three different

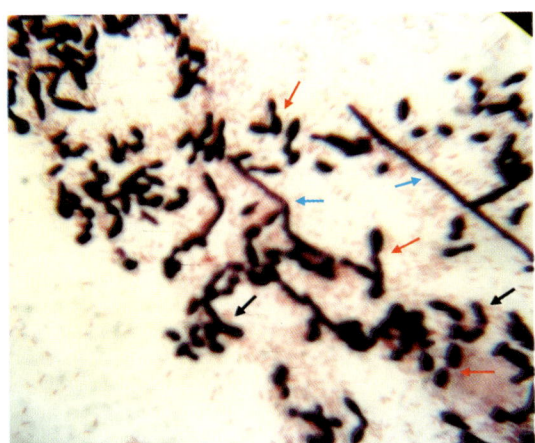

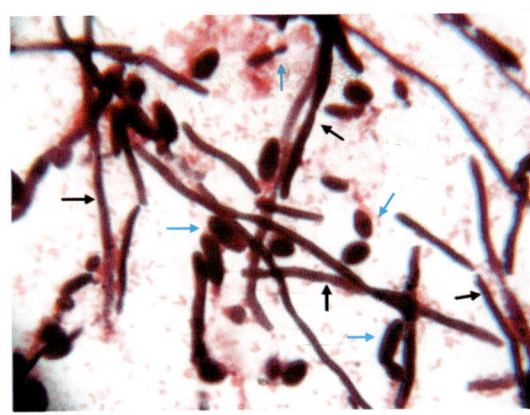

Fig. 4.7: *Candida albicans*. Oval to elongate budding yeast cells (blue arrow) with plenty of pseudomycelia (black arrow) are noticed in this smear prepared from colonies appeared on Sabouraud's dextrose agar following an inoculation of sputum sample at 37°C for 3 days. The sputum sample was obtained from a 21 years male patient of 'acute myeloblastic leukaemia' [Gram stain ×1000].

Fig. 4.5: Gram stained smear prepared from colonies appeared on Sabouraud's dextrose agar (SDA) at 37°C for 3 days. Yeast cells are oval to elliptical with budding (red arrow), a few cylindrical cells (black arrow) and also mycelial fragments (blue arrow) are noticed. *Candida tropicalis* [Urine sample of a 68 years old male patient with symptoms of UTI; ×1000].

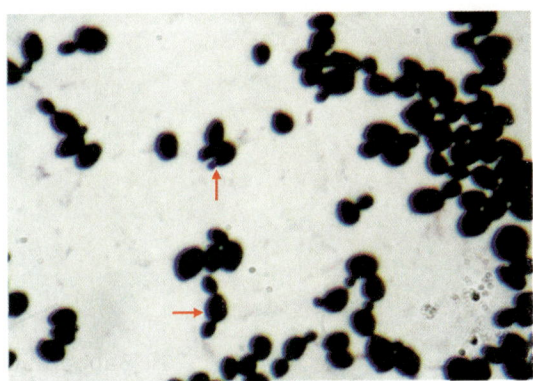

Fig. 4.6: *Candida guillermondii*. Ovoid to elongate yeast cells with single or multiple budding (red arrow) are produced when grown on Sabouraud's dextrose agar (SDA) for three days but pseudo or true hyphae are not produced [Gram stain ×1000].

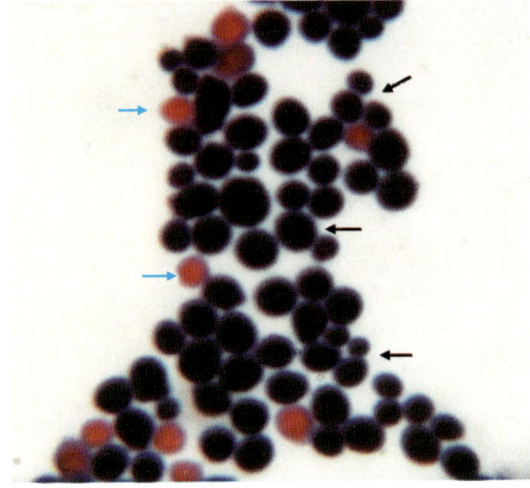

Fig. 4.8: *Candida glabrata*. Spherical to oval shaped yeast cells with budding (black arrow) are present in this smear prepared from culture. Mycelial structures (true or pseudo) are absent. Pink coloured cells (blue arrow) are nonviable (dead and degenerated) yeast cells [Gram stain ×1000].

morphogenetic processes, namely blasto-spores formation, mycelium and pseudo-myelium formation.

Generally, the pH and chemical composition of the growth media as well as inoculum size and incubation temperature, affects the growth forms.

Masses of blastoconidia (1–4 μ) at inter-nodes, terminal, thick-walled (8–12 μ) thallic conidia (chlamydoconidia) are formed by

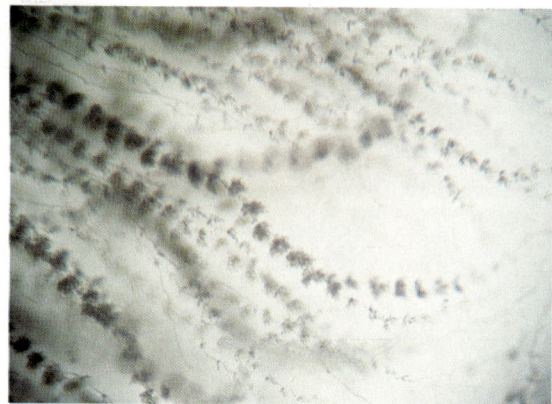

Fig. 4.9: *Candida albicans*. Clusters of blastospores along pseudohyphae at regular intervals (cornmeal agar morphology ×200).

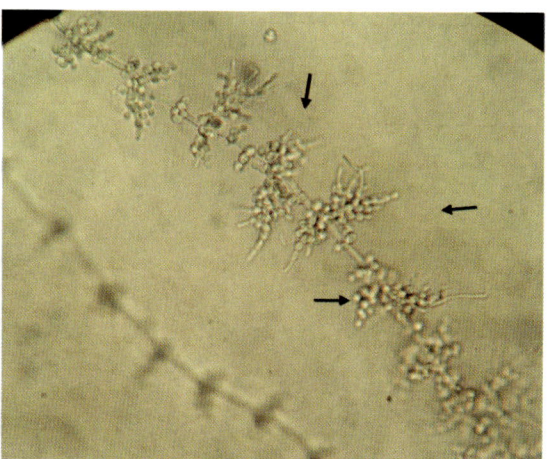

Fig. 4.10: *Candida albicans* grown on cornmeal agar. Blastospores are arranged in clusters (black arrow) on pseudohyphae at regular intervals (×400).

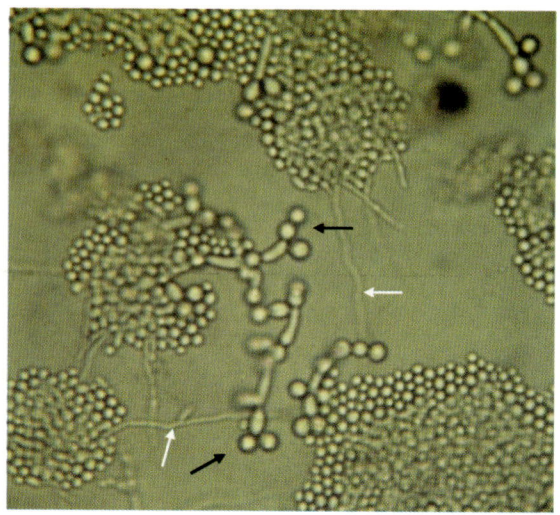

Fig. 4.11: *Candida albicans*. Large, thick-walled, round resting spores borne terminally. Chlamydospores are not produced at 30–35°C (×600).

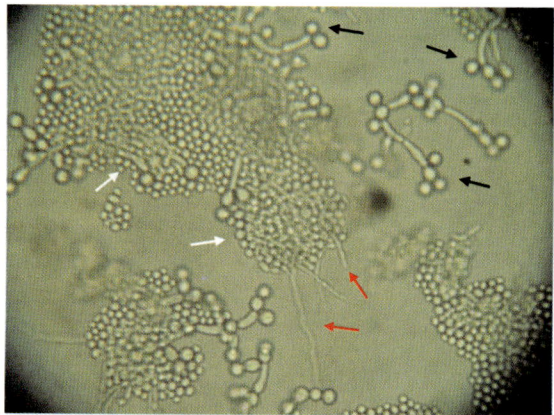

Fig. 4.12: *Candida albicans*. Chlamydospores (black arrow) produced mostly at the tip of pseudohyphae in pairs; clusters of blastospores (white arrow) produced from the side of pseudohyphae (red arrow; ×400).

most strains when inoculated by Dalmau technique or streak technique on Cornmeal-Tween 80 agar at 22 to 25°C within 48 to 72 hours. Chlamydospores are spherical, thick-walled (8–12 µ) are produced on supporting cells that occur along pseudohyphae or at the tip of hyphae (Figs 4.11 and 4.12). Clusters of blastospores are produced on pseudohyphae at regular intervals (Fig. 4.10).

Germ tube formation and the chlamydospore formation are the two most reliable morphologic criteria diagnostic for *Candida albicans* and *Candida dubliniensis*.

Candida tropicalis

Colony morphology

Colonies grown on SDCA at 25°C for 3 days are white to cream coloured, glistening to dull, soft, smooth, reticulated or wrinkled often with overgrowth of mycelium (Fig. 4.4). Old cultures become hairy and tough.

Microscopic morphology

The cells grown on Sabouraud's agar (SDCA) are globose, ovoid to elongated, measuring 4 to 7 × 5 to 11 µm (Figs 4.13 and 4.14). Pseudohyphae are long and branched, bearing blastospores singly or in small chains at the septa. A few oral isolates of *Candida tropicalis* form germ tube in serum when they were first isolated but on repeated subculture, their ability to form 'germ tube' is lost.

Candida kefyr

Colony morphology

Colonies grown on Sabouraud's dextrose agar are cream coloured, semi-dull to glistening and indistinguishable from other species of *Candida*.

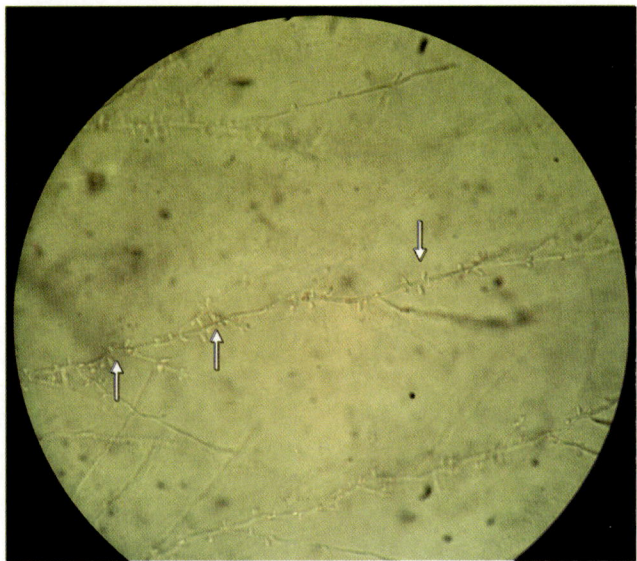

Fig. 4.13: *Candida tropicalis*. Sparse blastospores borne singly or in very small group along long pseudohyphae (morphology on CMA ×200).

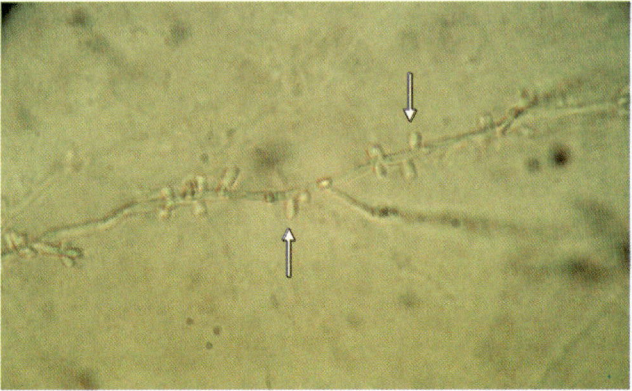

Fig. 4.14: *Candida tropicalis*. Ovoid to elongate blastospores borne singly along long pseudohyphae (morphology on CMA ×600).

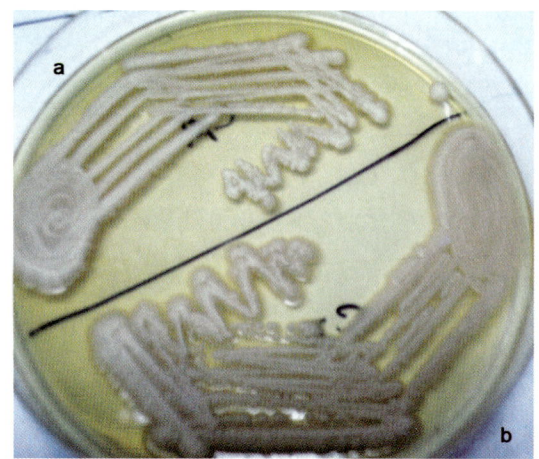

Fig. 4.15: Colony morphology on Sabouraud's dextrose agar; (a) *Candida parapsilosis;* (b) *Candida guilliermondii.*

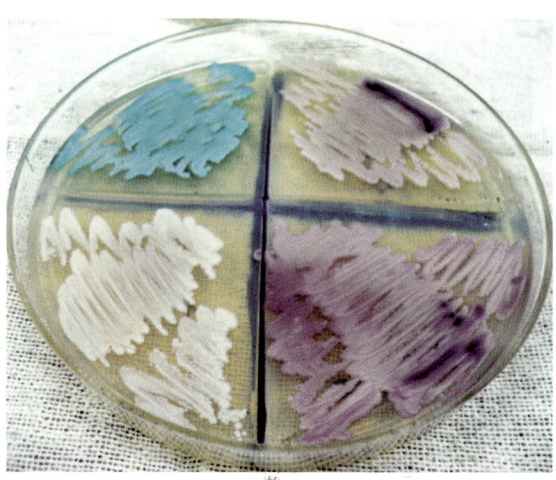

Fig. 4.17: Different *Candida* species in HiChrom candida differential agar. Green colonies—*Candida albicans*; Cream colonies—*Candida parapsilosis*; Purple colonies—*Candida glabrata*; Light pink colonies—*Candida krusei.*

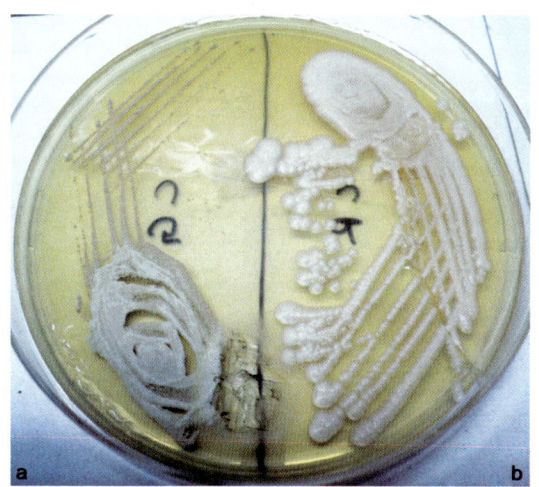

Fig. 4.16: Colony morphology on Sabouraud's dextrose agar; (a) *Candida glabrata;* (b) *Candida rugosa.*

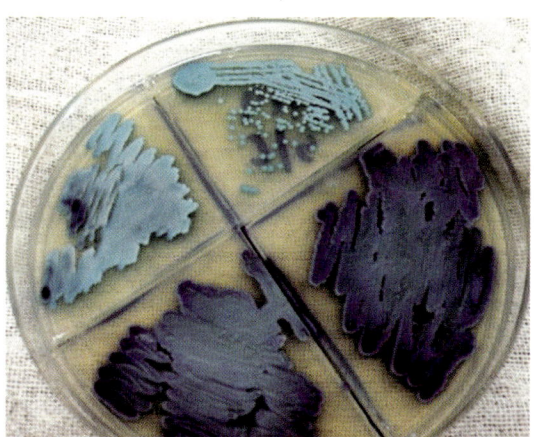

Fig. 4.18: HiChrom candida differential agar. Colonies of different species. *Candida tropicalis*—blue colony with pink halo, *Candida dubliniensis*—dark green colony, *Candida albicans*—light green.

Microscopic morphology

The yeast cells are long ovoid, blastospores are scanty, pseudomycelia lie parallel to each other like logs in stream.

The colony morphology and also microscopic morphology of other species of *Candida* are described in detail with figures.

ASPERGILLOSIS

The diseases caused by *Aspergillus* species are relatively uncommon and the severe invasive form is almost always confined to immunosuppressed host. *Aspergillus fumigatus* is the most common cause of both invasive and noninvasive aspergillosis. *Aspergillus flavus* is the second most common species causing invasive

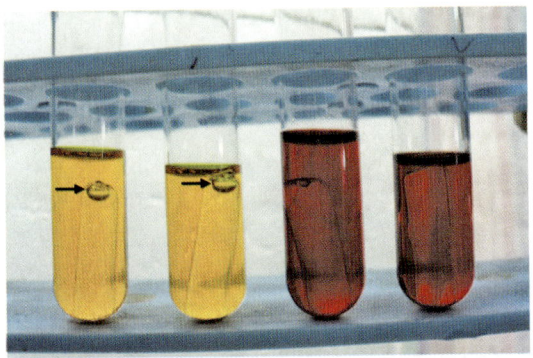

Fig. 4.19: Sugar fermentation by *Candida* species (*C. guilliermondii*). G—glucose, S—sucrose, M—maltose, L—lactose. Fermentation is indicated by production of acid and gas. Accumulation of gas at the top of the Durham's tube (black arrow) is more important feature than mere acid production.

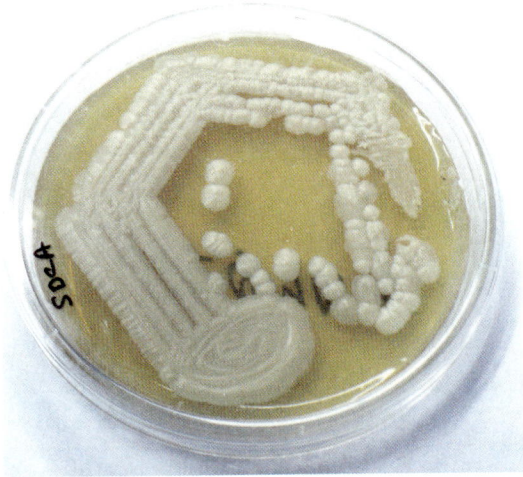

Fig. 4.21: *Candida guilliermondii.* Colonies grown on SDCA at 37°C after 3 days of incubation.

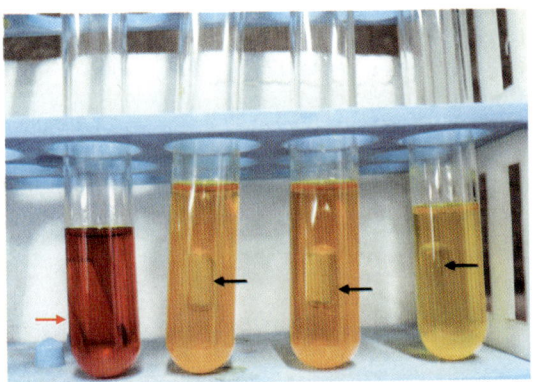

Fig. 4.20: *Candida tropicalis.* Glucose, sucrose and maltose are fermented with production of acid and gas (black arrow). Lactose is not fermented (red arrow).

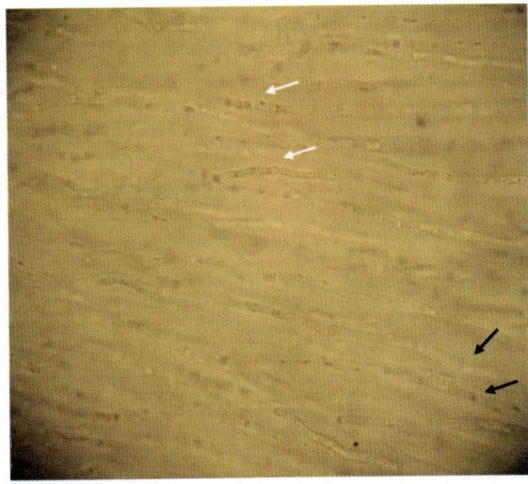

Fig. 4.22: *Candida kefyr.* Fragile pseudohyphae of long cells. These fall apart and lie parallel like "logs in a stream" (black arrow; ×400).

aspergillosis in immunosuppressed patients and lesions originating in nasal sinuses in immunocompetent patients. *Aspergillus niger* is the third most common cause of invasive pulmonary aspergillosis. *Aspergillus fumigatus* and *Aspergillus flavus* are the two most common species known to produce a 'fungus ball'. Other species of *Aspergillus* involved in producing lesions in different tissues of human host are *A. versicolor, A. nidulans, A. terreus, A. amstelodami, A. sydowi,* etc. *Aspergillus flavus* (aflatoxin) and *Aspergillus parasiticus* is notorious in causing mycotoxicosis.

Clinical entities caused by *Aspergillus* species:
1. Allergy to *Aspergillus* antigen.
   - Allergic bronchopulmonary aspergillosis
   - Sprophytic colonization of air spaces (otomycosis, fungal ball of paranasal sinuses, fungal ball of lung, endobronchial colonization).

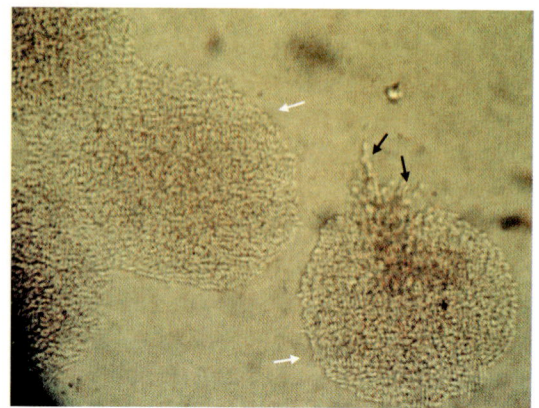

Fig. 4.23: *Candida guilliermondii.* Cells are ovoid and small in size. Few short filamentous pseudohyphae (black arrow) and small segments of blastospores (white arrow) are seen [Cornmeal agar morphology ×400].

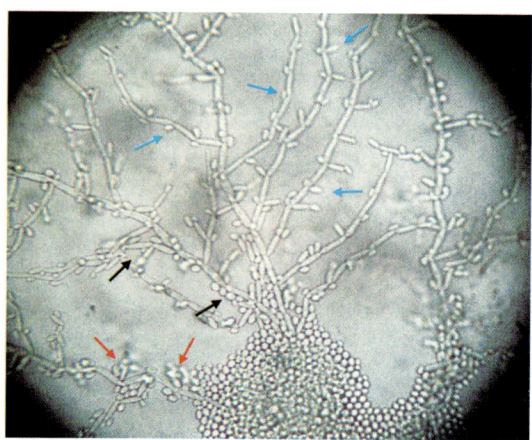

Fig. 4.25: *Candida guilliermondii.* Morphology on cornmeal agar at 25°C after 3 days of incubation. Many of the isolates produce sparing amount of pseudomycelium. The pseudomycelium elongates with a few branches, sometimes bearing ramified chains of small ovoid cells or stalagtoid (black arrow) and verticillated blastoconidia (red arrow); small ovoid cells are seen at septa (blue arrow) [×400].

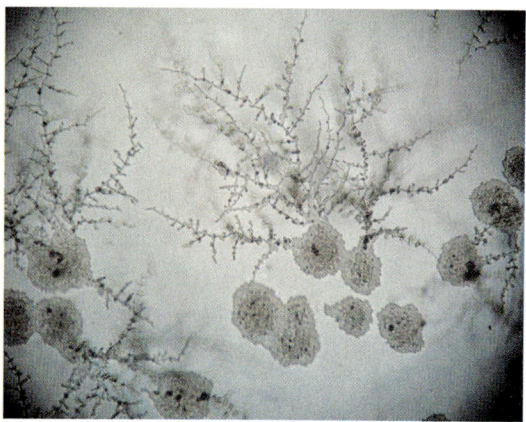

Fig. 4.24: *Candida guilliermondii.* Yeast cells are small, ovoid and sometimes cylindrical. Pseudomycelia are thin, short and elongates with a few branches. [Morphology on CMA ×200].

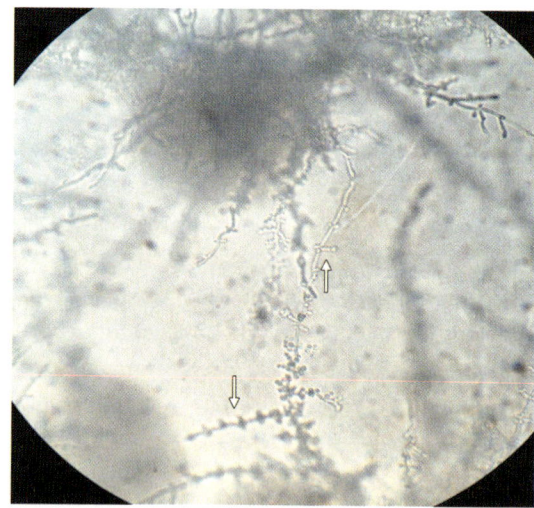

Fig. 4.26: *Candida krusei.* Oval to elongated blastospores are found at the tip of the pseudohyphae (Cornmeal agar morphology ×200).

2. Invasive aspergillosis.
  • Nonpulmonary portal of entry
    Eye—keratomycocis, exogenous end-ophthalmitis
    Paranasal sinus, cardiac or vascular surgery, intravenous drug addiction, skin
  • Pulmonary portal of entry
    Lung abscess, pneumonia.

Laboratory Diagnosis

Direct examination

Aspergillus hyphae in clinical specimens of sputum, sinus drainage, or bronchial washings can be readily detected by direct

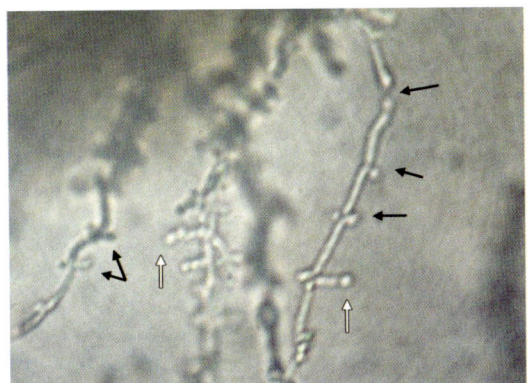

Fig. 4.27: *Candida krusei.* Cross matchsticks appearance (white arrow) of blastospores; oval to elongated blastospores are found at the tip of the pseudohyphae (black arrow) [on CMA ×400].

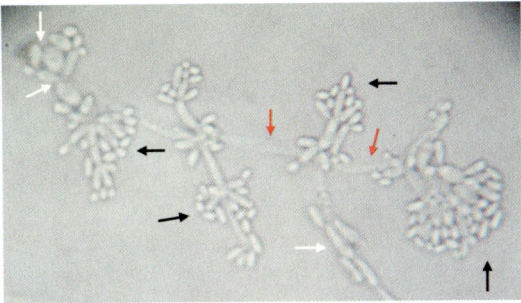

Fig. 4.30: *Candida viswanathii.* Yeast cells are globose, ovoid to cylindrical (white arrow) measuring 2.5 to 7 × 4 to 12 μm. On cornmeal agar, wavy pseudohyphae (red arrow) bearing verticillated branched chains of blastospores (black arrow) are produced (×400).

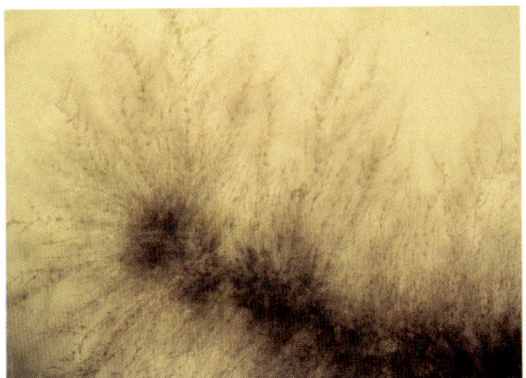

Fig. 4.28: *Candida parapsilosis.* Short, straight or slightly curved pseudohyphae spreading in all directions. Spider shape appearance is a characteristic feature [CMA ×200].

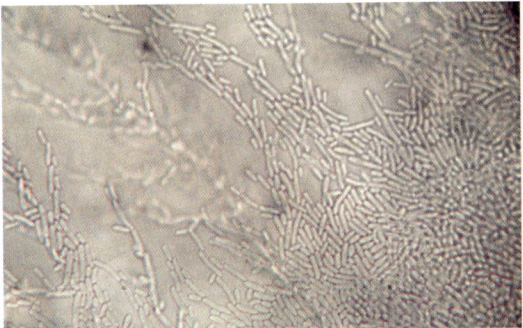

Fig. 4.31: *Candida rugosa.* Simple to elaborate pseudohyphae are produced on cornmeal agar. Budding yeast cells are also seen [Morphology on CMA ×400].

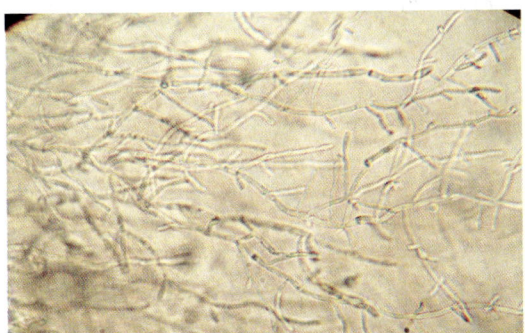

Fig. 4.29: *Candida parapsilosis.* Short, straight or slightly curved pseudohyphae are seen. Giant pseudohyphae may be found occasionally [CMA ×400].

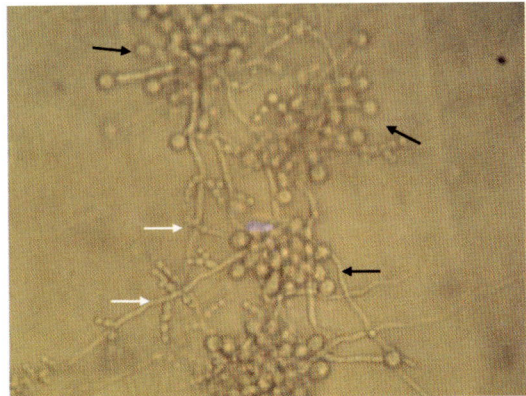

Fig. 4.32: *Candida dubliniensis.* Chlamydospores are arranged in clusters (black arrow); blastospores are arranged in short chains on pseudohyphae (White arrow) [Morphology on CMA ×400].

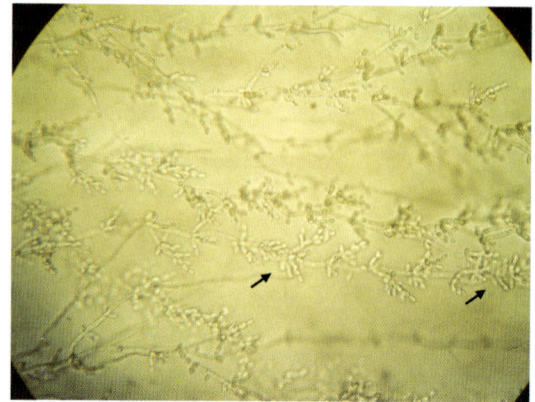

Fig. 4.33: *Candida lusitaniae*. Pseudohyphae are slender, curved and branched. Elongated blastospores are arranged in chains [Morphology on Cornmeal agar ×400].

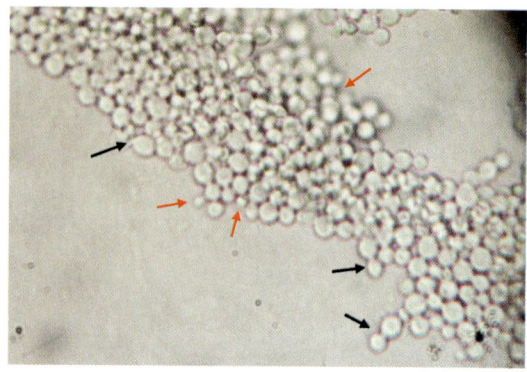

Fig. 4.36: *Candida glabrata*. Single, oval and terminal budding (black arrow); small cell size (red arrow) and absence of pseudohyphae are characteristic features for identification [Cornmeal agar morphology ×600].

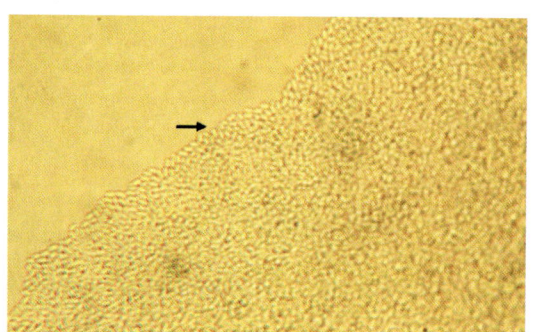

Fig. 4.34: *Candida glabrata*. Yeast cells are oval, single terminal budding is present usually. No pseudohyphae are produced [Cornmeal agar morphology ×400].

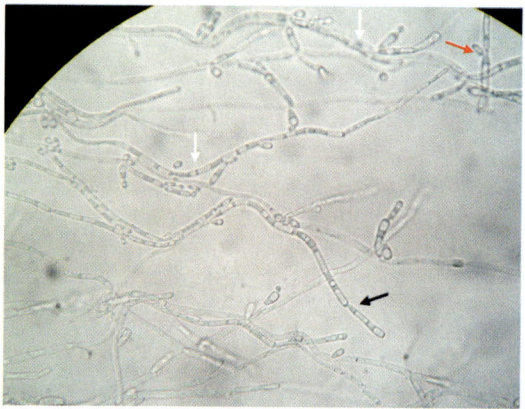

Fig. 4.37: *Candida lipolytica*. Both true septate hyphae (white arrow), pseudohyphae (black arrow), are present. Elongated blastospores are in short chains (red arrow). Sometimes short segments of arthroconidia are also noticed [CMA ×200].

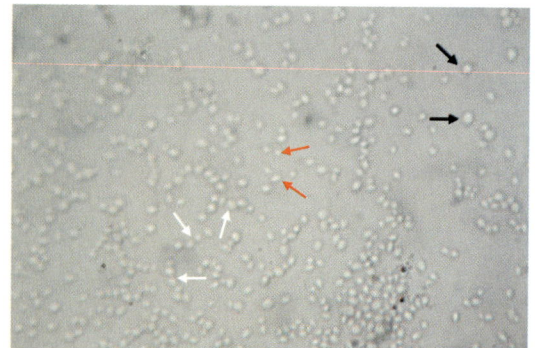

Fig. 4.35: *Candida haemulonii*. Yeast cells are ovoid (red arrow) to globose (black arrow); short chains of globose cells may be produced (white arrow) but true or pseudohyphae are absent [Morphology on CMA ×400].

microscopic examination. Purulent or blood tinged, thick sputum may be digested with 10% potassium hydroxide before examination.

Long strands of hyphae with dichotomous branching and regular septation may be present. Occasionally whole conidial structures may be seen which indicates that *Aspergillus* is colonizing an area in contact with air (Fig. 4.42). In invasive aspergillosis cases hyphae are rarely observed in sputum. Small pieces of biopsy material from invasive

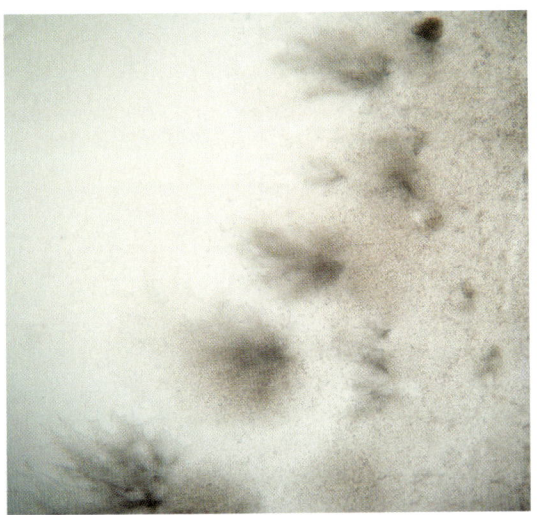

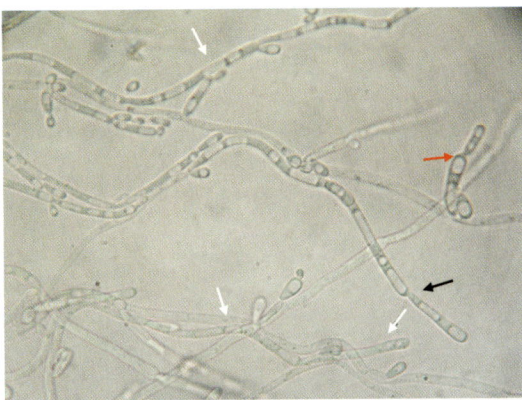

Fig. 4.40: *Candida lipolytica*. Pseudohyphae (black arrow), septate hyphae (white arrow) and elongated blastospores arranged in chains (red arrow) are characteristic features [Morphology on CMA ×400].

Fig. 4.38: *Candida zeylanoides*. "Feather-like appearance" of blastospores and curved pseudohyphae are identifying features [Cornmeal agar morphology ×200].

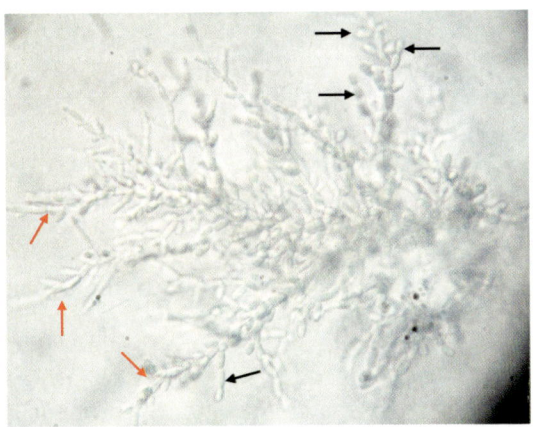

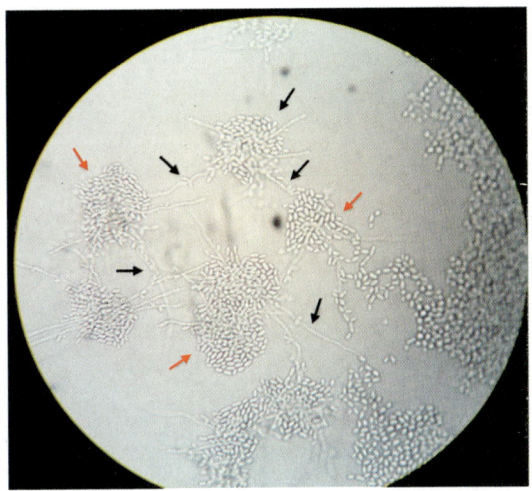

Fig. 4.39: *Candida zeylanoides*. Oval to elongated blastospores are arranged in small clusters or short chains (black arrow) and curved pseudohyphae (red arrow) together make a "feather-like appearance" [CMA morphology ×400].

Fig. 4.41: *Candida stellatoidea*. Blastospores (red arrow) are arranged in clusters. Elaborate pseudohyphae (black arrow) which appears as if they are communicating with each other [Morphology on CMA ×200].

aspergillosis can be examined for promising results both in direct microscopy and culture isolation. Biopsy material is minced and digested with 10% KOH solution. The preparation is warmed gently over a low flame which facilitates clearing of tissues and debris.

Isolation in culture

Aspergillus grow well on a variety of conventional agar media. The most useful media Sabouraud's dextrose agar with antibiotic chloramphenicol (SDCA), **cyclohexamide should not be used as majority of the species of *Aspergillus* are sensitive to it**.

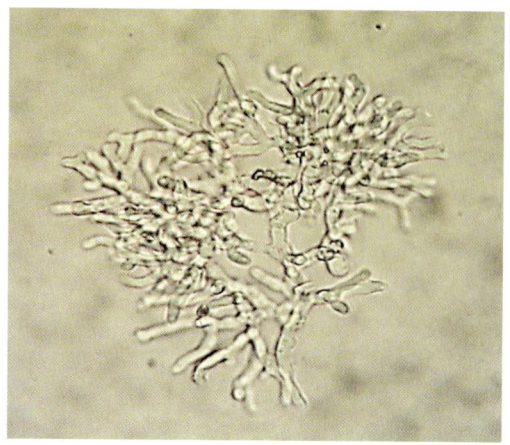

Fig. 4.42: Bronchopulmonary aspergillosis. Direct microscopy of sputum sample after digestion with 10% KOH (potassium hydroxide). Clumps of aspergillus are seen that demonstrate finger-like dichotomous branching [×400].

Aspergillus fumigatus

Colony morphology

The colonies have a velvety texure and spread broadly over the surface of Sabouraud's dextrose agar. The colour for the colony for the first 2 to 3 days is white, gradually turns into greenish blue to grayish green as the conidial heads mature (Fig. 4.43).

Reverse is usually colourless. The conidia masses of the conidial heads are columnar, compact and often crowded.

Microscopic morphology

Conidiophore is short, smooth and has a slightly green or brownish colouration especially towards the upper part near the vesicle. The conidiophores enlarge to form the flask-shaped vesicle. The vesicle produces a series of phialides on the upper half. The phialides bend upward paralleling the axis of conidiophores. The conidia are globose to subglobose, grayish green, smooth (Fig. 4.44).

Aspergillus flavus

Colony morphology

Colony grows rapidly on Sabouraud's dextrose agar and consists of a close textured basal

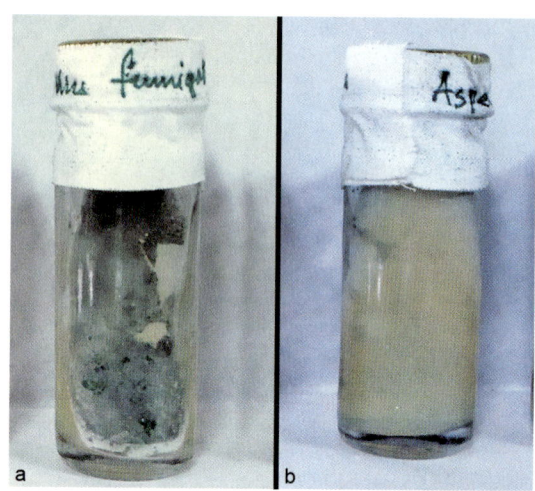

a   b

Fig. 4.43: Colony morphology of *Aspergillus fumigatus* grown on Sabouraud's dextrose agar at 25°C for 1 week; (a) obverse—flat, white for the first 2 to 3 days but soon become velvety in texture, greenish blue to grayish green with maturation of conidial heads and production of conidia, (b) reverse is colourless.

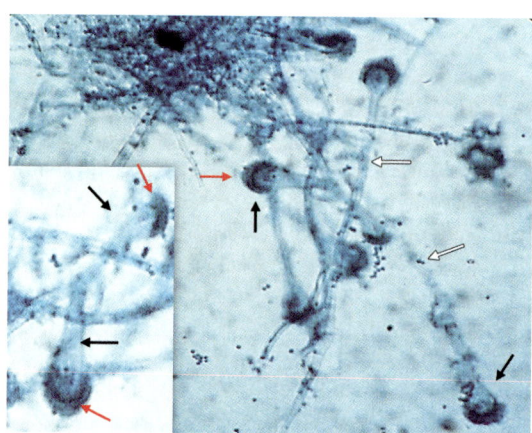

Fig. 4.44: Microscopic morphology of *Aspergillus fumigatus*. Conidiophores are smooth walled, colourless (white arrow), vesicles are flask-shaped (black arrow), phialides uniseriate and are arranged parallel to the conidiophore (inset: Red arrow) [LPCB mount ×200].

mycelium which is flat or radially furrowed or wrinkled (Fig. 4.56). Conidial heads are abundant and of intense yellow to yellowish green in colour. Reverse is colourless.

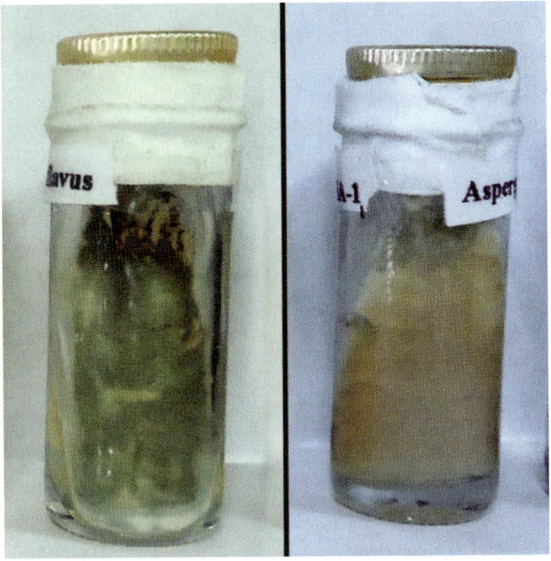

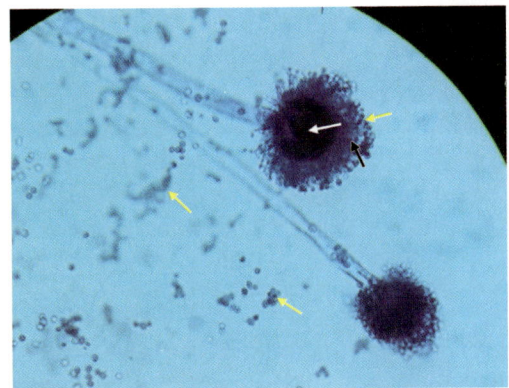

Fig. 4.46: Microscopic morphology of *Aspergillus flavus*. Vesicles (white arrow) are globose, sterigmata biseriate and radiating (black arrow), conidia are round to oval smooth greenish yellow (yellow arrow) [LPCB mount ×400].

Fig. 4.45: Colony morphology of *Aspergillus flavus* at 28°C for 5–6 days. Colonies grow rapidly as white flocculent at first and gradually become velvety, yellowish green when conidial heads mature and produce conidia, reverse is colourless; (a) obverse, (b) reverse.

Microscopic morphology

Conidiophores are thick-walled, unpigmented, coarsely roughened, long and ends in a vesicle which is globose to subglobose and produce phialides covering the entire surface. Phialides are biseriate or sometimes uniseriate. Primary phialides are up to 10 µ in length and the secondary phialides are about 5 µ in length. The conidia are elliptical at first, but later they are mostly globose and conspicuously echinulate (Fig. 4.46).

Aspergillus terreus

Colony morphology

On Sabouraud's dextrose agar at 25°C to 30°C the colony grows rapidly. The consistency of the colony is floccose to velvety, sometimes furrowed or tufted and the colony conidiates profusely. The massed conidial heads are columnar and the colour is cinnamon-buff to wood brown which is revealed in colony colour. Reverse is usually colourless (Fig. 4.47).

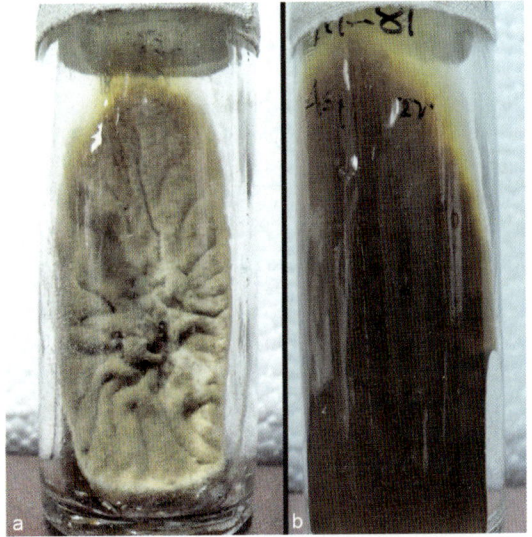

Fig. 4.47: Colony morphology of *Aspergillus terreus* grown on Sabouraud's dextrose agar at 25°C for 2 weeks; (a) obverse is velvety, furrowed, cinamon-buff to wood brown in colour, (b) reverse is dark brown.

Microscopic morphology

The conidiophores are long and slender, smooth and uniform diameter throughout. The vesicles are hemispherical or dome-like and merge in perceptively with the conidiophore. The phialides are in two series. The primaries are longer and wider than secondaries. The conidia

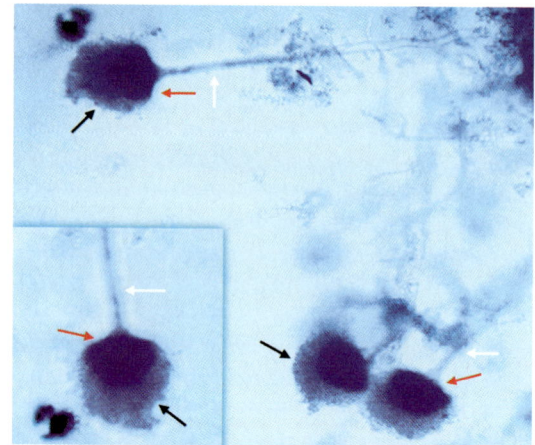

Fig. 4.48: *Aspergillus terreus.* Microscopic morphology showing conidiophores long, smooth and colourless (white arrow), vesicles are hemispherical to subglobose (red arrow), phialides are radiating, arranged in two rows (biseriate, black arrow) [LPCB mount ×400].

are smooth to somewhat elliptical in shape. Spherical to oval hyaline cells (aleuroconidia) which are produced laterally on the mycelia submerged on the agar (Fig. 4.48).

HISTOPLASMOSIS

Histoplasmosis is a granulomatous disease of worldwide distribution caused by the dimorphic fungus *Histoplasma capsulatum.* Infection is initiated after inhalation of conidia of the fungus and result in a variety of clinical manifestations. Approximately 95% cases are inapparent, subclinical or completely benign. In the vast majority of patients, the infection is aborted, leaving only residual calcification in the lung and sometimes the spleen. Resolution of the disease confers a certain degree of immunity to reinfection and also varying degrees of hypersensitivity to the antigenic component of the organism.

Clinical forms of histoplasmosis
1. *Benign infection*
   - *Endemic histoplasmosis* (primary cutaneous disease; 'fungus flu' in adults; summer sickness in children; subclinical disease)

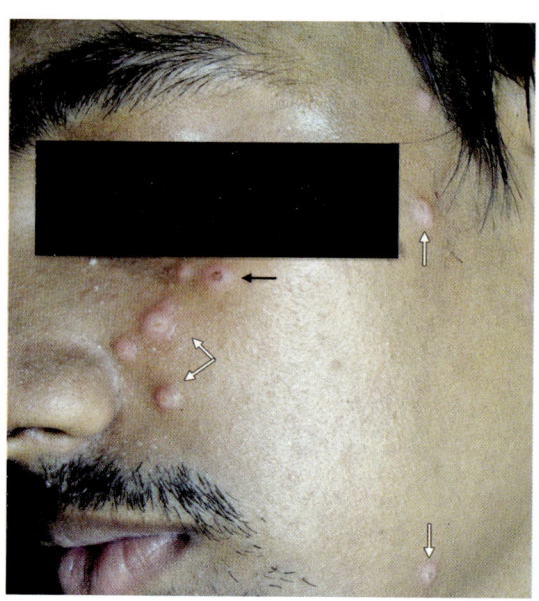

Fig. 4.49: Secondary cutaneous lesions in disseminated histoplasmosis in HIV reactive patient. Papular skin lesions (white arrow) are suggestive of histoplasmosis while the papulopustular lesions (black arrow) are very much suggestive of cutaneous manifestation of disseminated blastomycosis.

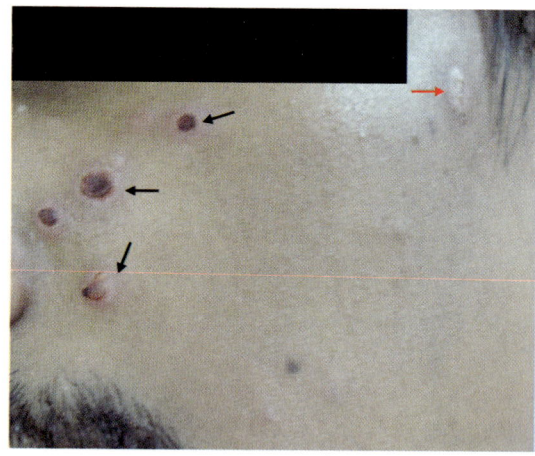

Fig. 4.50: Cutaneous lesions in blastomycosis. These are papulopustular lesions which gradually become necrotic (black arrow) with some scarring in the center (red arrow).

- *Epidemic histoplasmosis* (acute pulmonary histoplasmosis and acute disseminated histoplasmosis)

2. *Opportunistic infection*

- *Chronic pulmonary histoplasmosis* (cavitary histoplasmosis; smokers emphysema; colonization of preexisting structural anomalies)
- *Disseminating histoplasmosis* (fulminant disease in children; fulminant disease of adults associated with immuno-suppression)

3. *Aberrant fibrosis and hypersensitivity disease*

- Histoplasmoma
- Mediastinal fibrosis.

Laboratory Diagnosis

Direct examination

The KOH procedure, which is useful in other fungal diseases, is usually negative in histoplasmosis. Sputum is more useful specimen when cultured.

Sputum, the buffy coat of centrifuged blood specimens, the sediment of such specimens, biopsy material and sternal puncture material are best examined following staining.

The material is spread on a slide and fixed for 10 minutes with methyl alcohol. The fixed material is stained by Wright or Giemsa stain method.

Yeast cells are predominantly within macrophages or monocytes but may appear extracellular because of destruction of phagocytic cells.

Yeast cells are ovoid, 2 to 4 µ in diameter with the bud at the smaller end and **budding is characteristically with a 'narrow base'** (Fig. 4.51).

Culture method

Samples are planted directly on blood agar and Sabouraud's dextrose agar with antibiotic (chloramphenicol) and incubated at 25°C. In sputum sample, areas that are purulent or blood streaked should be selected for culture.

Gastric lavage is centrifuged and the sediment is planted on the same media as mentioned above. Other pathologic material

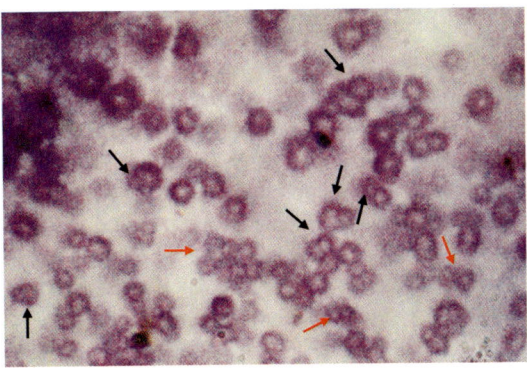

Fig. 4.51: Giemsa stained smear (superimposed) prepared from punch biopsy (skin) material dipped in KOH solution. Broad based budding yeast cells (black arrow) are suggestive of yeast cells of *Blastomyces dermatitidis*. A few yeast cells (red arrow) with narrow based budding are suggestive of yeasts of *Histoplasma capsulatum* [Giemsa stain ×1000].

such as biopsy specimens, sternal punctures, aspirations are minced aseptically and spread over blood agar or Sabouraud's dextrose agar with chloramphenicol.

Colony morphology

On Sabouraud's dextrose agar, the colony develops initially as white that gradually turns into buff-brown (Fig. 4.52). These two

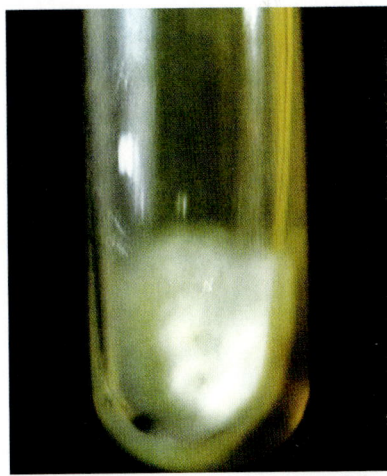

Fig. 4.52: Colony morphology of *Histoplasma capsulatum* grown on Sabouraud's dextrose agar at 25°C for two weeks. White to buff colonies appear which on repeated transfer produce white dense aerial hyphae.

morphologic types have been termed albino and brown. Both types may be isolated from the same patient and with subculture the brown type shows sectoring and eventual conversion to albino type.

Microscopic morphology

The characteristic tuberculate macroconidia are seen on hyphae. They are round to pyriform, 8 to 14 μ in diameter and are borne on narrow tubular conidiophores. The tubercle or fingerlike projections are quite variable in size and morphology (Figs 4.53 and 4.54). In subculture, only about 50% of the macroconidia show tubercles. Microconidia are also produced and are particularly abundant in fresh isolates of *H. capsulatum*. These conidia are spherical, 2 to 4 μ in diameter, borne at the tip of short narrow conidiophores and at right angle to the vegetative hyphae. Occasionally there is a secondary lateral conidium that sometimes appears to bud, giving a unit of dumbbell shape. The walls are smooth but often somewhat roughened.

Mycelium to yeast conversion (M → Y):
At 37°C on blood agar with 10% glucose, yeast form of *H. capsulatum* arises from within the mycelium itself or conidia (both types), first germinate and then convert to the yeast phase.

The colony produced is at first glabrous and tenacious. Examination shows it to be mixture hyphae in the process of conversion or freely budding yeast cells. On subsequent transfer the colony becomes white, smooth and yeast like. Yeast cells are oval, 2 to 3 × 3 to 4 μ in size, budding occurs at the narrow end of the oval cyst cell. **The buds have a narrow neck (0.2 to 0.3 μ) and the attachment is often drawn out as a narrow thread (Fig. 4.55). This characteristic is useful in differentiating it from small forms of *Blastomyces dermatitidis* that have a broad based bud.**

BLASTOMYCOSIS

Blastomycosis is a chronic granulomatous and suppurative disease having a primary pulmonary stage that is frequently followed by dissemination to the other body site, chiefly the skin and bone. The primary infection in lung is often inapparent. The causative agent is the dimorphic fungus *Blastomyces dermatitidis* which has been assumed to be a soil saprophyte in nature.

The clinical disease can be divided into five categories:

- Primary pulmonary blastomycosis— inapparent infection resolves spontaneously or disseminates to another form.
- Chronic cutaneous and osseous blasto-mycosis.
- Single organ system blastomycosis—may remain occult for many years.
- Systemic blastomycosis.
- Inoculation blastomycosis.

Laboratory Identification

Direct examination

Examination in a potassium hydroxide preparation is the easiest and most rapid procedure for diagnosis. In cutaneous disease, aspirated material from pustules at the outer edge of the lesions or pus from the open lesion are examined in KOH mount to identify the presence of yeast cells in the samples. The yeast of *Blastomyces dermatitidis* is a thick walled spherical cell, 8 to 15 μ in diameter. The young bud has a thin wall, which thickens as it grows. The bud on the parent cell has a characteristic broad base (Fig. 4.51). Buds may grow to the size of the parent cells and sometimes do not detach easily resulting in a cluster of cells (Fig. 4.52). The most important diagnostic aid for differentiation of *Blastomyces dermatitidis* from other yeast cells (spherical fungi) is the width of the bud attachment base which is 4 to 5 μ.

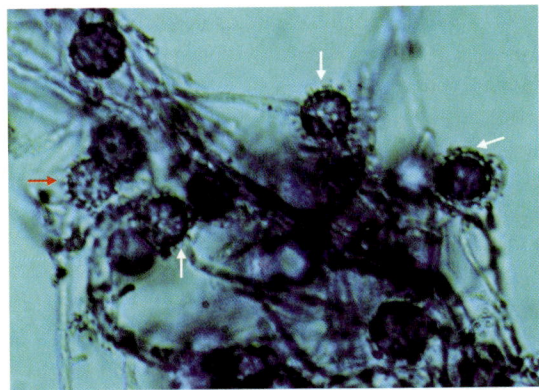

Fig. 4.53: Characteristic macroconidia of *Histoplasma capsulatum*. Large, thick walled, spherical (occasionally oblong or pear shaped) macroconidia (white arrow) with finger-like projections (red arrow); also called 'tuberculate' conidia [LPCB mount ×600].

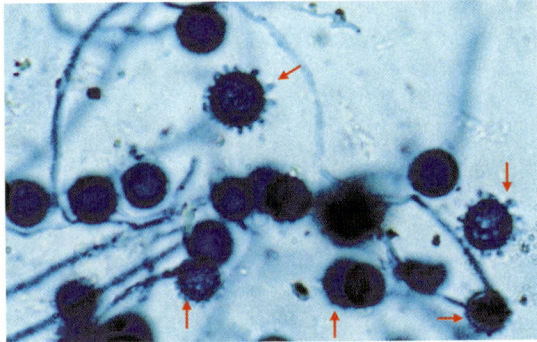

Fig. 4.54: Characteristic tuberculate macroconidia of *H. capsulatum*. Tubercles or finger-like projections are quite variable in size and morphology (red arrow) [LPCB mount ×600].

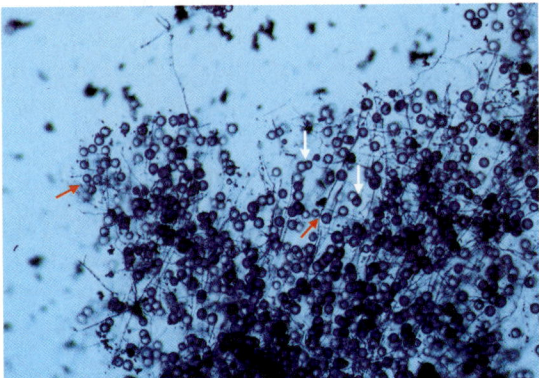

Fig. 4.55: Yeast conversion of *Histoplasma capsulatum* (M→Y). Microscopic morphology of yeast form cells from culture. Mixture of hyphae in the process of conversion and freely budding yeast cells are seen. Yeast cells are small (2–3 μ × 3–4 μ), oval to round and have a narrow neck of budding. The attachment is often drawn out as a narrow neck (red arrow). Some broad based budding yeast cells (white arrow) indicate yeast conversion of *Blastomyces dermatitidis*; might be the lesion is caused by dual pathogenic fungi [LPCB mount ×400].

Culture method

Demonstration of the characteristic broad-based bud of the yeast cells in tissue is usually sufficient to make the diagnosis of blastomycosis. Culture should always be done particularly when the KOH examination is negative or doubtful.

Samples are inoculated onto blood agar and Sabouraud's dextrose agar with chloramphenicol (SDCA) at 25°C for a week or more.

Cyclohexamide should not be added into the cultivating media as both yeast form and to some extent, the mycelial form of the fungus is sensitive to it.

Colony morphology

At 25°C colony morphology and growth rate of *Blastomyces dermatitidis* are quite variable. Some strains grow rapidly producing fluffy white mycelium; others grow slowly as glabrous, tan non-conidiating colonies. Some strains have a dark brown colony consisting of concentric rings that conidiate heavily. Most strains become pleomorphic when maintained in culture.

At 37°C colony morphology on blood agar, Sabouraud's dextrose agar with chloramphenicol (SDCA) or brain heart infusion agar (BHIA) with 10% glucose supplement in each

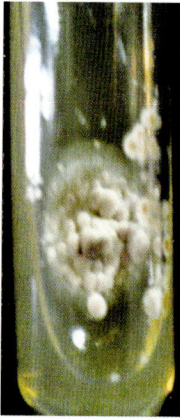

Fig. 4.56: Colony morphology of *B. dermatitidis* grown on SDCA (+ 10% glucose) at 37°C for two weeks (M→Y conversion is usually done on blood agar with 10% glucose supplement).

type produce wrinkled, folded, glabrous and yeast like colonies (Fig. 4.56).

Microscopic morphology

The conidia produced are ovoid or dumbbell shaped, 2 to 10 μ in diameter and are borne on short lateral or terminal branches of the mycelium. They may resemble microconidia of *Histoplasma* but these are usually roughened with echinulations. **Conidia of *Histoplasma* (both macroconidia and microconidia) are roughened with echinulations which is not an usual feature of *Blastomyces dermatitidis*.** The production of lateral globose conidia intermixed with dumbbell or double conidia (Figs 4.57 and 4.58) is fairly characteristics of *Blastomyces dermatitidis*.

Mycelium to yeast conversion (M → Y)

Blastomyces dermatitidis when grown at an elevated temperature of 37°C the organism produces characteristic yeast forms with broad based buds. The cells again vary in size from 8 μ to 13 μ in diameter and sometimes yeast cells up to 30 μ in diameter can be seen in tissue (Fig. 4.59).

MUCORMYCOSIS

Mucormycosis is a clinical entity which is caused by the agents belonging to the order Mucorales.

The etiological agents of mucormycosis in human are:

- *Mucor species*
- *Rhizopus oryzae (arrhizus)*
- *Rhizopus microspores* **var.** *rhizopodiformis*
- *Cunninghamella bertholletiae*
- *Lichtheimia corymbifera*
- *Rhizomucor pusilus*
- *Apophysomyces elegans*
- *Cokeromyces recurvatus*
- *Syncephalastrum racemosum*
- *Saksenaea vasiformis*

Members of the family Mucoraceae are more frequently isolated from cases of mucormycosis

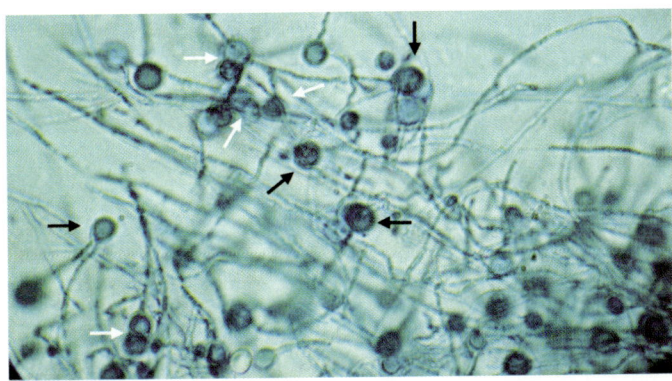

Fig. 4.57: *Blastomyces dermatitidis.* Mycelial form at 25°C. The conidia are of *Chrysosporium* type, ovoid (black arrow) to dumbbell shaped (white arrow) and may vary from 2 to 10 μ in diameter. Conidia are borne on short lateral (white arrow) or terminal branches of the mycelium (black arrow) [LPCB mount ×400].

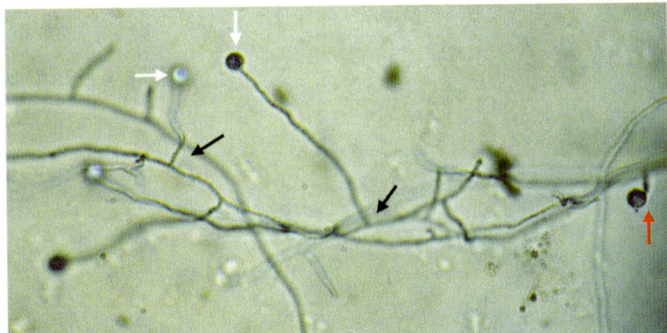

Fig. 4.58: *Blastomyces dermatitidis.* Typically smooth, round conidia (white arrow) produced on long branched (black arrow) and short lateral unbranched (red arrow) conidiophores [LPCB mount ×200].

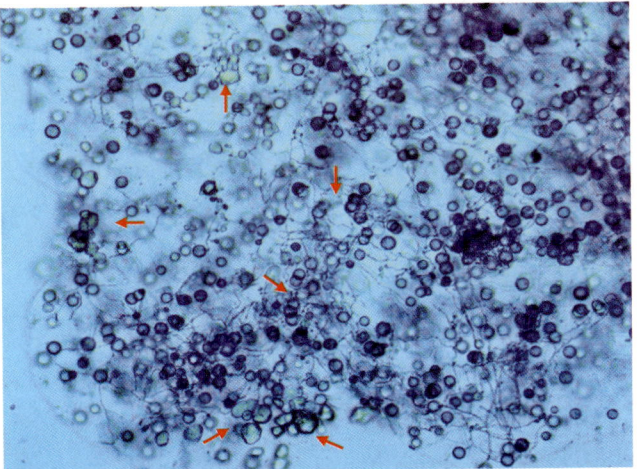

Fig. 4.59: Yeast conversion (M→Y) in *Blastomyces dermatitidis.* Culture mount showing mycelial conversion to yeast cells and freely budding yeast cells characteristically having a broad base (red arrow) [LPCB mount ×200].

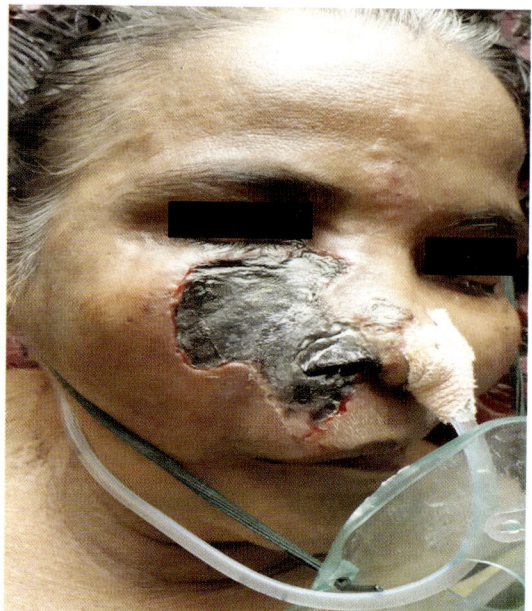

Fig. 4.60: Rhinocerebral mucormycosis in a patient with uncontrolled diabetic mellitus of many years duration.

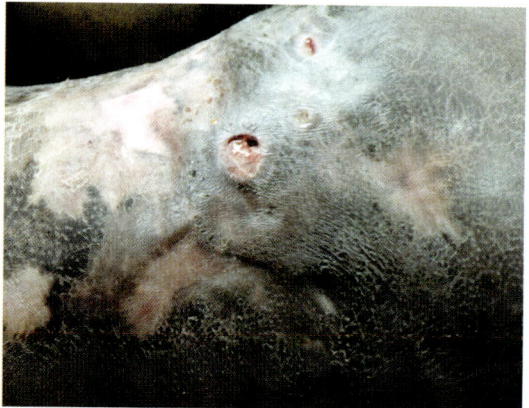

Fig. 4.61: Primary cutaneous mucormycosis over the left gluteal region in a diabetic patient with renal compromization. Necrosis, eschar formation, central ulceration and sloughing are seen. *Rhizopus oryzae* was cultured from the lesion.

than any other family of Mucorales. *Rhizopus oryzae* is the most frequent agent of the human mucormycosis followed by *Rhizopus microspores* ver. *rhizopodiformis* and *Mucor species,* however, discrete reports of mucormycosis caused by *Cunninghamella*

bertholletiae, Apophysomyces elegans, Lichthemia corymbifera, and *Saksenaea vasiformis* have also been documented in the literature. Various clinical types of mucormycosis depending upon the location of the lesions and the system involved are paranasal sinus mucormycosis, cutaneous mucormycosis, pulmonary mucormycosis, rhino cerebral mucormycosis and disseminated mucormycosis (Figs 4.60 and 4.61).

Laboratory Diagnosis

Direct examination

In samples like sputum, skin scrapings or aspirated material from sinuses, demonstration of broad, infrequently septate hyphae of Mucorales in these materials is considered more significant than culture isolation because many species of order Mucorales (*Rhizopus, Mucor,* etc.) are common contaminant in the laboratory. Hence isolation of these species in culture should be interpreted with caution. However, if the patient is diabetic or immunocompromised, culture isolation has greater validity.

In pulmonary mucormycosis cases, sputum and bronchial washings (after centrifugation)

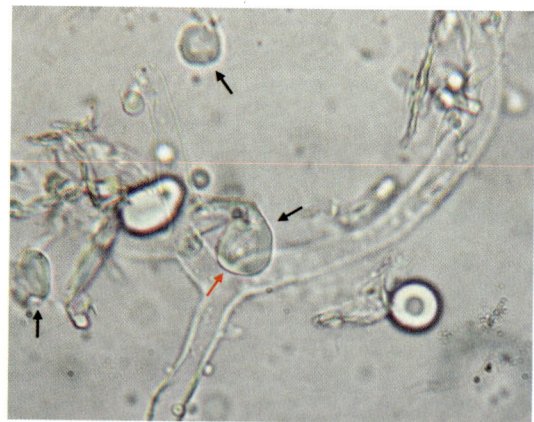

Fig. 4.62: Direct mount of punch biopsy from the lesion in the nasal area in a case of rhinocerebral mucormycosis. Sparsely septate broad ribbon-like hyphae with wide angle branching (red arrow) are noticed in this KOH preparation. Black arrow shows columella of the ruptured sporangium [×400].

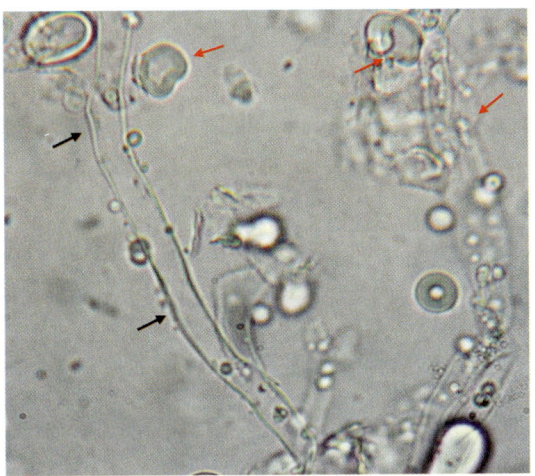

Fig. 4.63: Direct microscopy of a nasal scrapings after potassium hydroxide digestion in a case of rhino-cerebral mucormycosis. Broad, sparsely septate, thick walled, refractile hyphae (black arrow) are noticed. Some swollen cells and distorted hyphae (red arrow) are also seen [KOH preparation ×400].

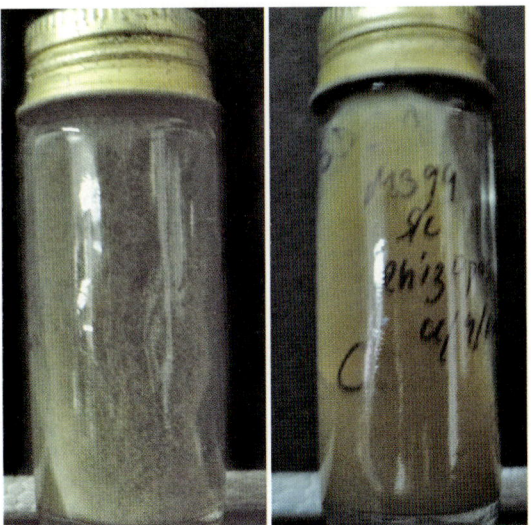

Fig. 4.64: Colony morphology of *Rhizopus oryzae* grown on SDCA at 30°C for 7 days of incubation. Colony is fast growing, white at first and become yellowish-brown with age. When sporangia are produced, the colony gradually turns into more dark-brown. The reverse is dark brown.

are used and in rhino cerebral cases, specimens are obtained from scrapings of the upper turbinates or from aspirated sinus material for microscopic examination. Biopsied necrotic tissue from cutaneous and other lesions can also be used.

Specimens are mounted on 10% potassium hydroxide solution and examined under low power and high power objective. Biopsied material is minced aseptically and a few pieces are put into 10% KOH solution. Gentle heating of the solution will clear the tissue rapidly and the fungal element can be visualized properly. Broad (7–15 μm), sparsely septate, 90° branching hyphae may be seen under the microscope. Occasionally hyphae of lesser width are also visible (Figs 4.73 and 4.74).

Direct culture
Specimens of sputum, scrapings or sinus aspirates are planted on Sabouraud's dextrose agar with chloramphenicol and incubated at 37°C or 25°C. Biopsy tissue material should be minced aseptically rather than grinding with a tissue grinder because grinding may cause cytoplasmic leakage in the hyphae, which are largely coenocytic in Mucorales and thus making the hyphae nonviable. Almost all the pathogenic Mucorales are easily isolated from such material. The media may contain antibacterial antibiotics, but **almost all isolates are sensitive to cyclohexamide**.

The Mucorales that are involved in human disease all grow on standard laboratory media without cyclohexamide. The growth is rapid and usually noticeable 12 to 18 hours after planting of the specimen.

Establishing a diagnosis on culture evidence alone is difficult. **The pathogenic species of the Mucorales are constant inhabitants of the environment, contaminants of skin, discharges and sputum and grow well on almost all moist organic substrates. An uncritical diagnosis of mucormycosis cannot be given on culture basis alone and conversely the isolation of a Mucorales from a patient cannot be discarded**

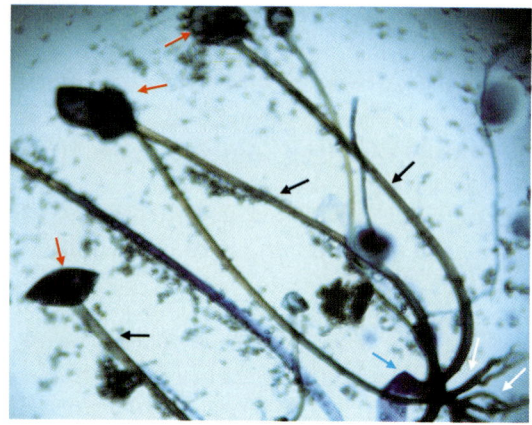

Fig. 4.65: *Rhizopus* species. Several sporangiophores (black arrow) arising from a node above the rhizoides (white arrow). Sporangia (red arrow) and broken stolon (blue arrow) are also seen [LPCB ×400].

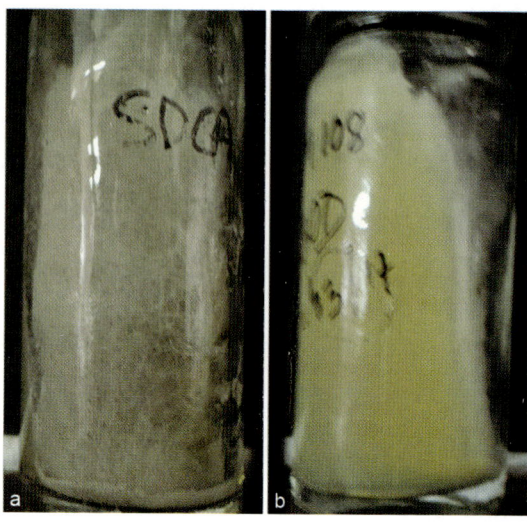

Fig. 4.67: Colony morphology of *Mucor* species on Sabouraud's dextrose agar at 37°C for 48 hours. Good growth is achieved at this temperature. Colonies are fast growing, white at first and become smoky gray with age. The reverse is cream to yellow; (a) obverse, (b) reverse.

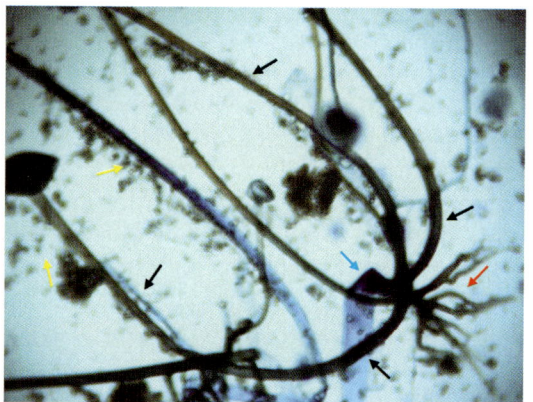

Fig. 4.66: *Rhizopus oryzae*. Sporangiophores are simple or branched (black arrow), rhizoids are yellow-brown (red arrow) and sporangiospores (yellow arrow) are light brown, striated, round to oval sometimes irregular in shape [LPCB mount ×600].

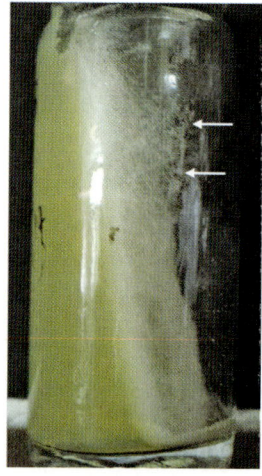

Fig. 4.68: Colony morphology of *Mucor* species on Sabouraud's dextrose agar at 30°C for 48 hours. Colonies are fast growing, smoky gray, aerial mycelium reaches up to 2–3 cm height (white arrow) and odoriferous. The reverse is cream to yellow.

as transient flora or a contaminant. All forms and sources of evidence must be marshaled and critically judged for an accurate diagnosis.

Rhizopus oryzae

Colony morphology

The colony on SDCA at 37°C is fast growing, white at first, becoming yellowish brown with age (Fig. 4.64). Sporangia are dark brown.

Microscopic morphology

The sporangiophores are simple or branched, up to 4 mm in length. Rhizoids are yellow brown (Fig. 4.65). Sporangiophores arise in

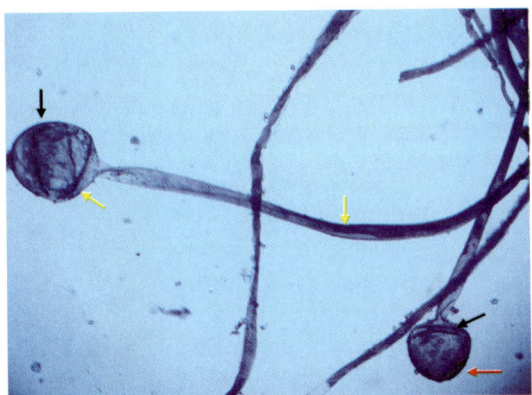

Fig. 4.69: *Mucor* species. Exposed columella (red arrow) are spherical to ellipsoidal with a distinct collarette (black arrow). These are visible following rupture of sporangium. Yellow arrow shows sporangiophore [LPCB mount ×400].

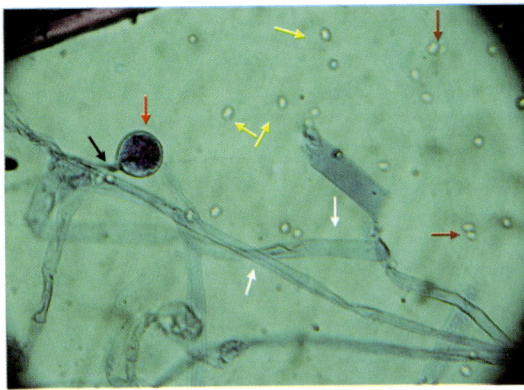

Fig. 4.71: *Mucor* species. Simple or branched, short or elongate sporangiophores arise randomly along the aerial mycelium. Short sporangiophore (black arrow) bear small sporangium (red arrow). Spores (yellow arrow) are short, oval and when free they are often seen as budding yeasts (brown arrow) [LPCB mount ×400].

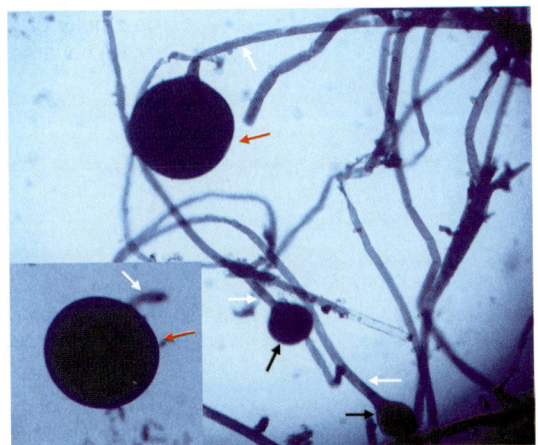

Fig. 4.70: *Mucor* species. Sporangia (black arrow) are in the process of maturation. Mature sporangium (red arrow) are dark brown, spherical and without any apophysis. Sporangiophores are indicated by white arrow [LPCB mount ×400].

groups directly above the rhizoids (Fig. 4.66). Sporangia are 100 to 350 μ in diameter and dark brown in colour. The sporangiospores are light brown, striated, irregularly shaped (6–8 μ × 7–9 μ in size). This species of *Rhizopus* is thermo tolerant and grows at a temperature of 40°C.

Mucor Species

Two members of this genus that cause human disease are *Mucor circinelloides* and *Mucor ramosissimus*.

Colony morphology

Colonies are fast growing, smoky gray, up to 2 cm in height; the reverse is yellow to cream coloured and odoriferous (Figs 4.67 and 4.68).

Microscopic morphology

Sporangiophores are of two types—elongate sporangiophores bear large sporangia (40 to 80 μ) and are brown (Figs 4.69 and 4.70), filled with granules, sympodially branched, with tapering branches. The second type of sporangiophore is short and grows haphazardly near the substrate with small sporangia (20 to 25 μ) (Fig. 4.71). The large sporangia are at first white, then greenish brown, globose or dorsoventrally compressed, circinately borne and characterized by 'bobbing heads'. The smaller sporangia have persistent walls that are smooth and hyaline. Hyaline columellae are variable in shape with well-developed collars. Spores are oval (4 to 7 μ) and are often seen as budding yeasts when they are free. Occasionally chlamydoconidia are seen which are heavy walled round structures. Good growth is achieved at 37°C.

Rhizomucor pusillus

The genus is similar to *Mucor* but has some poorly developed rhizoids.

Colony morphology

Similar to *Mucor* species. The colony is rapidly growing, smoky gray at first and becomes grayish brown to dark brown with age (Fig. 4.72).

Microscopic morphology

Sporangiophores are short and less than 3 mm in size and they arise from stolons. A few rhizoids are present and they are irregularly branched. Sporangia are spherical and black and have spines. Columellae are smooth and variable in shape and have a collar. They are thermophilic and common in heated environment.

Lichtheimia corymbifera

Colony morphology

The colonies are rapidly growing, floccose, light olive gray coloured. The colour fades in time (Fig. 4.73).

Microscopic morphology

Sporangiophores are very long, light gray in colour and arise from stolons. Numerous smaller and irregularly shaped sporangiophores are also produced (Fig. 4.74). Presence of rhizoids at the nodes and branching sporangiophores arise from stolons in between the nodes (Fig. 4.75). This is characteristic of genus *Lichthemia* which is in contrast to the location of sporangiophores in genus *Rhizopus*. The sporangiophores branch repeatedly to form corymbs. Sporangia are 20 to 35 μ in diameter and grayish. Columellae are 10 to 27 μ in diameter, ovoid to spatulate and may have a few spines (Fig. 4.76). The spores are formed by internal cleavage in a manner similar to that found in Coccidioides. Mature spores are globose to oval. Rhizoids

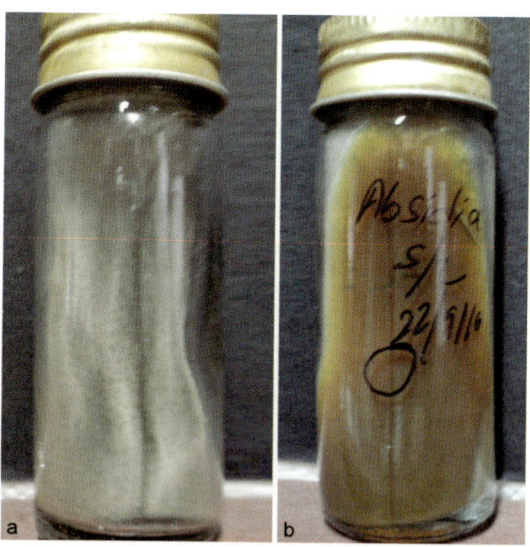

Fig. 4.72: Colony morphology of *Rhizomucor pusillus* grown on Sabouraud's dextrose agar at 30°C for five days; (a) obverse, (b) reverse.

Fig. 4.73: *Lichtheimia corymbifera*. On SDCA a rapidly growing floccose light gray colony appears. Reverse is often light brownish; (a) obverse, (b) reverse.

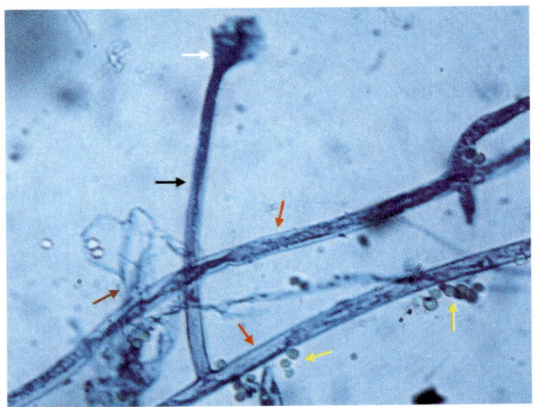

Fig. 4.74: *Lichtheimia corymbifera*. Sporangiophores (black arrow) are long, light gray colour, branched and arise from stolons (red arrow) between the nodes. Sporangia (white arrow) are pyriform and grayish. Rhizoids (brown arrow) are hyaline, arise from swollen areas on stolons called 'nodes.' Spores (yellow arrow) are globose to oval [Culture mount with LPCB ×400].

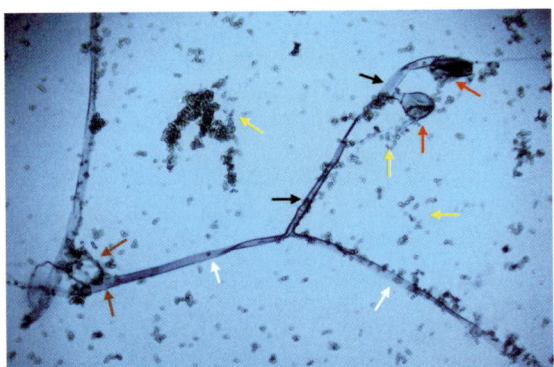

Fig. 4.75: Presence of rhizoids (brown arrow) at the nodes and branching sporangiophores (black arrow) which arise in between the nodes on stolons (white arrow) are the characteristic features of genus *Lichtheimia*. In *Lichtheimia corymbifera*, numerous smaller, irregular shaped sporangiophores are produced which branch repeatedly to form corymbs. Mature spores (yellow arrow) are oval to round, small, light gray in colour [Culture mount in LPCB ×200].

arise from swollen areas (nodes) along a stolon.

The colony morphology and also micro-scopic morphology of other members of family of Mucorales are described in detail with figures below.

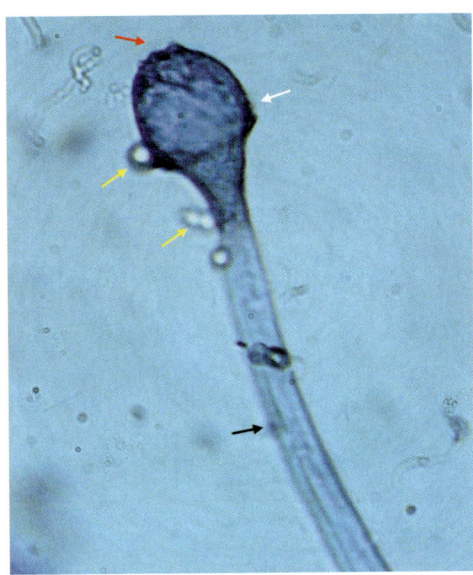

Fig. 4.76: *Lichtheimia corynbifera*. The columella is exposed after the rupture of sporangium. The columella (white arrow) is 16 to 27 μ in diameter, ovoid to spatulate and have a few spines (red arrow). The spores (yellow arrow) are lying dispersed in the surrounding area. Black arrow shows sporangiophore. [LPCB ×600]

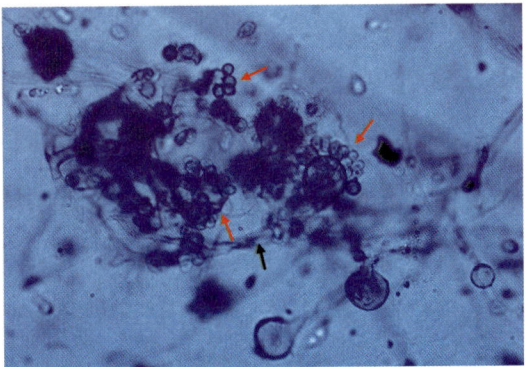

Fig. 4.77: *Cunninghamella bertholetiae*. Sporangiola atop a vesicle at the tip of sporangiophore (black arrow). One spored Sporangioles are attached by a short denticle and covering the entire surface of the vesicle (black arrow). Sporangiospores are oval to 'tear drop' shaped [LPCB mount ×400]

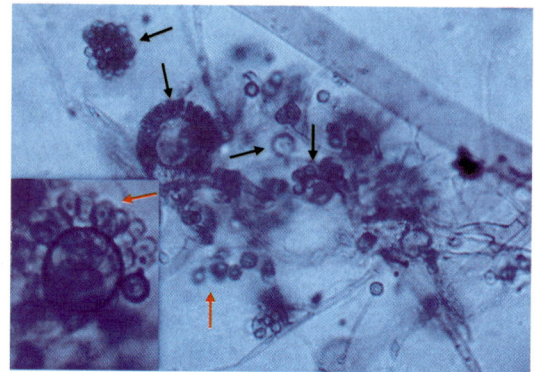

Fig. 4.78: *Cunninghamella bertholletiae.* Sporangioles cover the entire surface of the vesicle (black arrow). Sporangiospores are oval to tear shaped (inset—red arrow).

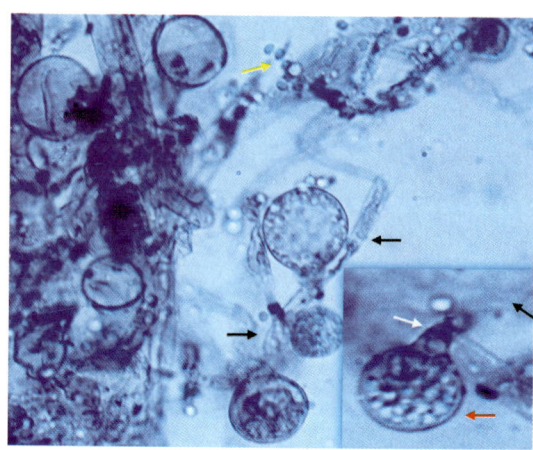

Fig. 4.80: Sporangiophores of *Apophysomyces elegans* arise from hyphal segments resembling 'foot cells'. Sporangia (inset—red arrow) are pyriform with prominent funnel-shaped apophyses (inset—white arrow) and are produced singly at the tip of sporangiophores (black arrow). Sporangiospores are oblong (yellow arrow) [LPCB mount ×400].

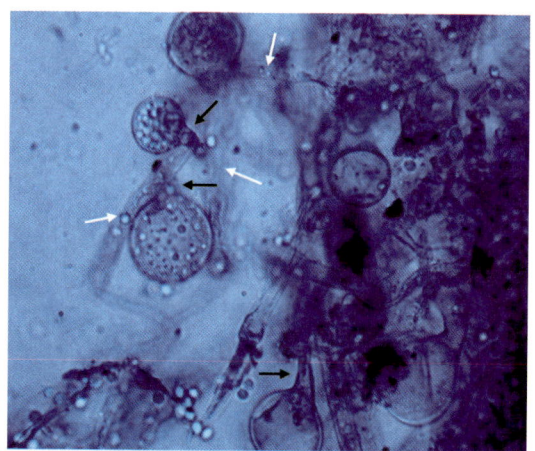

Fig. 4.79: *Apophysomyces elegans.* Sporangiophores (white arrow) are erect, unbranched. Pyriform sporangia with funnel or bell shaped apopysis (black arrow) at the tip of sporangiophore is a characteristic feature. Collumella is hemispherical. Sporangiospores are round to oval in shape [LPCB mount ×400].

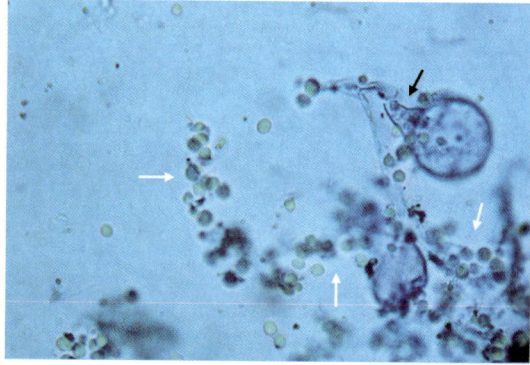

Fig. 4.81: *Apophysomyces elegans.* Sporangia are pyriform with prominent funnel or champagne glass-shaped apophyses (black arrow) and hemispherical columellae. Sporangiospores are smooth, mostly oblong, occasionally globose and subhyaline (white arrow), although appear brown in mass [LPCB mount ×400].

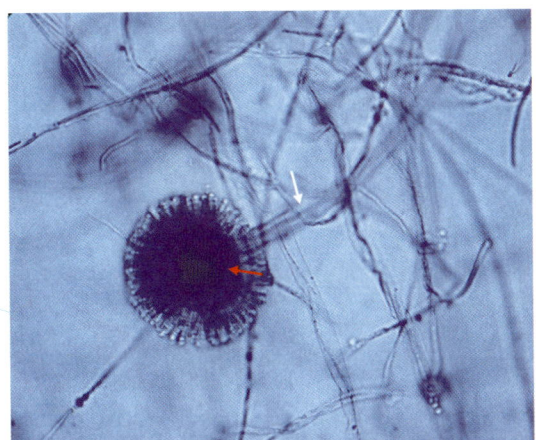

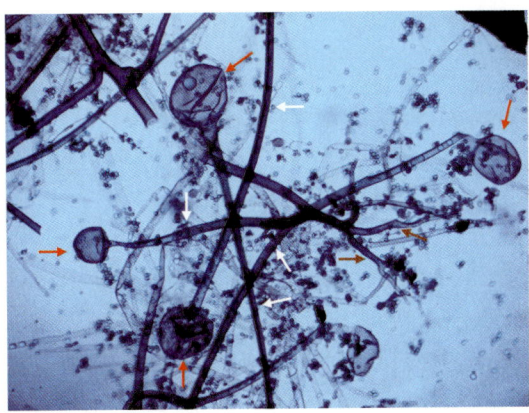

Fig. 4.82: *Syncephalastrum* species. Mycelia are arranged sympodially with many branches. Septations within mycelia are sparse. Sporangiophores (white arrow) arise irregularly and develop an ovoid to globose vesicle (red arrow) at the apex. The vesicle bears many finger-like radiating merosporangia that encloses many spores stacked like marbles in a tube [LPCB mount ×400].

Fig. 4.84: *Rhizomucor pusillus.* Sporangiophores (white arrow) are short, dark brown and arise from stolons. Few poorly developed rhizoids with irregular branching (brown arrow) are present. Columellae (red arrow) are smooth, variable in shape and have a collar [LPCB mount ×200].

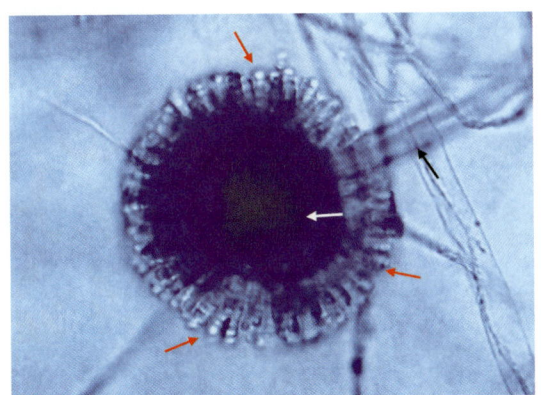

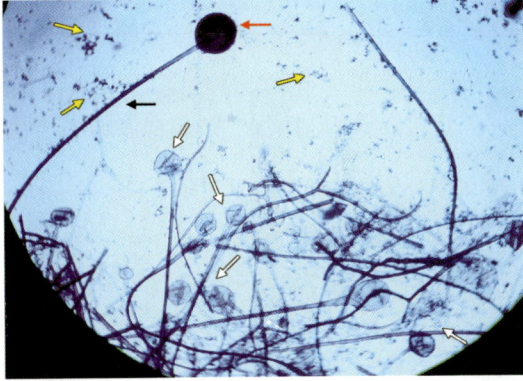

Fig. 4.83: *Syncephalastrum* species. Merosporangia (red arrow) radiating from the vesicle (white arrow). Stack of sporangiospores are visible within merosporangium. Black arrow indicates sporangiophore [LPCB mount ×600].

Fig. 4.85: An intact sporangium (red arrow) is seen at the tip of a brown sporangiophore (black arrow). Sporangia are black and spherical and have spines. Sporangia deliquesce on maturity dispersing spores (yellow arrow) and columellae (white arrow) become exposed. Columellae (white arrow) are smooth with varied shapes. *Rhizomucor pusillus* [LPCB mount ×100].

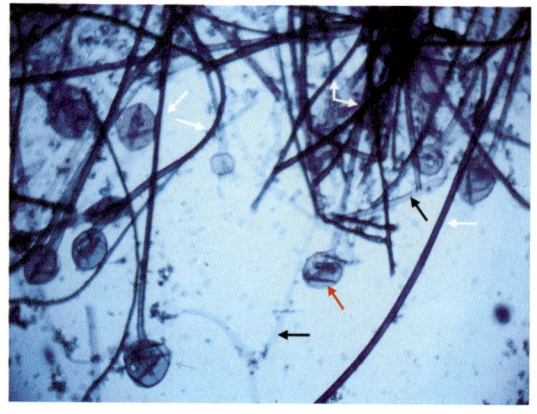

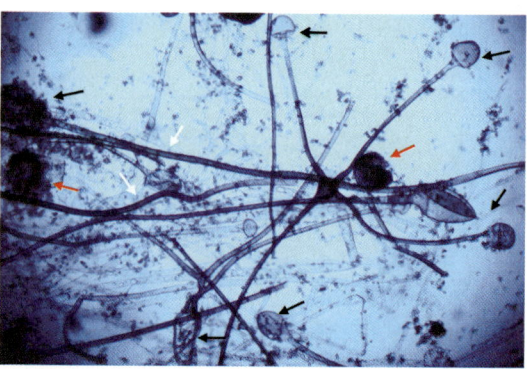

Fig. 4.87: Both intact sporangia (red arrow) and emptied sporangia (black arrow) are seen. Sporangiophores are brown pigmented. *Rhizomucor* species [LPCB mount ×200].

Fig. 4.86: *Rhizomucor pusillus.* Plenty of columellae (red arrow) are noticed. These are exposed due to rupture of mature sporangia. Sporangiophores (white arrow) are brownish, whereas mycelia and stolons (black arrow) are hyaline. [LPCB mount ×200]

CRYPTOCOCCUS

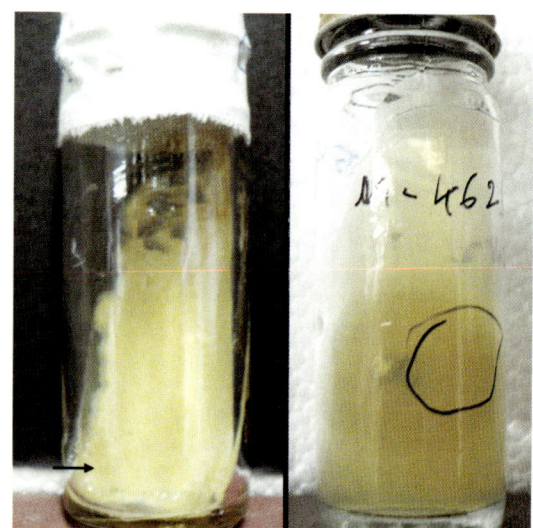

Fig. 4.88: Colony morphology of *Cryptococcus* species on SDCA at 37°C after 3 weeks. Colonies are cream coloured to yellowish, mucoid and may flow to the bottom of the slant (black arrow). The edges are entire and without pseudomycelium; (a) obverse, (b) reverse.

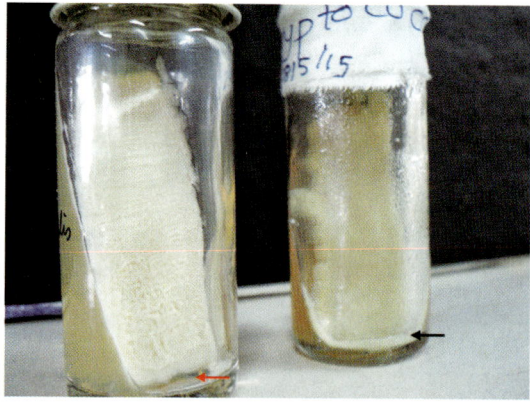

Fig. 4.89: (a) Colony of *Candida* species on SDCA. Colonies are creamy smooth, waxy, glistening and soft, gradually changes from smooth to reticulated surface as the colony ages but the bottom of the slant remains free (red arrow); (b) *Cryptococcus species:* colony texture is mucoid, creamy and the colonies flow to the bottom of the slant (black arrow).

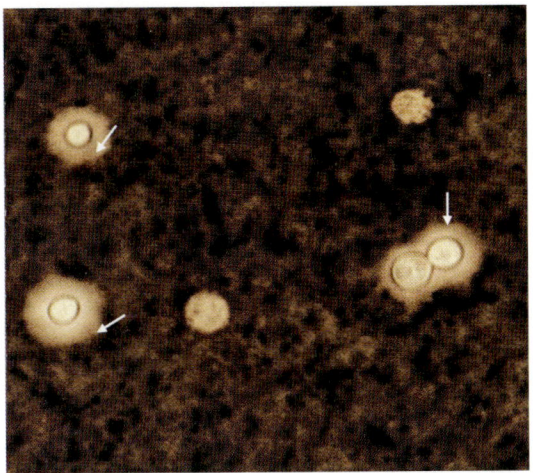

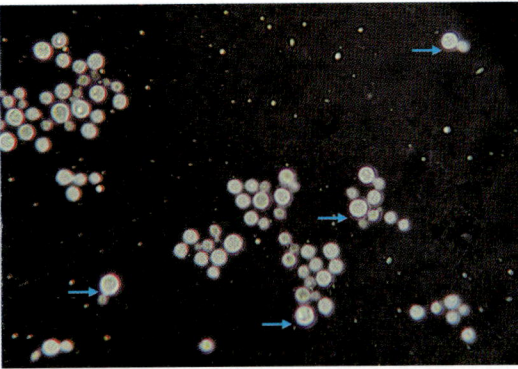

Fig. 4.91: Yeasts of *Cryptococcus neoformans* are seen in wet mount with a drop of India ink. The capsule is not so much distinctive here as it is prepared from a laboratory maintained strain where the capsule has become thinned out due to repeated subculture [×400].

Fig. 4.90: Yeasts of *Cryptococcus neoformans* are seen in wet mount with a drop of India ink. The capsule is so distinctive that it can be easily outlined by negative contrast. The thick polysaccharide capsule appears as a 'halo' surrounding the cell (white arrow). This clinical strain was isolated from a HIV reactive 14 years old boy and was clinically diagnosed as a case of 'meningitis'.

TRICHOSPORON

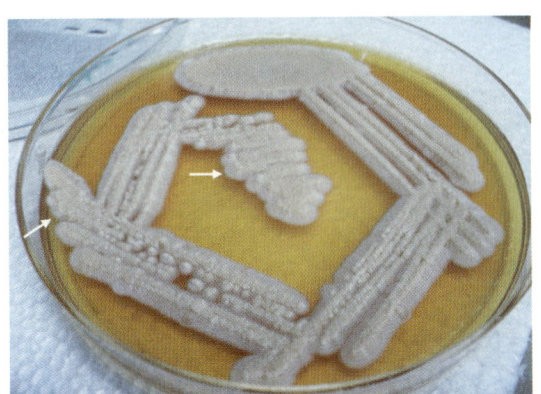

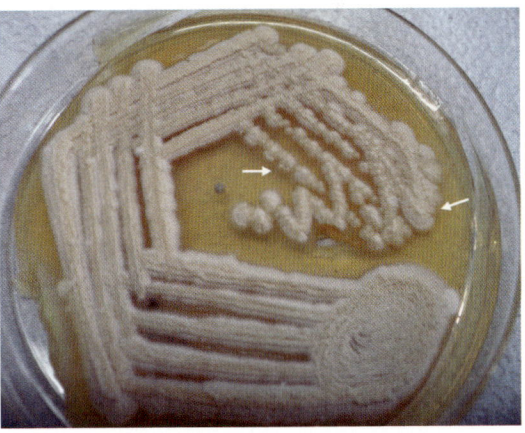

Fig. 4.92: White to cream coloured soft, wrinkled, folded, friable colonies which develop a farinose covering (covered with a whitish mealy dust) and has a fissured marginal zone (white arrow) of *Trichosporon asahii* grown on Sabouraud's dextrose agar at 37°C for 3 days.

Fig. 4.93: Colony of *Trichosporon asahii* grown on Sabouraud's dextrose agar, 72 hours at 37°C. Soft, wrinkled, folded, friable off-white colonies with crenated margins (white arrow) are characteristic that differs from smooth, moist, pasty, butyrous with entire margin, colonies of *Candida* species.

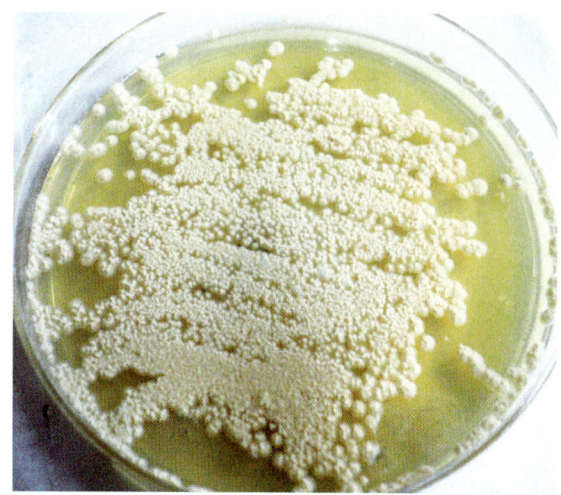

Fig. 4.94: *Trichosporon mucoides.* Colonies grown on Sabouraud's dextrose agar at 37°C after 3 days of incubation.

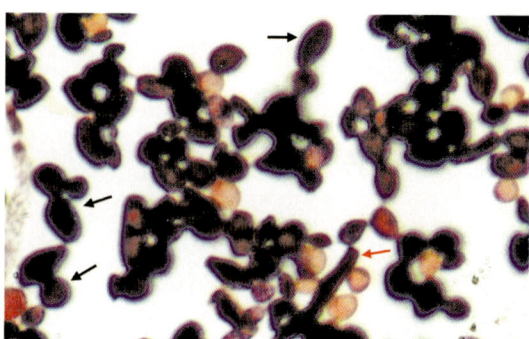

Fig. 4.96: *Trichosporon mucoides.* Globose, ellipsoidal, ovoid to elongate budding yeast cells (black arrow) along with presence of true hyphae (red arrow) are seen when grown on Sabouraud's dextrose agar (SDA). [Gram stained smear prepared from colonies appeared on SDA ×1000]

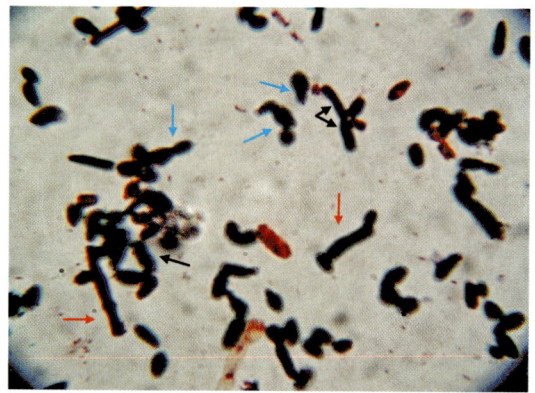

Fig. 4.95: *Trichosporon asahii.* Presence of true hyphal fragments (red arrow), free arthroconidia (black arrow) and oval to elliptical budding yeast cells (blue arrow) of varied sizes are suggestive. [Gram stain from colony grown on SDA ×1000].

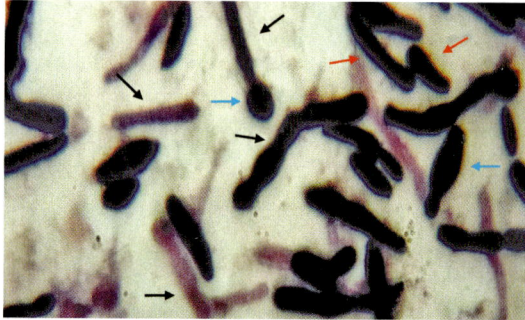

Fig. 4.97: *Trichosporon asahii.* Presence of true hyphal fragments (black arrow), free arthroconidia (red arrow) and a few oval to elliptical budding yeast cells (blue arrow) are seen. [Gram stain from colony grown on SDA ×1000].

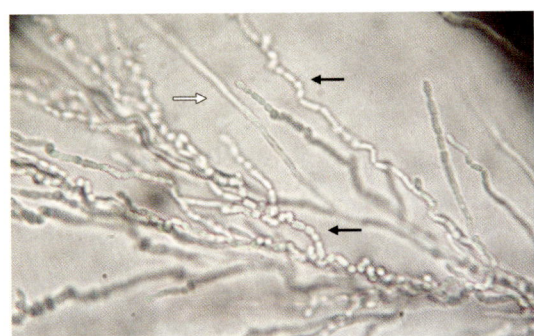

Fig. 4.98: *Trichosporon asahii.* Long chains of arthroconidia produced by fragmentation of true hyphae are seen (black arrow) but some true hyphae are unfragmented (white arrow) [Morphology on Cornmeal agar ×400].

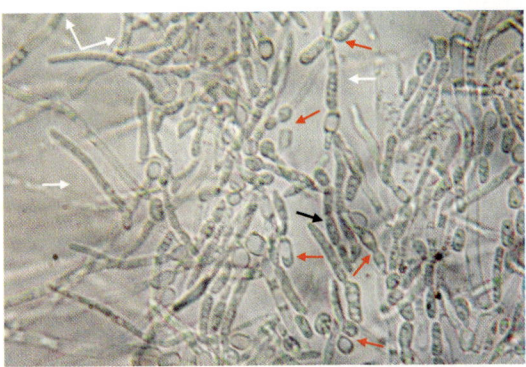

Fig. 4.100: *Trichosporon beigelii.* Morphology on Cornmeal agar reveals presence of true hyphae with regular septation (white arrow); a chain of arthroconidia (black arrow) and also oval to elongate, cylindrical blastoconidia (red arrow) are noticed [CMA ×400].

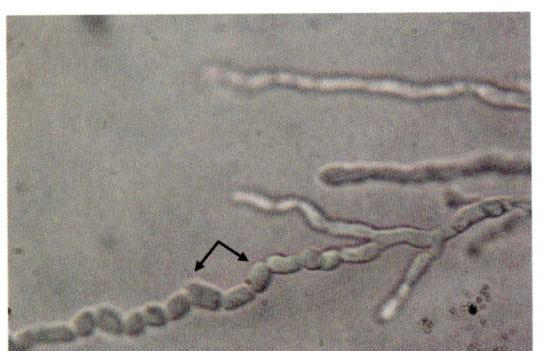

Fig. 4.99: *Trichosporon asahii.* Barrel-shaped arthroconidia are produced in chain (black arrow) on Cornmeal agar [×600].

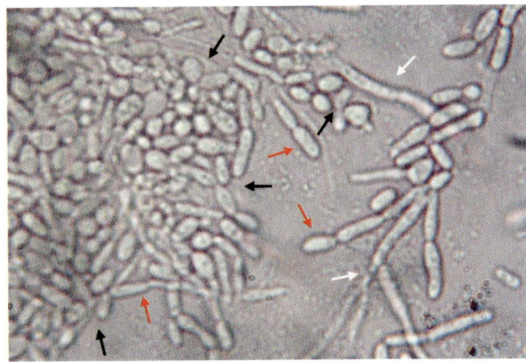

Fig. 4.101: *Trichosporon mucoides.* Presence of septate hyphae (white arrow); masses of round, oval and cylindrical blastoconidia (black arrow) and single blastoconidia at the hyphal tips (red arrow) are important features. The latter characteristic is specific for this species [Morphology on CMA ×400].

TALAROMYCES (PENICILLIUM) MARNEFFEI

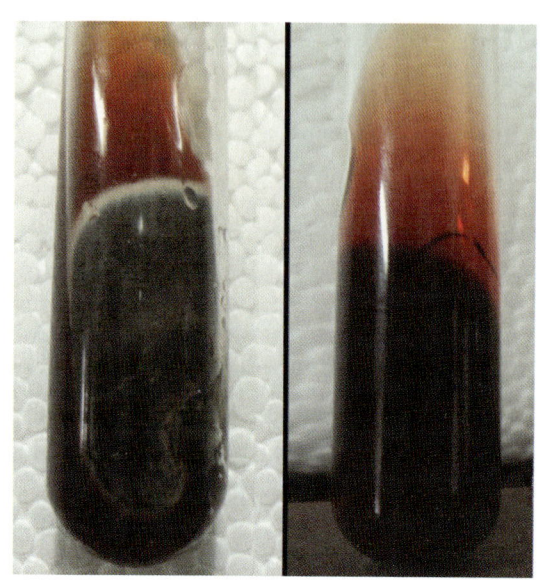

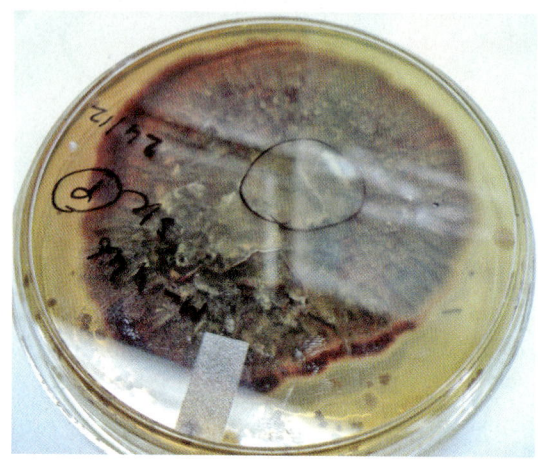

Fig. 4.104: Colony morphology (reverse) grown on blood agar with 10% glucose supplement, incubation at 37°C for 3 weeks. *Talaromyces marneffei*.

Fig. 4.102: Colony morphology of *Talaromyces marneffei* grown on Sabouraud's dextrose agar at 25°C after 2 weeks of incubation; (a) obverse, (b) reverse

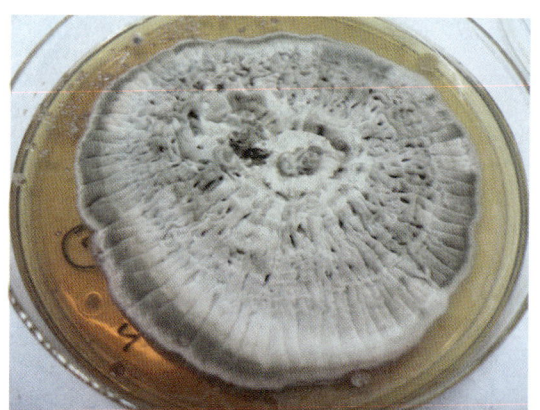

Fig. 4.103: *Penicillium marneffei*. Mycelium to yeast conversion done on blood agar with glucose (10–20%) supplement, incubation at 37°C for 3 weeks.

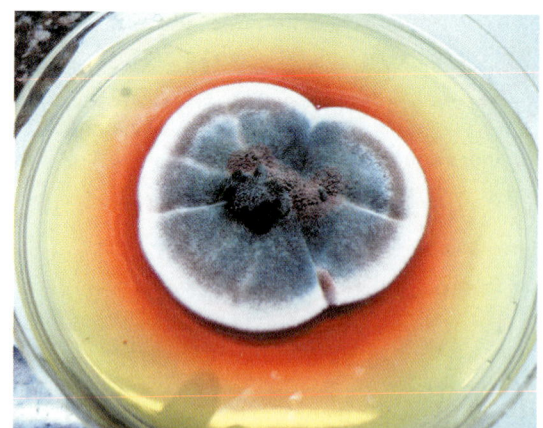

Fig. 4.105: Colony morphology of *Penicillium marneffei* grown on Sabouraud's dextrose agar at 25°C for two weeks.

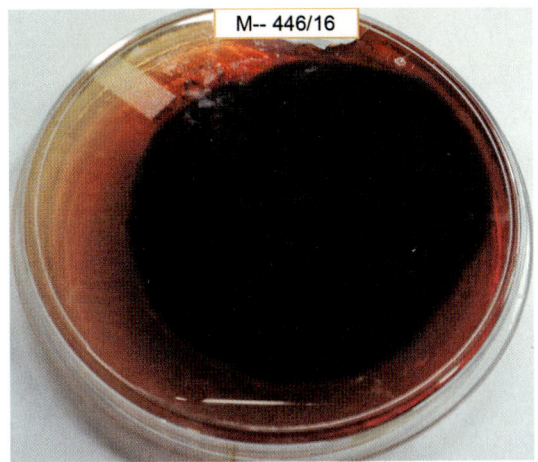

Fig. 4.106: *Talaromyces marneffei*. Red diffusible pigment on the underside of the colony when grown on Sabouraud's dextrose agar at 25°C.

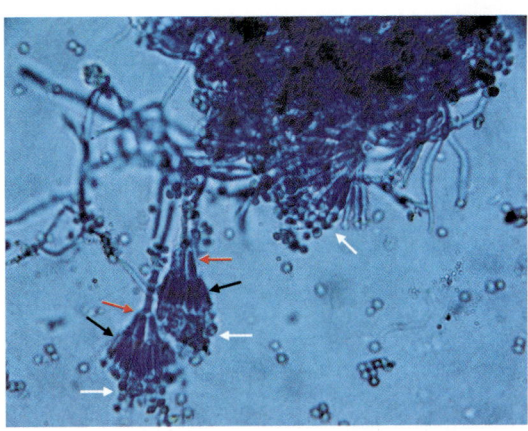

Fig. 4.108: Microscopic morphology of *Talaromyces marneffei*. Brush-like conidiophore showing primary branches and metulae (red arrow) which ends in phialides (black arrow) that bear chains (basocatenulate) of conidia (white arrow) with youngest at the base [LPCB mount ×400].

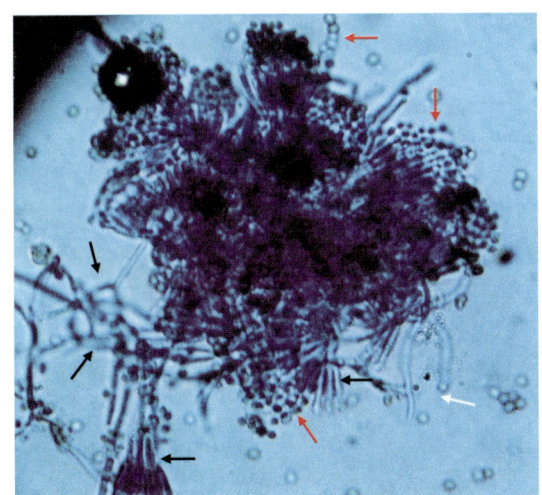

Fig. 4.107: Culture mount of *Talaromyces marneffei*. Mycelia are white, septate and multibranched (white arrow). Conidiophores produce branched metulae (black arrow) and phialides in groups giving a brush-like appearance. Conidia are single celled (ameroconidia) and in chains (red arrow) with youngest conidia at the base of the chain (or tip of the phialide) [LPCB mount ×400].

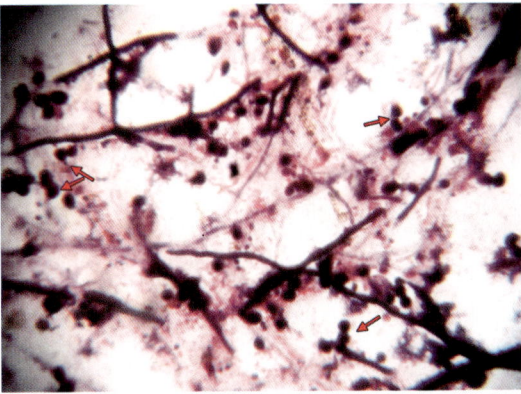

Fig. 4.109: Mycelium to yeast conversion (M→Y) in *Talaromyces marneffei*. Gram stained smear prepared from colonies appeared on blood agar with 10% glucose supplement. Budding yeast cells (red arrow) are seen. The process of mycelium conversion to yeast is similar to that of *H. capsulatum* and *B. dermatitidis* [Gram stain ×1000].

PNEUMOCYSTIS JIROVECII

We have found PAS stain to be a cheaper, faster and equally good substitute for GMS in our laboratory (Figs 4.112 and 4.113).

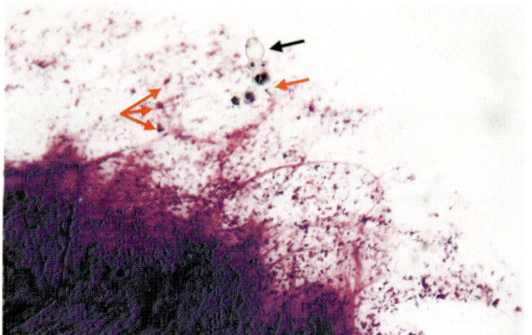

Fig. 4.110: Giemsa stained smear of deep tracheal aspirate (DTA) obtained from a HIV reactive patient having CD4 count grossly reduced (10/mm^3). A small clump of trophic forms (red arrow) and a 'ghost' cell (black arrow) which is devoid of nucleus are noticed. *Pneumocystis jirovecii* [× 200].

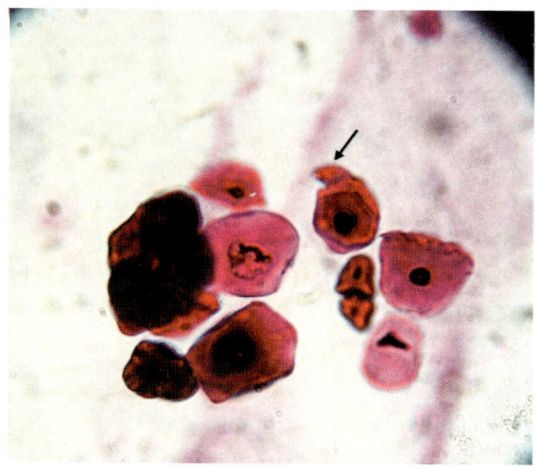

Fig. 4.112: *Pneumocystis jirovecii*. Black arrow shows tubular projections [PAS stain ×600].

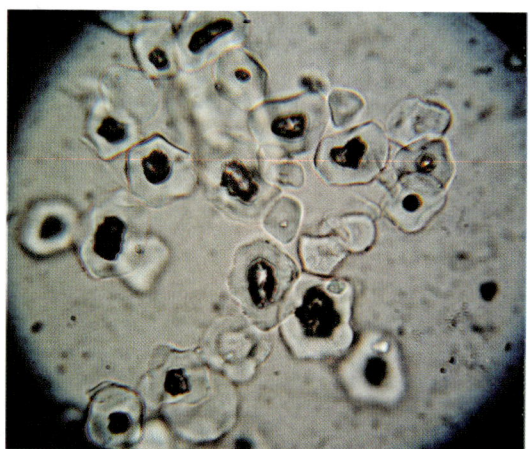

Fig. 4.111: Trophic forms of *Pneumocystis jirovecii*. These are tiny (4–6 μ), pleomorphic, contain basophilic cytoplasm (blue) and reddish purple nucleus. They have tubular surface projections from the cell surface [Giemsa stain ×600].

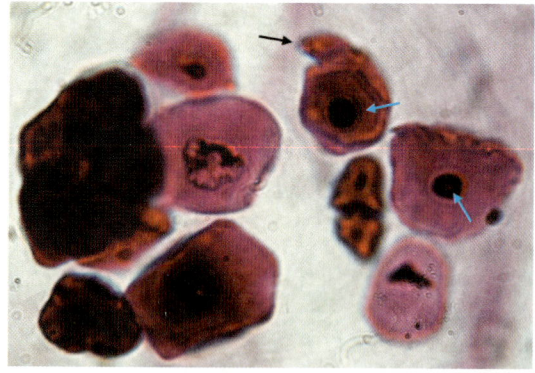

Fig. 4.113: PAS stained smear of DTA sample obtained from HIV reactive patient showing clumps of cysts which are pleomorphic and have characteristic tubular projection (black arrow) and intracystic bodies (blue arrow) *Pneumocystis jirovecii* [×1000].

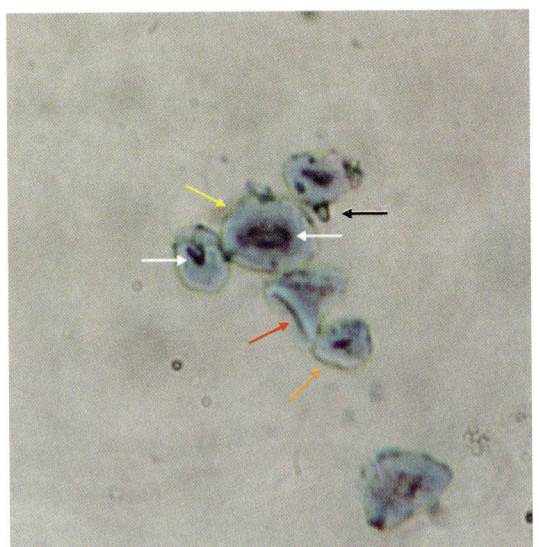

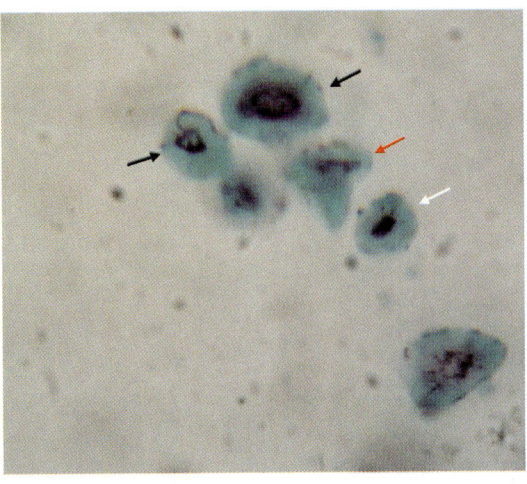

Fig. 4.116: Direct smear of DTA sample of a HIV reactive patient having CD4 count less than 10/mm³. Cysts of different stages and shapes are noticed here; black arrow indicates mature cyst with parentheses but white arrow indicates small immature cyst with intracystic bodies. Red arrow indicates 'cup-shaped' cells. *Pneumocystis jirovecii* [Giemsa stain ×1000].

Fig. 4.114: *Pneumocystis jirovecii.* Mature cysts (yellow arrow) contain intracystic bodies and many show "parentheses" within the round cysts (white arrow). The crescent-shaped cells (red arrow) represent cysts from which small cells have escaped and these are thin-walled immature cyst (brown arrow). Black arrow shows tubular projections [Giemsa stain ×600].

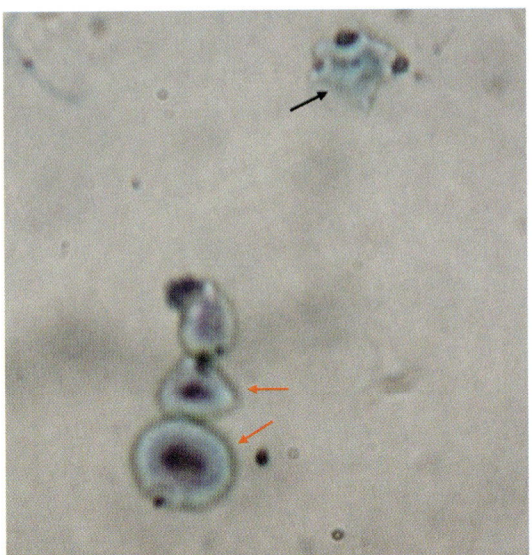

Fig. 4.115: Mature cysts of *Pneumocystis jirovecii.* Mature cysts are round, thick walled containing intracystic bodies (red arrow). Sometimes crescent, cup-shaped and wrinkled cells (black arrow) are also noticed [Giemsa stain ×600].

SELF ASSESSMENT

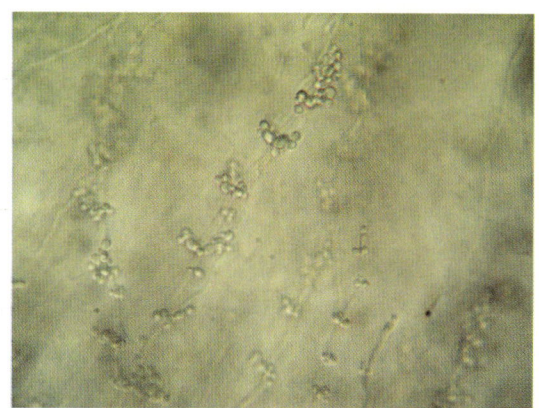

Fig. 4.117: Morphology on cornmeal agar; Identify the fungus (yeast).

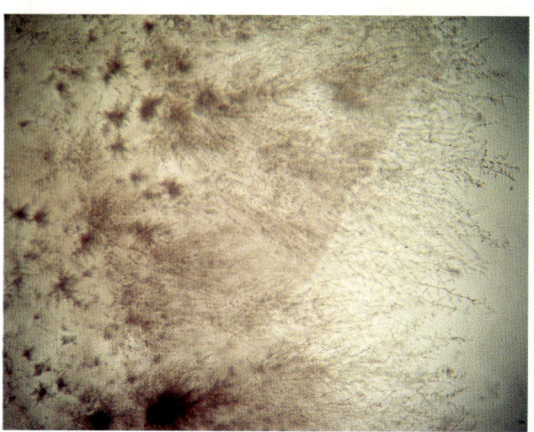

Fig. 4.119: Identify the fungus (yeast). Morphology on cornmeal agar ×200.

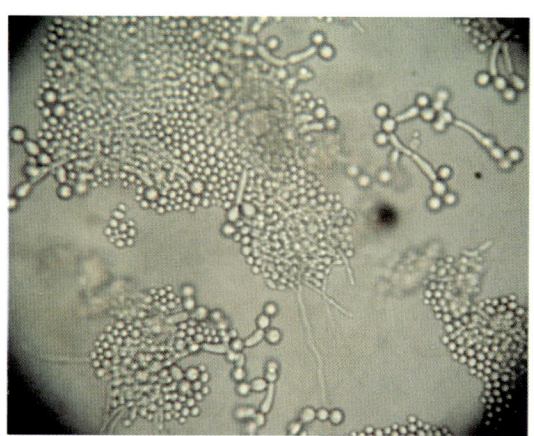

Fig. 4.118: Morphology on cornmeal agar after incubation at 37°C for 3 days. Identify the structures and the relevant fungus (yeast) [×400].

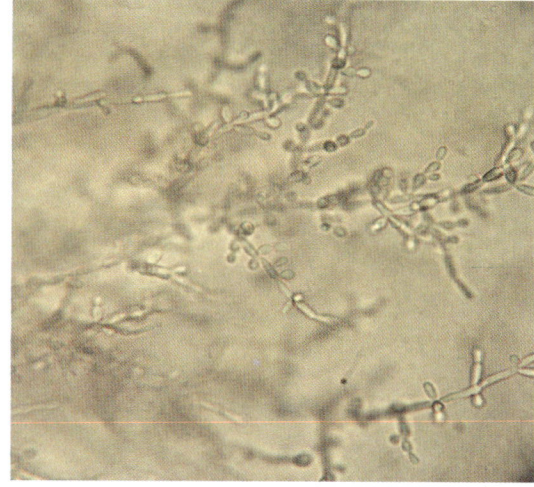

Fig. 4.120: Identify the fungus [Cornmeal agar morphology ×400].

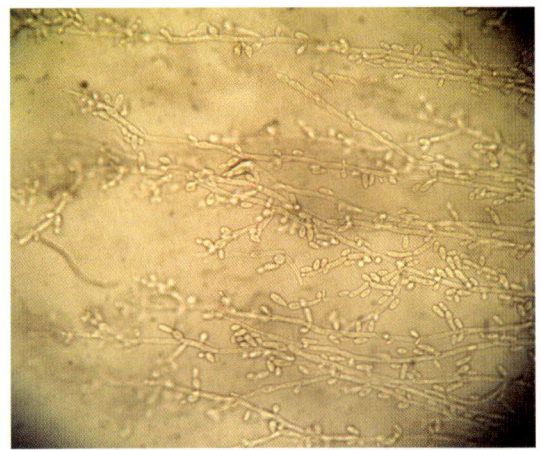

Fig. 4.121: Morphology on cornmeal agar. Identify the fungus [×400].

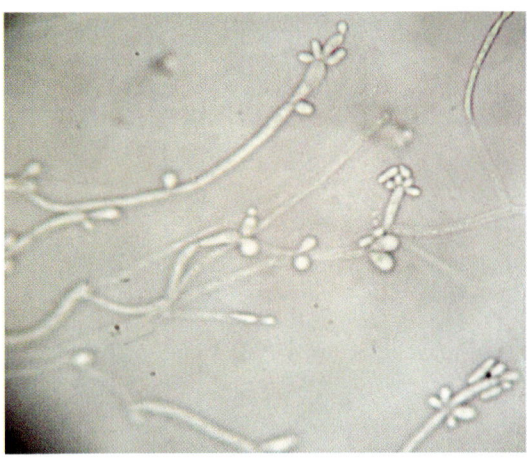

Fig. 4.123: Morphology on cornmeal agar. Identify the fungus [×400].

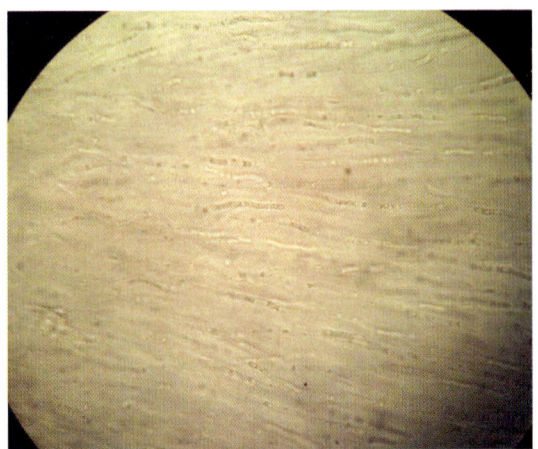

Fig. 4.122: Morphology on cornmeal agar [×200]. Identify the yeast.

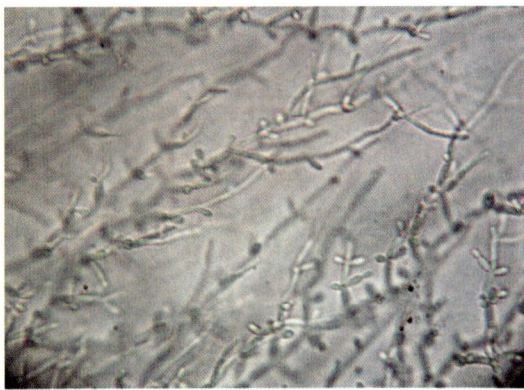

Fig. 4.124: Identify the *Candida* species [Morphology on cornmeal agar ×400].

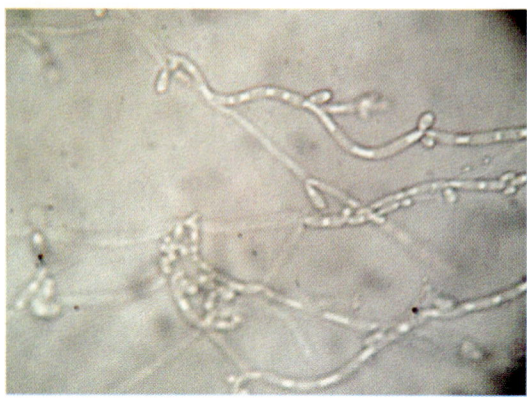

Fig. 4.125: Morphology on cornmeal agar. Identify the *Candida* species. [×400]

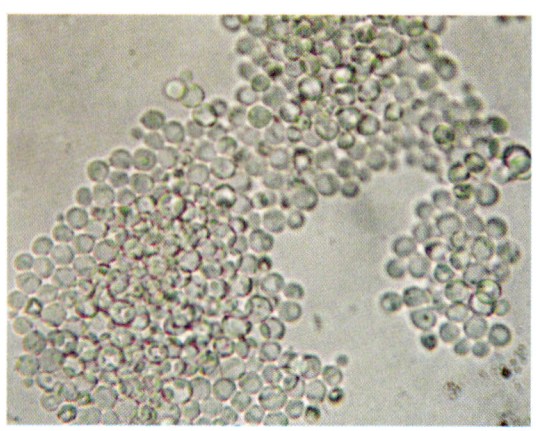

Fig. 4.127: Morphology on cornmeal agar. Identify the *Candida* species. [×400]

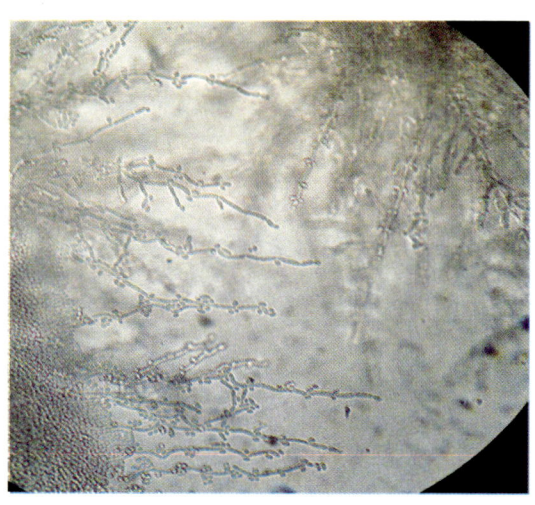

Fig. 4.126: Morphology on cornmeal agar. Identify it. [×200]

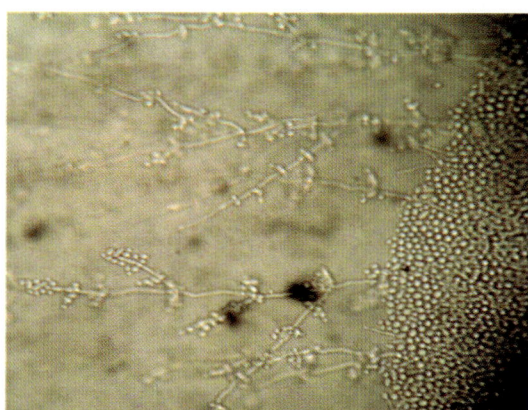

Fig. 4.128: Morphology on cornmeal agar. Identify the *Candida* species. [×200]

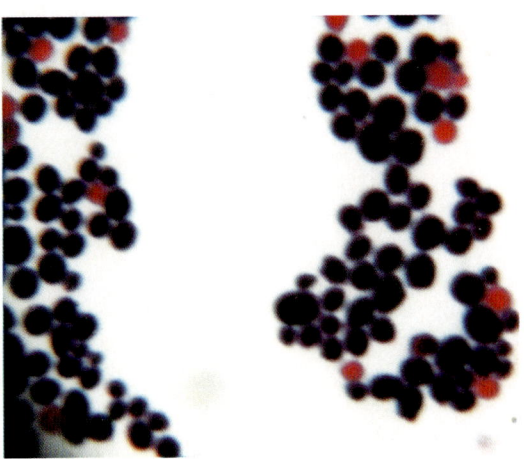

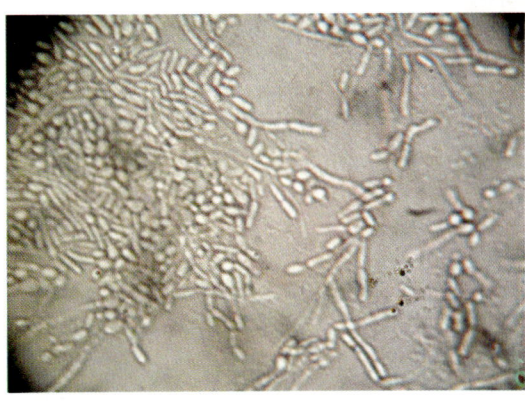

Fig. 4.131: Morphology on cornmeal agar. Identify the species of *Trichosporon* (based on morphology) [×200].

Fig. 4.129: Gram stained smear of colony grown on SDCA at 37°C. A pasty yeast like colony appeared on SDCA following a subculture of turbid blood culture. Turbidity appeared after 48 hours of incubation at 37°C. This was a blood sample of a 10-day-old preterm neonate clinically diagnosed as a case of 'neonatal septicaemia'. Identify the isolated yeast (based on morphology) [×1000].

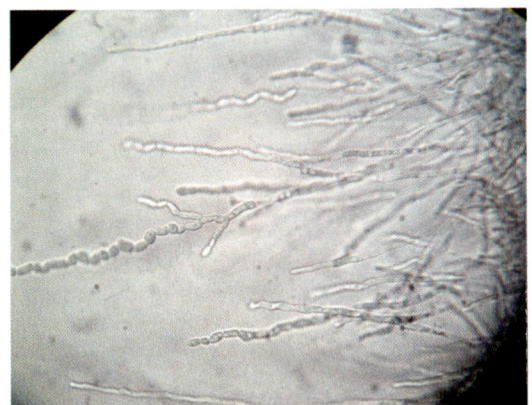

Fig. 4.130: Morphology on cornmeal agar. Identify the yeast [×200].

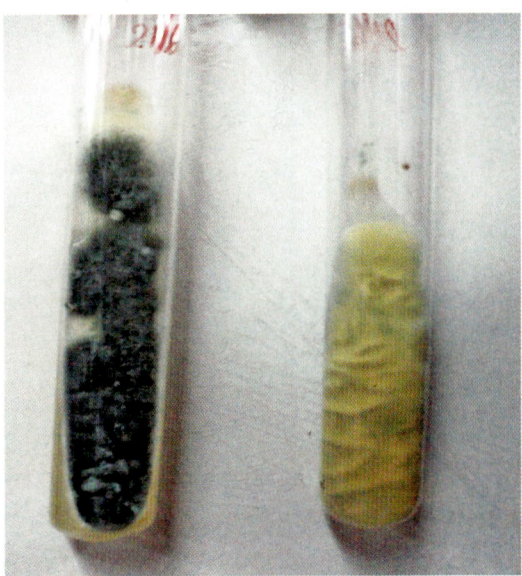

Fig. 4.132: The picture shows colony morphology of an *Aspergillus* species isolated from a DTA sample of a clinically diagnosed case of allergic bronchopulmonary aspergillosis (ABPA). Identify the species based on colony morphology.

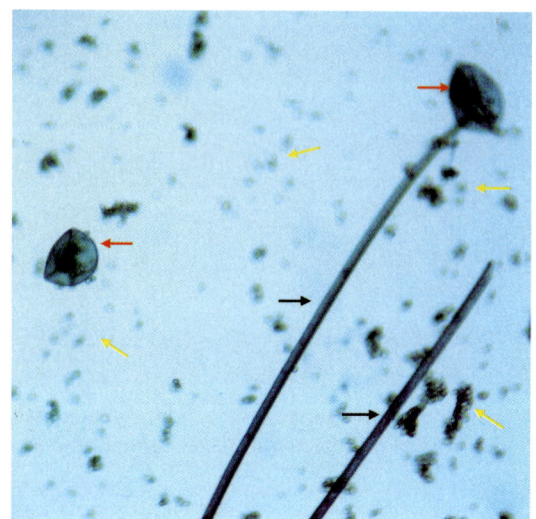

Fig. 4.133: Microscopic morphology of a fungus belonging to Mucorales. Identify the structures indicated by coloured arrows and the relevant fungus (up to species level) [LPCB mount ×400].

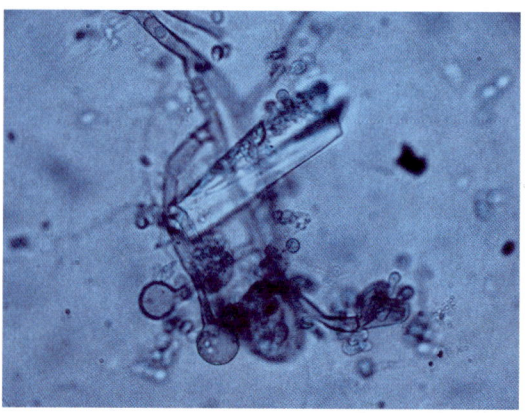

Fig. 4.135: Microscopic morphology of a fungal isolate obtained from a patient with thalassaemia major who had presented with lesions of multiple subcutaneous abscesses throughout the body. A clinical diagnosis of mucormycosis was confirmed by microbiological and histopathology examination. Identify the fungal isolate [LPCB mount ×400].

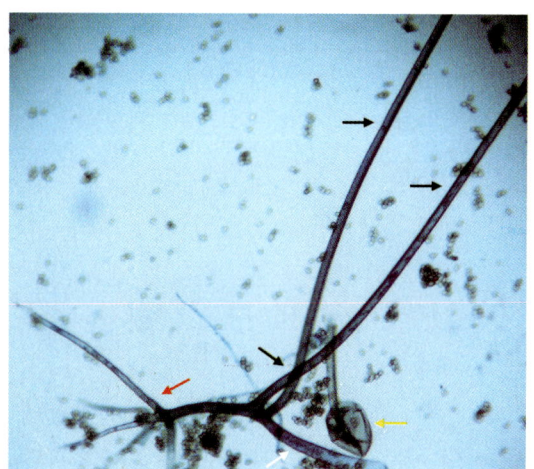

Fig. 4.134: Identify the fungus with its typical morphology (indicated by arrows), belonging to order Mucorales [Culture mount, LPCB ×400].

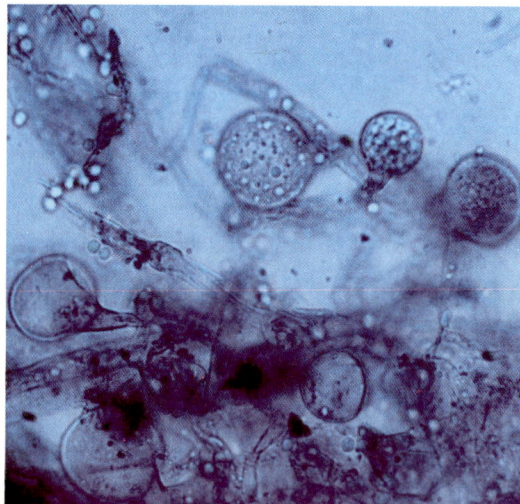

Fig. 4.136: Microscopic morphology of a fungus isolated from a patient with clinical diagnosis of 'fungal sinusitis' who had an underlying condition of diabetes mellitus for last 15 years. Microbiological and histopathology examination revealed the picture which confirmed the final diagnosis of Mucormycosis of the paranasal sinus. Identify the fungus with proper justification [LPCB mount ×400].

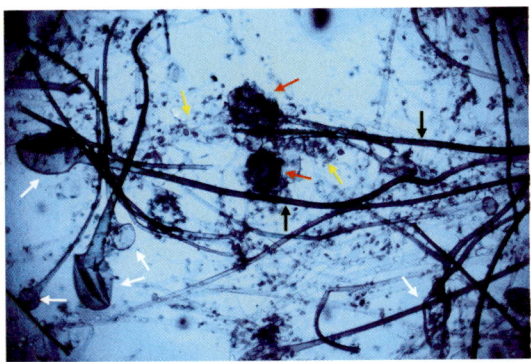

Fig. 4.137: Microscopic morphology of a fungus isolated from the lung biopsy specimen of a 65-year-old female suffering from diabetic ketoacidosis with pneumonia. Identify the structures marked and the likely fungus [LPCB mount ×400].

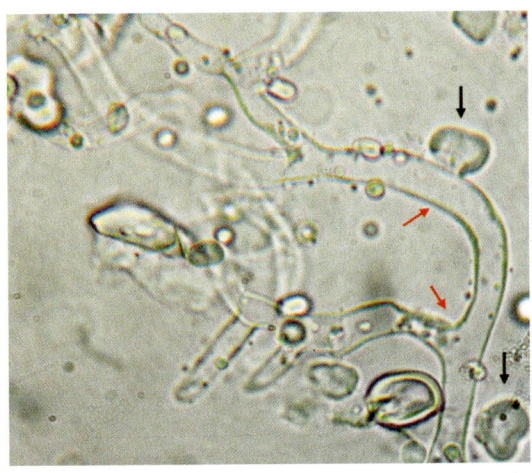

Fig. 4.139: KOH mount of skin (punch) biopsy material from an extensive ulcerated cutaneous lesion above the right medial malleolus of a leukemic patient. Identify the structures and also state the order/phylum of the etiologic agent [×400].

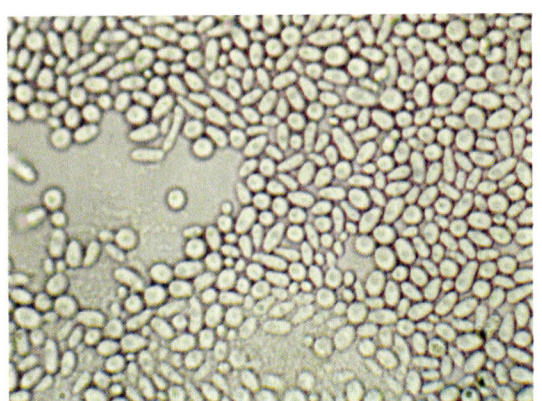

Fig. 4.138: Morphology on cornmeal agar of a fungus (yeast), isolated from the urine sample of a 78-year-old male with a history of diabetes over 25 years. The patient had a symptoms of urinary tract infection. The isolate was found to be urease positive. Identify the yeast (up to species level) based on microscopic morphology [×400].

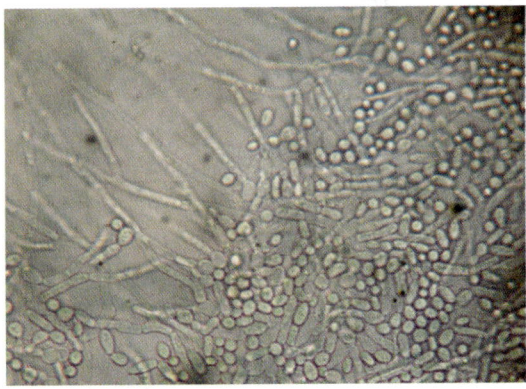

Fig. 4.140: Microscopic morphology of a fungus (yeast) grown on cornmeal agar, isolated from a 72-year-old male patient having symptoms of urinary tract infection. The isolate was urease positive. Identify the fungus [CMA ×400].

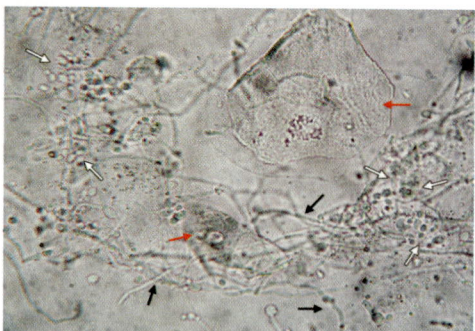

Fig. 4.141: Direct examination of a sputum sample of a 65-year-old male patient suffering from COPD for last 12 years and is put on continued steroid inhalation. Identify the structures visible and interpret the smear findings with proper justification [KOH preparation ×400].

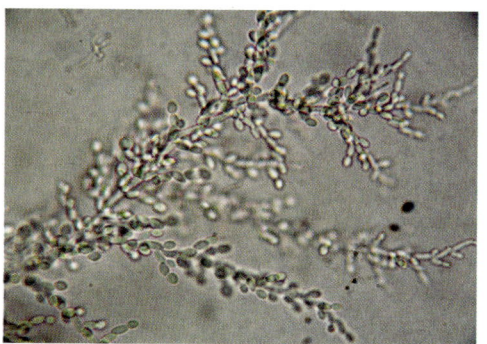

Fig. 4.142: Morphology on cornmeal agar (Dalmau plate culture) isolated from the deep tracheal aspirate (DTA) of a 41-year-old. HIV reactive patient having CD4 count 192/µL. Identify the yeast (species level) based on microscopic morphology [CMA ×400].

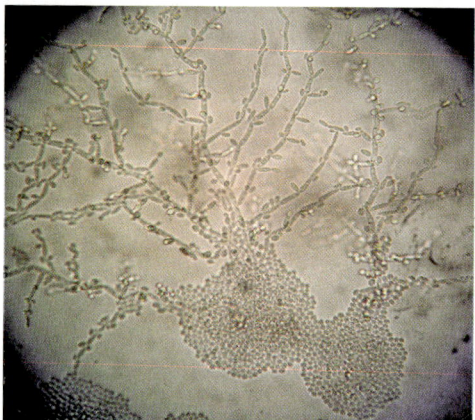

Fig. 4.143: Microscopic morphology of *Candida* species grown on cornmeal agar (Dalmau plate culture). Identify the species and mention the features for identification [×200].

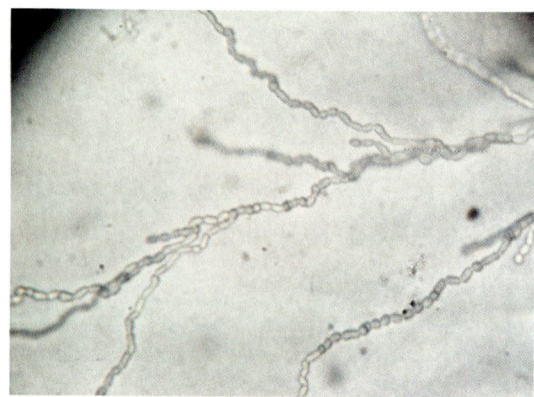

Fig. 4.144: Microscopic morphology of yeast, isolated from urine sample of a 5-year-old. Thalassaemic (major) male child having symptoms of urinary tract infection. The isolate is urease positive and does not ferment carbohydrates. Identify the yeast (species) and mention the special feature (shown here) in their morphology which might help in species identification [Morphology on CMA ×200].

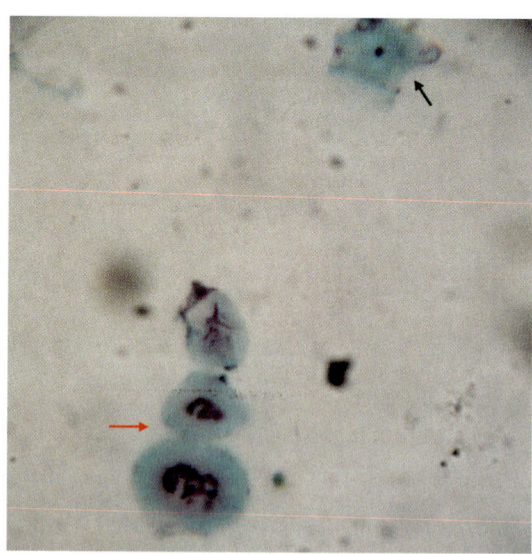

Fig. 4.145: Direct smear of DTA sample of HIV reactive patient . Identify the structure and the relevant fungi [Giemsa stain ×1000].

ANSWERS

- **Fig. 4.145:** Cyst of *Pneumocystis jirovecii*
- **Fig. 4.144:** *Trichosporon asahii*
- **Fig. 4.143:** *Candida guillermondei*
- **Fig. 4.142:** *Candida lusitaniae*
- **Fig. 4.141:** Epithelial cells (red arrow), budding yeast cells (white arrow), pseudohyphae (black arrow) of *Candida* species
- **Fig. 4.140:** *Trichosporon mucoides*
- **Fig. 4.139:** Broad aseptate coenocytic hyphae of *Zygomycetes* with wide angle branching (red arrow)
- **Fig. 4.138:** *Trichosporon mucoides*
- **Fig. 4.137:** Sporangiophore (black arrow), sporangium (red arrow), collumellae (white arrow), sporangiospores (yellow arrow); *Rhizomucor pusillus*
- **Fig. 4.136:** *Apophysomyces elegans*
- **Fig. 4.135:** *Cunninghamella bertholletiae*
- **Fig. 4.134:** Rhizoids (red arrow), sporangiophore (black arrow), collumella (yellow arrow), coencytic hyphae (white arrow); *Rhizopus* species
- **Fig. 4.133:** Sporangium (red arrow), sporangiophore (black arrow), sporangiospores (yellow arrow); *Rhizopus* species
- **Fig. 4.132:** *Aspergillus fumigatus*
- **Fig. 4.131:** *Trichosporon mucoides*
- **Fig. 4.130:** *Trichosporon asahii*
- **Fig. 4.129:** *Candida guillermondei*
- **Fig. 4.128:** *Candida viswanathii*
- **Fig. 4.127:** *Candida glabrata*
- **Fig. 4.126:** *Candida krusei*
- **Fig. 4.125:** *Candida lipolytica*
- **Fig. 4.124:** *Candida parapsilosis*
- **Fig. 4.123:** *Candida viswanathii*
- **Fig. 4.122:** *Candida keyfr*
- **Fig. 4.121:** *Candida parapsilosis*
- **Fig. 4.120:** *Candida tropicalis*
- **Fig. 4.119:** *Candida parapsilosis*
- **Fig. 4.118:** Chlamydoconidia of *Candida albicans*
- **Fig. 4.117:** *Candida albicans*

Mycotic Infections of Eye and Ear

Our environment is the normal habitat of too many microorganisms, hence the eye and the ear are continually subjected to challenge by these varieties of microorganisms such as fungus, bacteria, virus and many others. Any breach in the normal defenses preventing infections may lead to colonization and disease by the omnipresent potential invaders. Injury to the cornea of the eye is the most common predisposing factor leading to infection of this organ, whereas the accumulation of debris, particularly in the damp tropical environments, allows colonization and infection of the external ear.

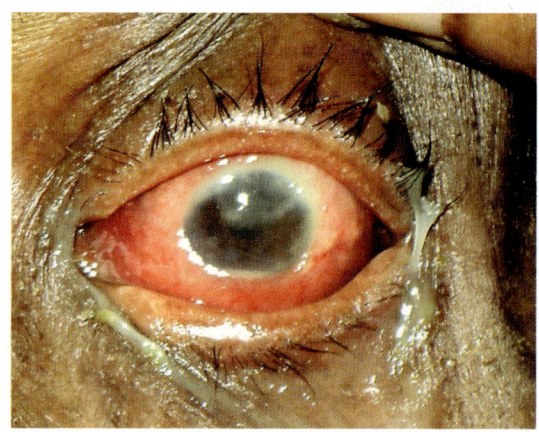

Fig. 5.2: Mycotic keratitis. Typical fungal ulcer with hyphate border and satellite lesion along with a small hypopyon.

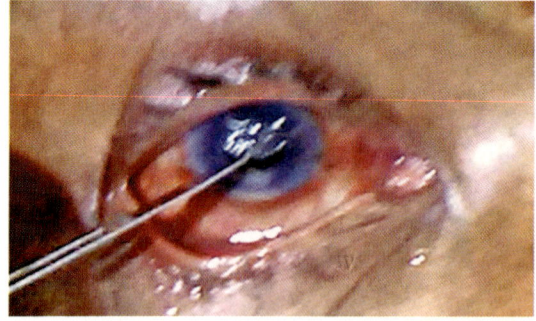

Fig. 5.3: Mycotic keratitis. Central ulcer with necrotic hyphate infiltrate within cornea underlying ulcer is seen. Development of hypopyon is also noticed.

Clinical specimens from keratomycosis cases such as corneal swabs need to be inoculated in a special manner to differentiate

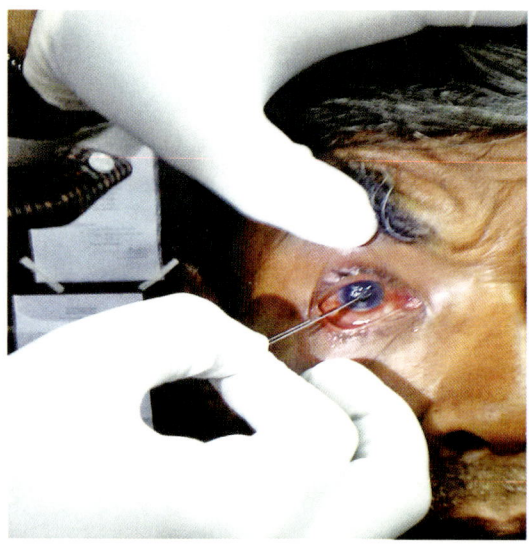

Fig. 5.1: Corneal scraping sample is being collected from a patient with corneal ulcer.

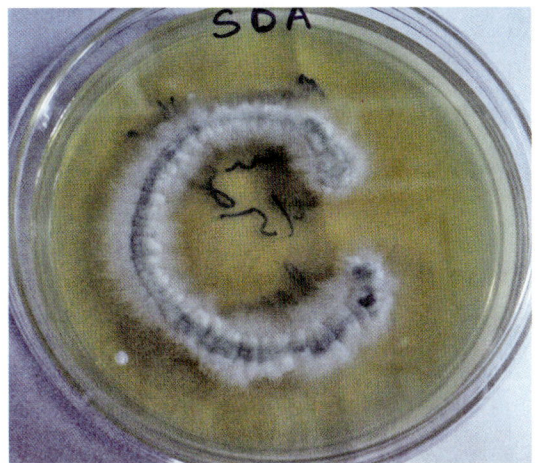

Fig. 5.4: 'C streak'. Filamentous fungi (*Aspergillus fumigatus*) grown on 'C' streak. A small colony outside the 'C' streak is laboratory contaminant.

inoculums from laboratory contaminants. A common method is to make 'C' streak on the plates (Fig. 5.4). Because keratomycosis is caused frequently by the fungi commonly found in the laboratory as contaminant, the growth in the form of 'C' streak ensures that the growth is from the inoculum rather than growth from laboratory contaminants.

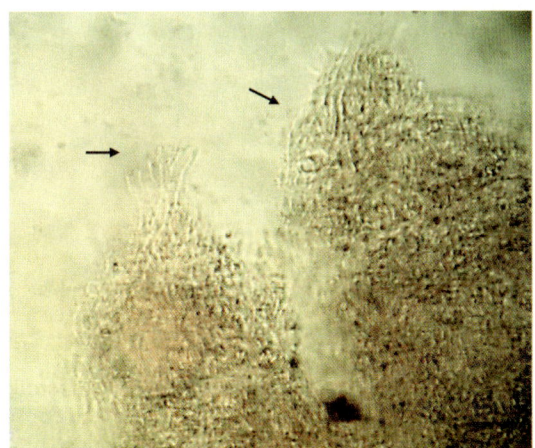

Fig. 5.5: Direct microscopy of corneal scraping in potassium hydroxide preparation. Thin, hyaline tangled mass of hyphae are seen within corneal tissue (black arrow) [×400].

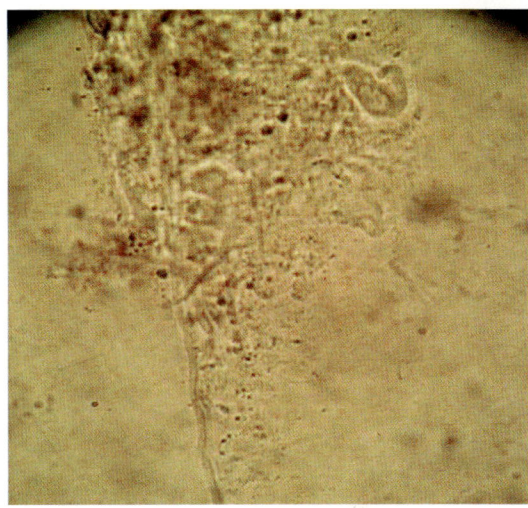

Fig. 5.6: Corneal scraping showing hyphal strands which are slightly thick, hyaline and having regular septation (black arrow) [KOH mount ×400].

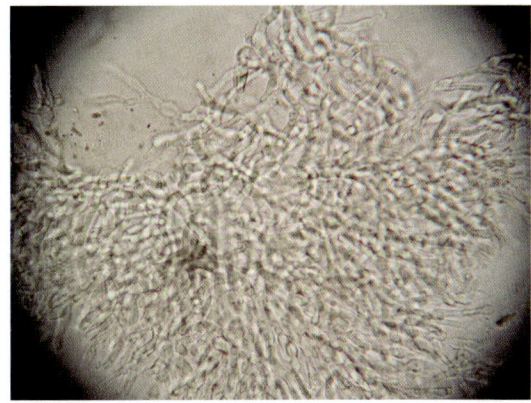

Fig. 5.7: Dense mass of dichotomously branched hyphae of *Aspergillus* species in corneal scrapings [KOH mount ×600].

The list of fungi isolated from patients with keratitis is long and varied. Members of genus ***Aspergillus*** are involved in majority of the cases.

Aspergillus fumigatus

Colony morphology

The organism grows rapidly on Sabouraud's dextrose agar with chloramphenicol (SDCA) or Czapek dox agar (25°C or 37°C) producing

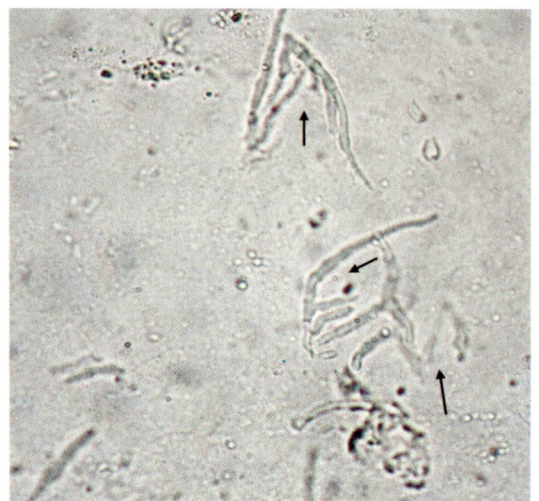

Fig. 5.8: Dichotomously branching hyphae (black arrow) of *Aspergillus* species in corneal scrapings [KOH mount ×400].

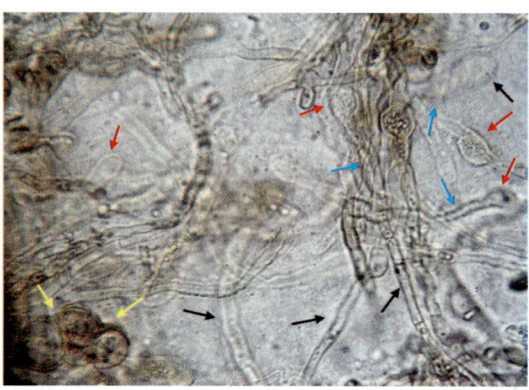

Fig. 5.10: KOH mount of corneal scrapings showing long septate hyaline hyphae (black arrow), brownish thick walled conidiophores (blue arrow), subglobose vesicle like structures (red arrow) and globose to oval cells (yellow arrow) which are suggestive of 'Hulle cells'. *Aspergillus nidulans* has been isolated and identified in culture from this sample obtained from a patient with 'mycotic keratitis' of more than 1 month duration [×400].

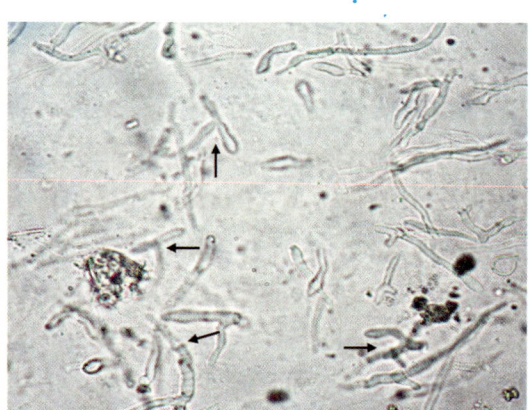

Fig. 5.9: Direct microscopical examination of corneal scrapings after 10% potassium hydroxide (tinted with ink) digestion. Numerous long and short strands of hyphae which are septate and some are dichotomously branched (black arrow) seen [×400].

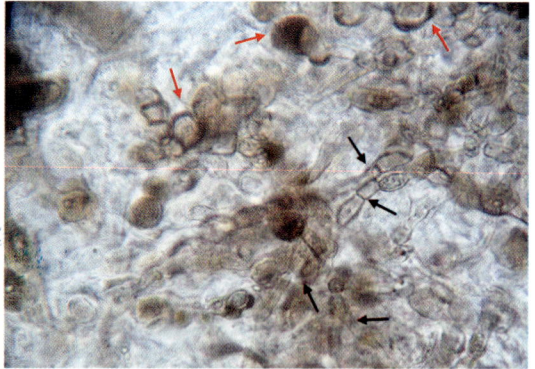

Fig. 5.11: Direct microscopical examination of corneal scrapings after 10% KOH digestion shows dark pigmented septate hyphae (black arrow), plenty of dark coloured round to oval cells (red arrow) arranged in clusters or lying singly. A 62 years old farmer had a pigmented corneal ulcer for more than 3 weeks duration, the pathogen is most likely a phaeoid fungi [×400].

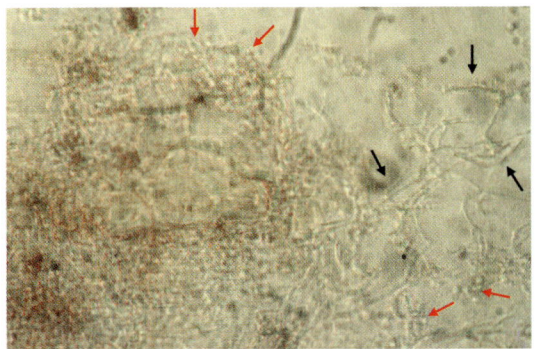

Fig. 5.12: Vitreous humor aspirated material in potassium hydroxide preparation showing tangled mass of mycelia which are hyaline, septate (black arrow); small clusters of conidia like structures are also noticed (red arrow). *Paecilomyces variotii* has been isolated and identified in pure culture in this case [×400].

a flat, white colony that quickly becomes gray-green with the production of conidia. The texture may vary from velvety to deep felt, floccose or somewhat folded.

Reverse is usually colourless. The conidia masses of the conidial heads are columnar, compact and often crowded.

Microscopic morphology

Conidiophore is short, smooth and have a slightly green or brownish colouration especially towards the upper part near the vesicle. The conidiophore enlarges to form the flask shaped vesicle. The vesicle produces a series of phialides on the upper half only. The phialides bend upward paralleling the axis of conidiophore. The conidia are globose to subglobose, grayish green, smooth (*see* Figs 4.43 and 4.44).

Aspergillus flavus

Colony morphology

Colony grows rapidly on Sabouraud's dextrose agar and consists of a close textured basal mycelium which is flat or radially furrowed or wrinkled. Conidial heads are abundant and of intense yellow to yellowish green in colour. Reverse is colourless.

Microscopic morphology

Conidiophores are thick-walled, unpigmented, coarsely roughened, long and ends in a vesicle which is globose to subglobose and produce phialides covering the entire surface. Phialides are biseriate or sometimes uniseriate. Primary phialides are up to 10 µ in length and the secondary phialides are about 5 µ in length. The conidia are elliptical at first, but later they are mostly globose and conspicuously echinulate (*see* Figs 4.31 and 4.46).

Aspergillus niger

Colony morphology

Colonies grow on SDCA at 25°C to 30°C within three to four days are compact basal mycelium, white to light yellowish white but soon turns into black due to abundant production of conidial structures (Fig. 5.13).

Microscopic morphology

Conidiophores are smooth, colourless and turning dark towards the vesicle. The vesicle is globose and produces phialides covering all the surface. The phialides are biseriate. The

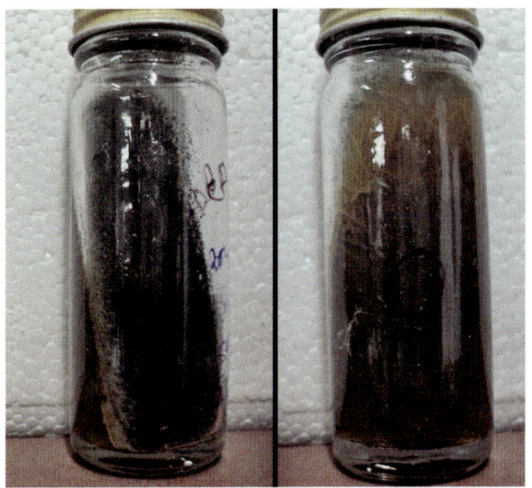

Fig. 5.13: Colony morphology of *Aspergillus niger* grown on Sabouraud's dextrose agar at 25°C for 5–6 days; (a) obverse—colony appears white, fluffy but soon becomes brownish black to intense black due to heavy conidiation, (b) reverse is colourless to black with increased conidiation.

primaries are long, brownish in colour and may be septate. The secondaries are short and produce conidia. These are globose, brown to black and very rough (Figs 5.14 and 5.15).

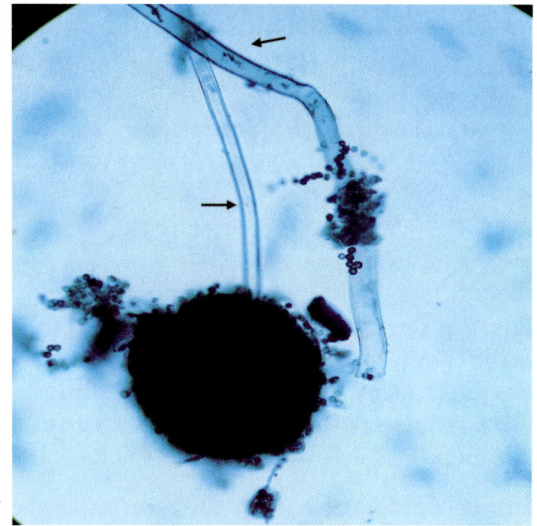

Fig. 5.14: Microscopic morphology of *Aspergillus niger*. Conidiophores (black arrow) are variable in size with thick, smooth walls, either hyaline or brownish near vesicle. The conidial heads (red arrow) are large and black or brownish black, appear globose at first but soon become radiate or splitting to form divergent spore columns [LPCB mount ×400].

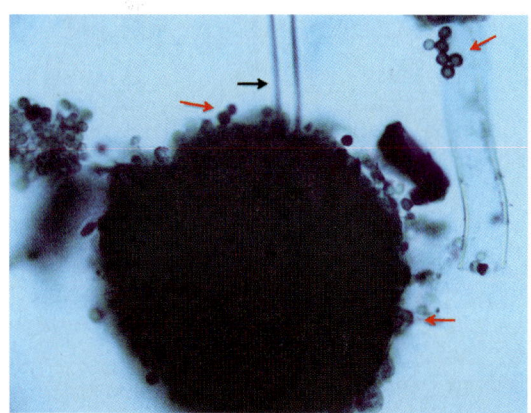

Fig. 5.15: *Aspergillus niger*. Conidiophores are brownish near the vesicle (black arrow). Vesicle is typically globose and produces brownish sterigmata on its entire surface. Sterigmata are biseriate and produce brown to black echinulate, globose conidia (red arrow) in chains [LPCB mount ×600].

Aspergillus terreus

Colony morphology

On Sabouraud's dextrose agar at 25° to 30°C the colony grows rapidly. The consistency of the colony is floccose to velvety, sometimes furrowed or tufted and the colony conidiates profusely. The massed conidial heads are columnar and the colour is cinnamon-buff to wood brown which is revealed in colony colour. Reverse is usually colourless (*see* Figs 4.47 and 4.48).

Microscopic morphology

The conidiophores are long and slender, smooth and uniform diameter throughout. The vesicles are hemispherical or domelike and merge inperceptively with the conidiophore. The phialides are in two series. The primaries are longer and wider than secondaries. The conidia are smooth to somewhat elliptical in shape. Spherical to oval hyaline cells (aleuroconidia) which are produced laterally on the mycelia submerged on the agar.

Aspergillus amstelodami

Colony morphology

Obverse of the colony is somewhat wrinkled or zonate, dark yellowish in colour because of the abundance of cleistothecia in most isolates. The conidial heads are a deep olive green, but this colouration does not affect that of the colony. A few isolates are primarily conidial type and the colony may appear as dark olive green colour (Fig. 5.16).

Microscopic morphology

Conidiophores appear hyaline or have a yellowish green tinge and ends in a subglobose vesicle. The vesicle produce only the primary series of sterigmata which covers either three-fourths of or the entire vesicle surface. The conidia appear finely rough, green, and subglobose to elliptical (Fig. 5.17). In **ascosporic** state it produces abundant cleistothecia (Fig. 5.18), which are globose to

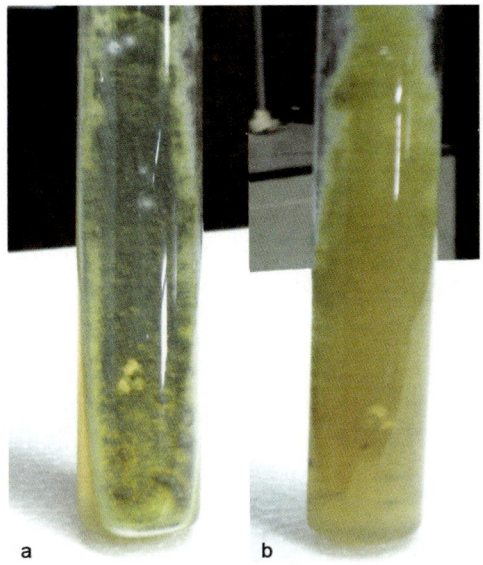

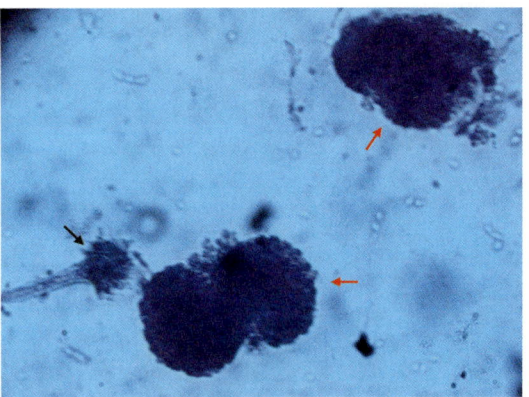

Fig. 5.18: Cleistotheicia (red arrow) of *Aspergillus amstelodami* produced abundantly in old culture. Flask-shaped vesicle with primary series of phialides and conidial attachments are also noticed (yellow arrow). [LPCB mount ×400].

Fig. 5.16: Colony morphology of *Aspergillus amstelodami* grown on Sabouraud's dextrose agar at 28°C for 7 days; (a) obverse, (b) reverse.

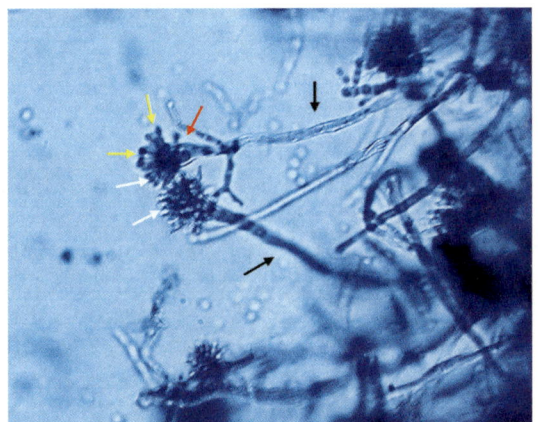

Fig. 5.17: *Aspergillus amstelodami*. Microscopic morphology. Conidiophores appear hyaline or have a yellowish green tinge (black arrow); subglobose to flask-shaped vesicle (red arrow); vesicle produces only the primary series of sterigmata (white arrow); conidia appears subglobose to elliptical (yellow arrow). [LPCB mount ×200].

subglobose, yellow, naked, thin walled and shiny. The asci, which are subglobose in shape, contain eight ascospores. The ascospores are

hyaline, lenticular and have a rough texture with a prominent 'V' shaped equatorial furrow flanked by two irregular ridges.

Aspergillus sydowi

Colony morphology

The colonies exhibit moderate growth on Sabouraud's dextrose agar and are blue green with narrow, white margins. The radiate conidial heads are abundantly produced.

Microscopic morphology

The conidiophores are long (up to 500 µm), hyaline with thick smooth walls and produce nearly globose vesicle. Conidiophores produced on aerial hyphae are often greatly reduced in length. The vesicles bear double series of sterigmata, the secondaries being longer than the primary series sterigmata. The conidia are green when seen as a mass, are globose to subglobose definitely rough appearance (Fig. 5.19). Other medically important *aspergillus* species are described in detail with figures.

Fusarium species

Fusarium species are well known plant pathogen and soil saprophytes, with a

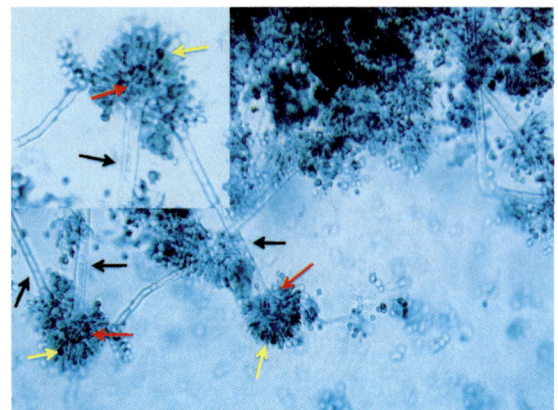

Fig. 5.19: *Aspergillus sydowi.* Microscopic morphology shows conidiophores smooth, colourless (black arrow), vesicles subglobose (red arrow), phialides biseriate and radiating which give rise to bluish green unicellular conidia (yellow arrow) [LPCB mount ×400].

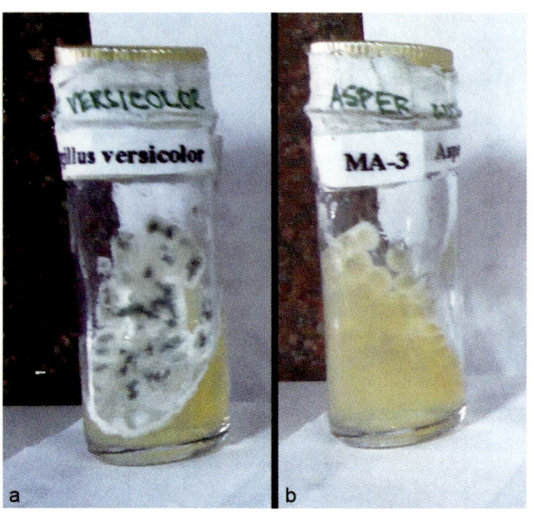

Fig. 5.20: *Aspergillus versicolor.* One-week-old colony of an isolate grown on Sabouraud's dextrose agar at 25°C. Variable colour of the colony as white, green, yellow green, buff are seen in the same culture, reverse is colourless; (a) obverse, (b) reverse

worldwide distribution. Several species of *Fusarium* are known to cause infections like keratomycosis, mycetoma and onychomycosis in human. In recent years, *Fusarium* have increasingly been reported from colonizing and disseminated infections in patients with underlying disease. *Fusarium* species most often causes human infections are **Fusarium solani, Fusarium oxysporum, Fusarium chlamydosporum, Fusarium dimerum, Fusarium moniliforme** and **Fusarium proliferatum.**

Colony morphology

Colonies of **Fusarium** species are fluffy to cottony owing to extensive mycelium. Colour of the colony differs from species to species. Sometimes diffusible pigments are produced on reverse and that helps in species identification to some extent (*see* Figs 3.42 and 3.46).

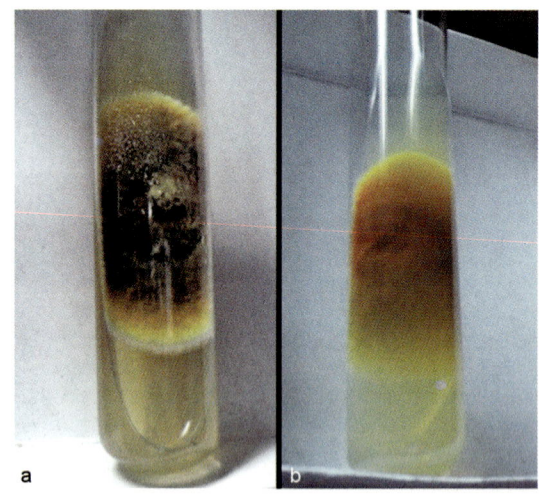

Fig. 5.21: *Aspergillus glaucus.* Colonies grown on Sabouraud's dextrose agar at 25°C are greenish yellow that turns to deep yellow and finally to dark brown as the colony ages. Reverse is yellow to maroon; (a) obverse, (b) reverse.

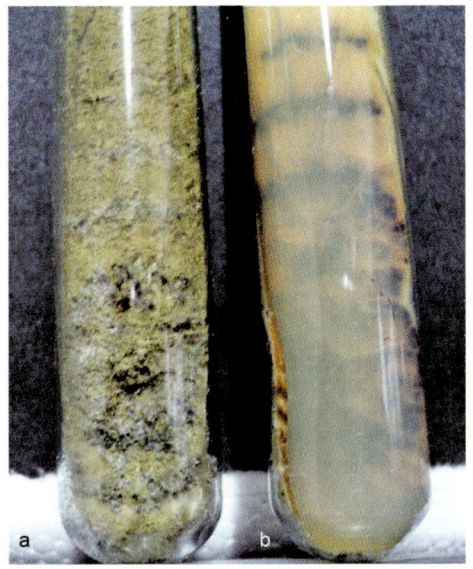

Fig. 5.22: Colony morphology of *Aspergillus parasiticus* grown on Sabouraud's dextrose agar at 28°C for 10 days; (a) obverse, (b) reverse.

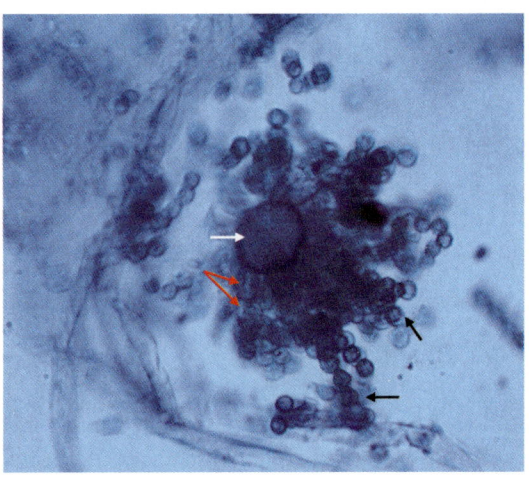

Fig. 5.24: Conidial structure of *Aspergillus parasiticus*. Vesicles are oval to subglobose (white arrow), sterigmata biseriate (red arrow) and radiating. Conidia (black arrow) are larger in size compared to other species, dark greenish brown, rough echinulated [LPCB mount ×400].

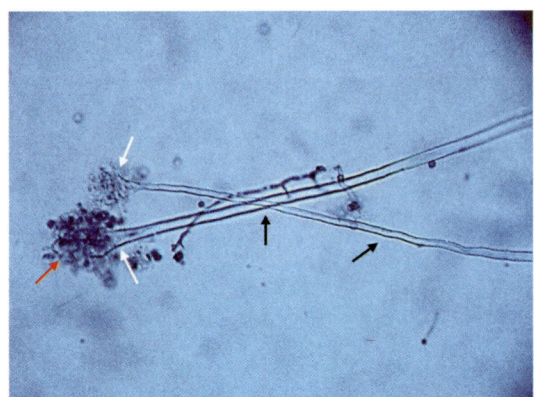

Fig. 5.23: *Aspergillus versicolor*. Microscopic morphology showing conidiophore rough walled (black arrow) although many strains have smooth conidiophore; globose to flask-shaped vesicle (white arrow); sterigmata (phialides) biseriate, radiate produce small, round, smooth conidia in chains (red arrow). Conidial heads are green, yellow green, buff and white in the same culture [LPCB mount ×200].

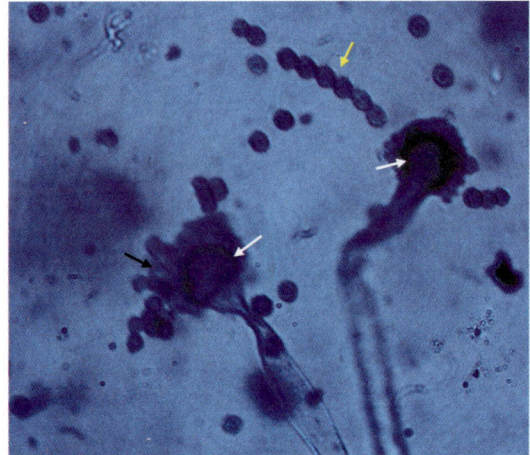

Fig. 5.25: Vesicles of *Aspergillus parasiticus* are globose to subglobose (white arrow) with phialidic arrangement in double series (black arrow). Conidia dark echinulated [LPCB mount ×400].

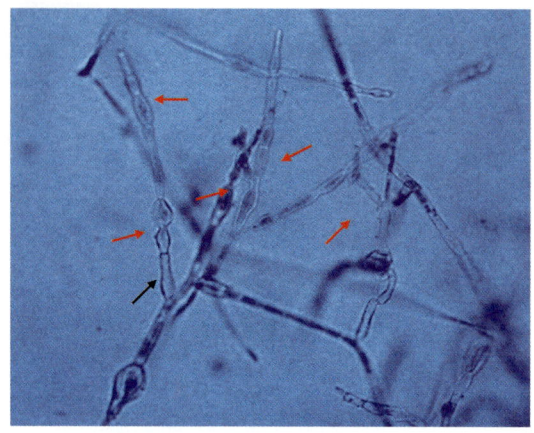

Fig. 5.26: *Fusarium moniliforme.* Fusoid macroconidia are infrequently produced. Microconidia (red arrow) with a flattened base arise in chains from monophialides (black arrow) [LPCB mount ×400].

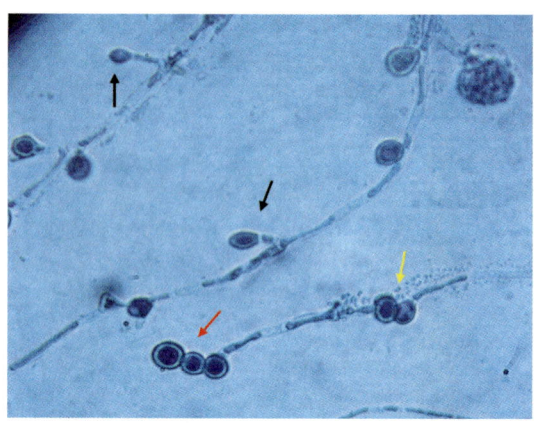

Fig. 5.28: *Fusarium chlamydosporum.* Characteristically very few macroconidia and microconidia are noticed instead chlamydoconidia are produced abundantly in young culture. Chlamydoconidia are spherical to oval, borne singly atop short conidiophore (black arrow), some are terminal in chains (red arrow) or intercalary (yellow arrow) [LPCB mount ×400].

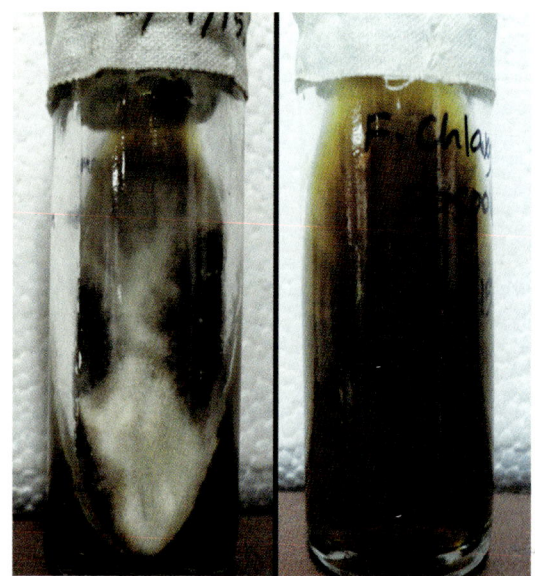

Fig. 5.27: *Fusarium chlamydosporum.* Colony grown on Sabouraud's dextrose agar at 25°C for 10 days. (a) obverse, (b) reverse.

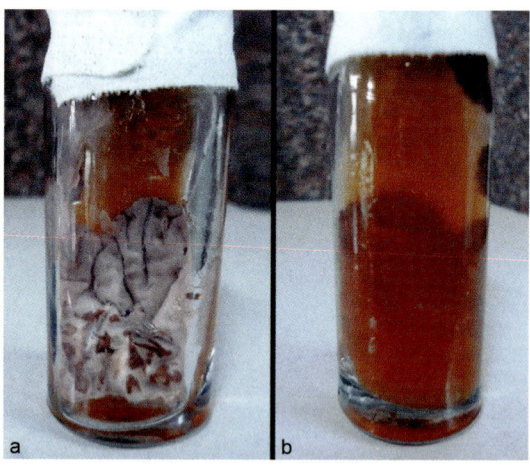

Fig. 5.29: Colony morphology of *Fusarium moniliforme* grown on Sabouraud's dextrose agar at 28°C for 3 weeks. Colony is rapidly growing, cottony and flat. The colour is at first white, soon develops light pink and gradually turns into dark pink smooth, folded and leathery colony. Rusty to brick red pigment diffuse into the media; (a) obverse, (b) reverse.

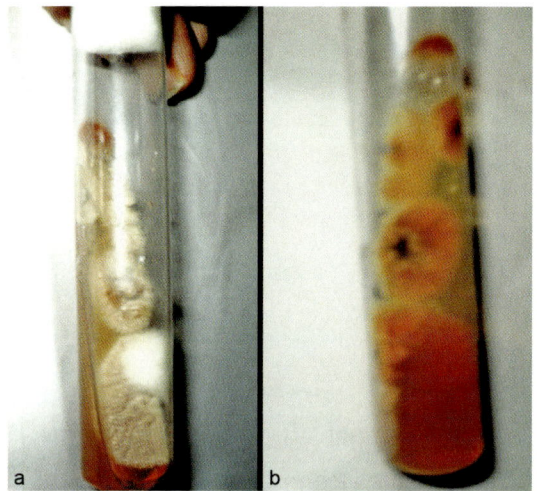

Fig. 5.30: Colony morphology of *Fusarium moniliforme* var. *verticelloides* grown on SDA at 28°C for 7 days; (a) obverse, (b) reverse.

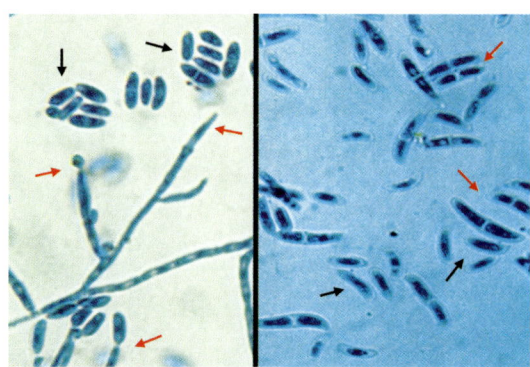

Fig. 5.32: (a) *Fusarium moniliforme (var. verticilloides)*. Microconidia are produced from monophialide (red arrow) and in verticillate arrangement (black arrow); (b) Fusiform macroconidia with a central septa (red arrow) are characteristic feature of *Fusarium dierum*. Microconibia are fusoid, small and single celled (black arrow) [LPCB mount ×600].

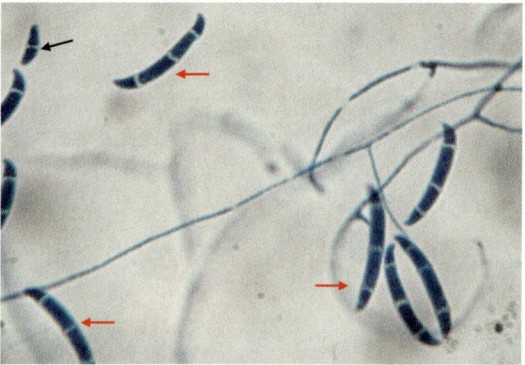

Fig. 5.33: Microscopic morphology of *Fusarium solani* showing abundant macroconidia (red arrow), microconidia (black arrow) and thin septate hyaline hyphae [LPCB mount ×400].

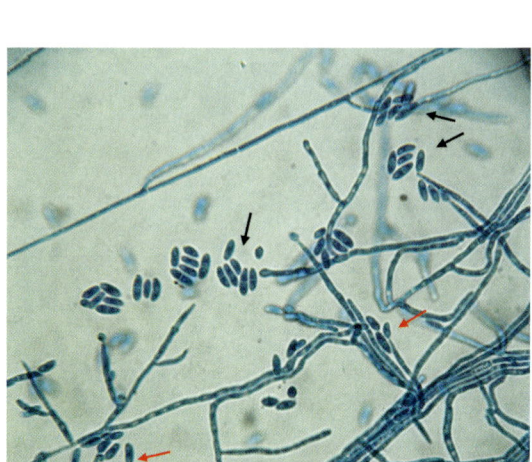

Fig. 5.31: *Fusarium moniliforme* var. *verticelloides*. Fusoid microconidia arise from monophialides (red arrow) and are in verticillate arrangement (black arrow), macroconidia if produced at all are scanty [LPCB mount ×400].

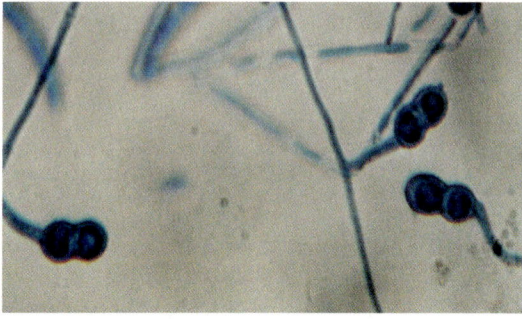

Fig. 5.34: Chlamydoconidia of *Fusarium solani* found in old culture [LPCB mount ×400].

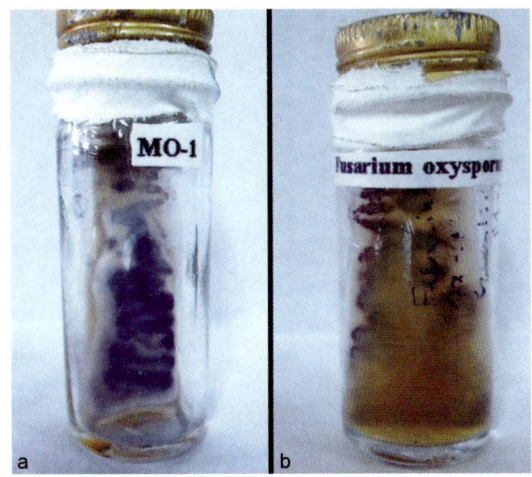

Fig. 5.35: *Fusarium oxysporum*. Colonies are grown on SDCA at 25°C for 4 to 7 days. White fluffy colony appears at first, it soon develops a cream colour to light pink and finally to mauve after 2–3 weeks (as shown in this picture); (a) obverse, (b) reverse.

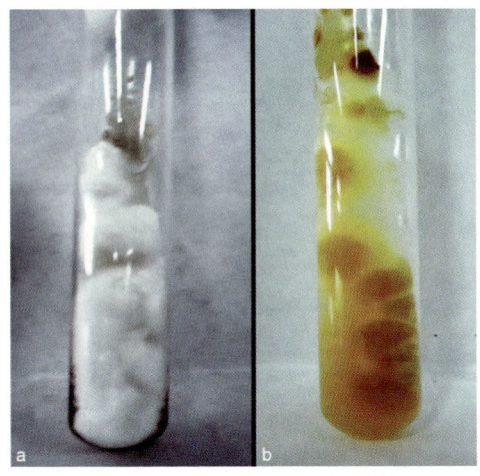

Fig. 5.37: Colony morphology of *Fusarium dimerum* grown on SDA at 28°C for 7 days; (a) obverse, (b) reverse.

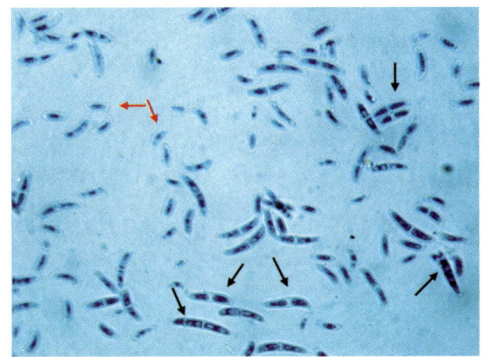

Fig. 5.38: Microscopic morphology of *Fusarium dimerum* showing numerous macroconidia with one/two septa (black arrow). Plenty of microconidia are also noticed (red arrow). [LPCB stain ×400]

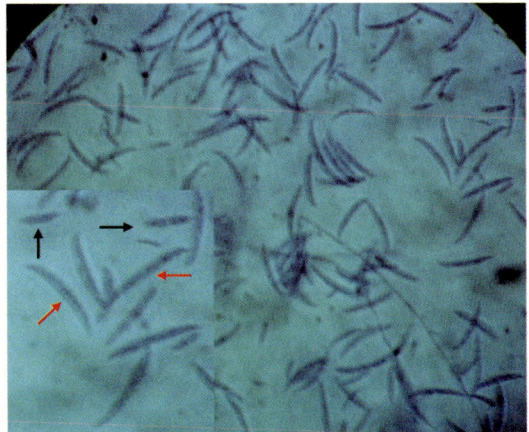

Fig. 5.36: *Fusarium oxysporum*. Macroconidia are crescent shaped, thin walled, multiseptate (red arrow) produced abundantly. Microconidia are single celled or single septate (black arrow) [LPCB mount ×400].

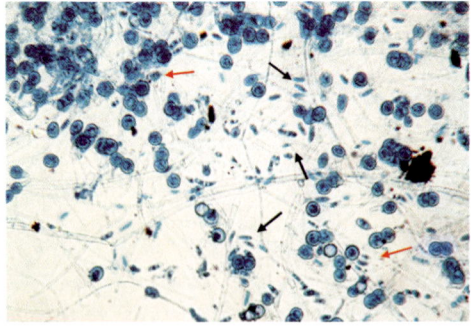

Fig. 5.39: *Fusarium dimerum*. Abundant thick walled chlamydoconidia (red arrow) are seen in old culture. Numerous fusoidl nonseptate single celled small in size microconidia are also noticed (black arrow) [LPCB mount ×400].

OTHER AGENTS OF FUNGAL KERATITIS

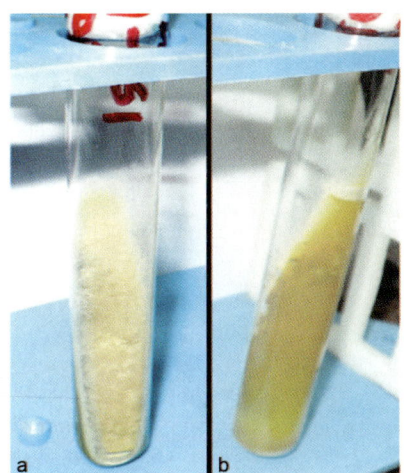

Fig. 5.40: *Paecilomyces lilacinous.* Colonies grown on Sabouraud's dextrose agar at 25°C for three days. Colonies are lilac or tan to golden yellow. Reverse is yellowish brown; (a) obverse, (b) reverse.

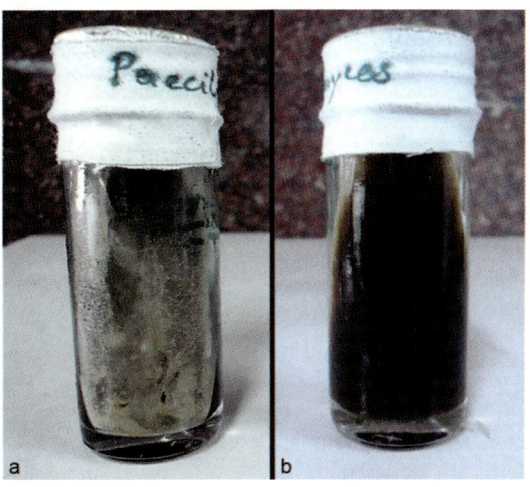

Fig. 5.42: *Paecilomyces variotii.* Colony grown on Sabouraud's dextrose agar at 25°C for 7 days; (a) obverse, (b) reverse.

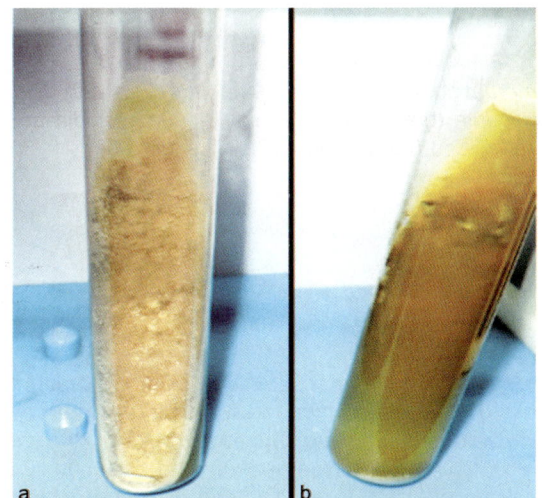

Fig. 5.41: *Paecilomyces lilacinous.* Colonies grown on Sabouraud's dextrose agar at 25°C for 7 days. Colonies become golden yellow to yellowish brown with aging. Reverse is brown; (a) obverse, (b) reverse.

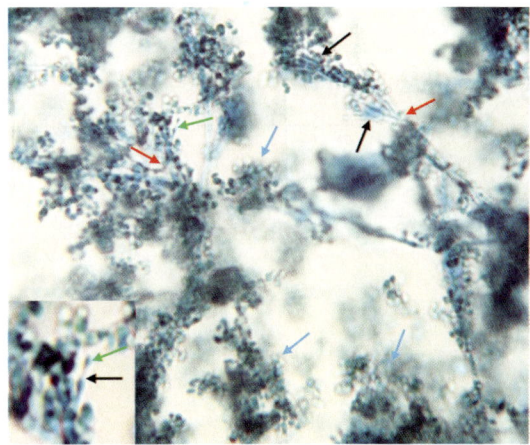

Fig. 5.43: *Paecilomyces variotii.* Phialides are long tapering tubes with long narrow neck (inset—black arrow) compactly arranged at the terminal part of conidiophores (red arrow) or sometimes directly from main hyphae. The tip of phialides bear small young conidium (basocatenulate;inset—green arrow). Conidia are arranged in clusters (in masses; blue arrow) but not in chains [LPCB mount ×400].

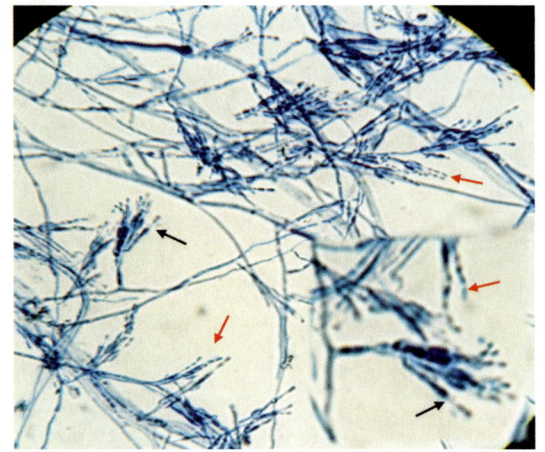

Fig. 5.44: *Paecilomyces lilacinus.* Slide culture shows compactly arranged phialides with long narrow neck (black arrow) and conidia are arranged in chains (red arrow) where small young conidium is produced at the tip of phialide which is attached to chain of older conidia (basocatenulate). Conidia are characteristically oval to elliptical (lemon shaped) in shape [LPCB mount ×400].

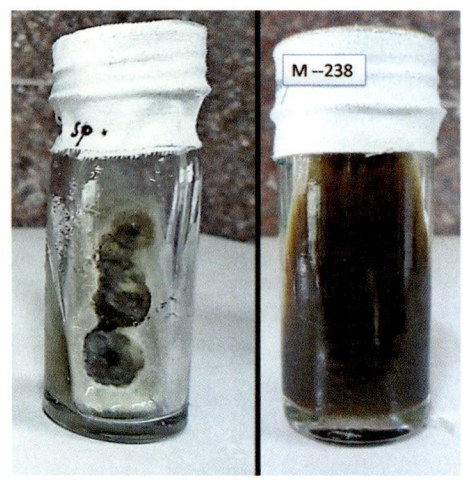

Fig. 5.46: Colony morphology of *Bipolaris spicifera* grown on SDCA at 28°C for 10 days. Colony of this dematiaceous fungi is initially floccose, grayish white but soon turns into shiny dark brownish black. Reverse of the colony is black.

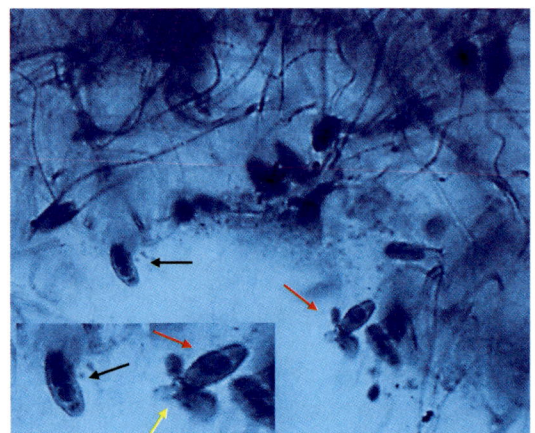

Fig. 5.45: *Curvularia lunata.* Conidia are dark, straight, elliptical to cylindrical in shape, multicelled with one or more central cells darker (black arrow). Conidia are produced in whorls arising through pores in the walls of conidiophore or at the apex (yellow arrow) of it (inset—red arrow) [LPCB mount ×400].

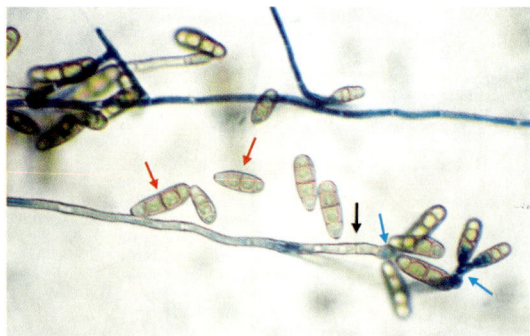

Fig. 5.47: *Bipolaris spicifera.* Conidia are straight, oblong to cylindrical, rounded at both ends (red arrow) with protruding truncate dark hilum (black arrow) and small hyaline area (blue arrow) just above the hilum are important features. Conidia with consistently 3 septa are characteristic feature of this species [LPCB mount ×400].

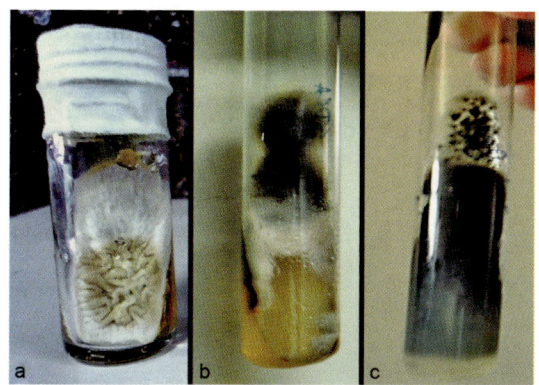

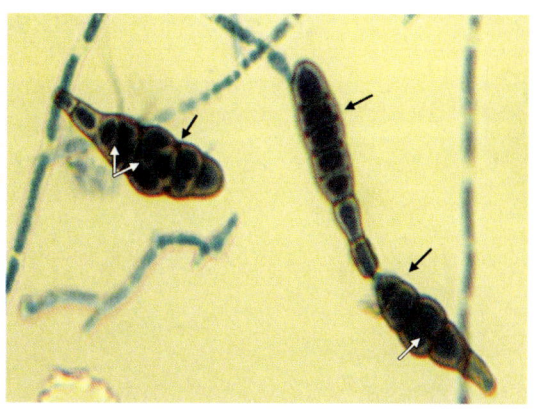

Fig. 5.48: Colony morphology of *Alternaria* species grown on Sabouraud's dextrose agar at 28°C; (a) colony morphology after 7 days of incubation (obverse), (b) colony morphology after 2 weeks (obverse) white fluffy colony is transformed to brownish-black pigmented colony (dematiaceous fungi), (c) reverse is brown to black pigmented.

Fig. 5.50: *Alternaria alternata.* Muriform macro-conidia have both transverse (black arrow) and also vertical septum (white arrow) [LPCB mount x 600].

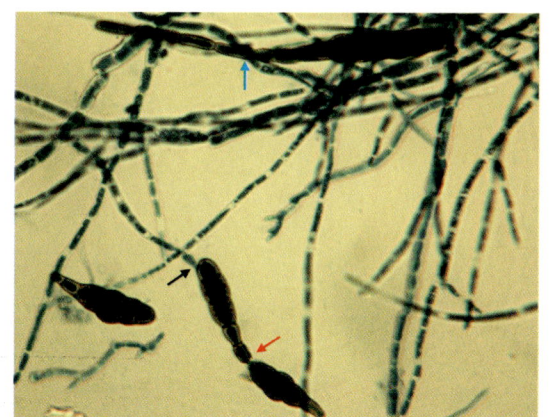

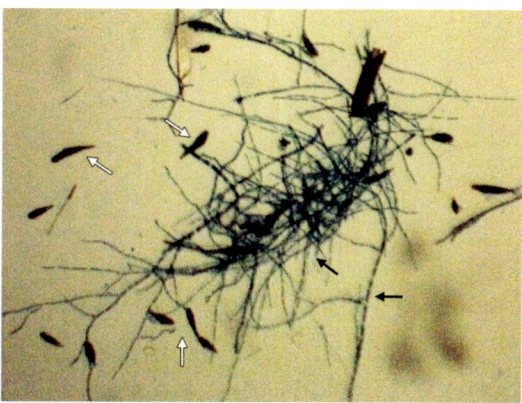

Fig. 5.49: Muriform conidia (also called dictyoconidia) of *Alternaria alternata*. One conidium is shown arising from a pore at the apex of conidiophore (black arrow). The long tube that can be seen at its apex into an appendage (a hypha-like structure; blue arrow) or into more conidia forming a chain of conidia (red arrow) [LPCB mount ×400].

Fig. 5.51: Numerous muriform conidia (white arrow) of *A. alternata* produced on cornmeal agar. Hyphae dematiaceous (black arrow) [LPCB mount ×200].

SELF ASSESSMENT

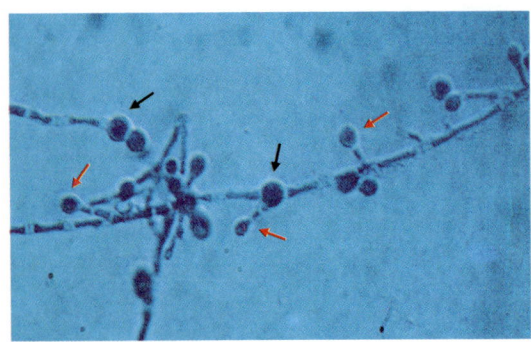

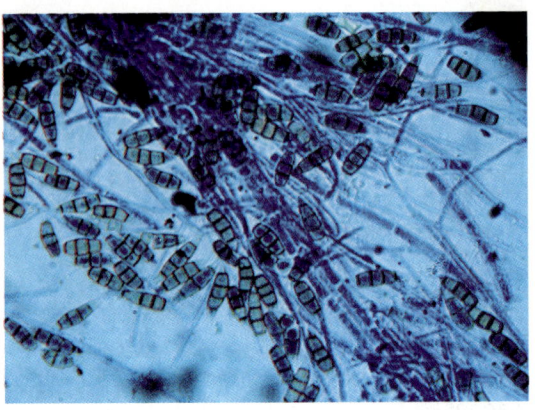

Fig. 5.52: Abundant smooth walled spherical to oval chlamydoconidia are produced atop a short conidiophore (red arrow) while a few are intercalary (black arrow) in young culture. The fungus was isolated from a corneal scrapping sample obtained from a 12 years old girl who had a history of injury in her left eye while playing on the ground. She was clinically diagnosed as a case of 'fungal keratitis'. Identify the fungal pathogen. This is a well-known plant pathogen and soil saprophyte [LPCB mount ×400].

Fig. 5.54: Microscopic morphology of a dematiaceous fungi isolated from a case of suspected mycotic keratitis. Identify the fungus (up to species level) [LPCB mount ×400].

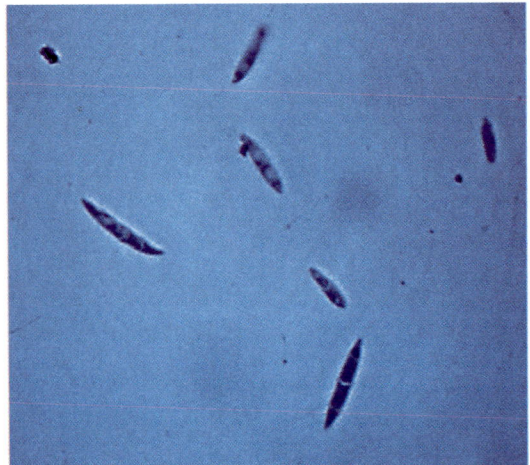

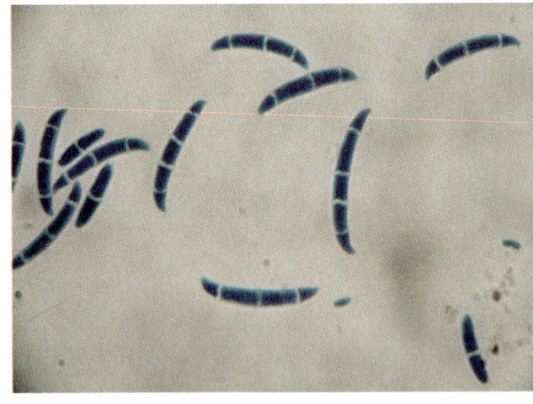

Fig. 5.53: Macroconidia of *Fusarium* species. Identify the species [LPCB mount ×400].

Fig. 5.55: Identify the structure and the relevant fungi, isolated from a 58 male farmers, with a clinical suspicion of 'fungal keratitis' of more than 1 month duration [LPCB mount ×400].

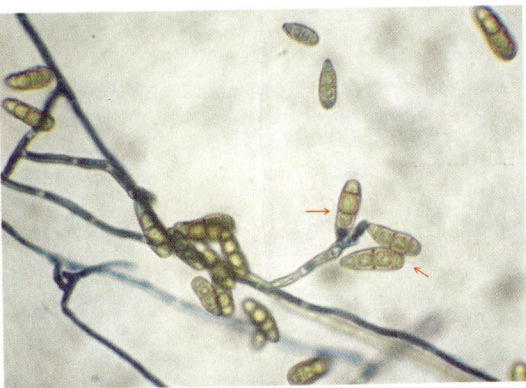

Fig. 5.56: Microscopic morphology of a phaeoid fungi isolated from a 52 years old male patient, clinically diagnosed case of 'fungal keratitis'. Identify the structure indicated and the likely fungus [LPCB mount ×400].

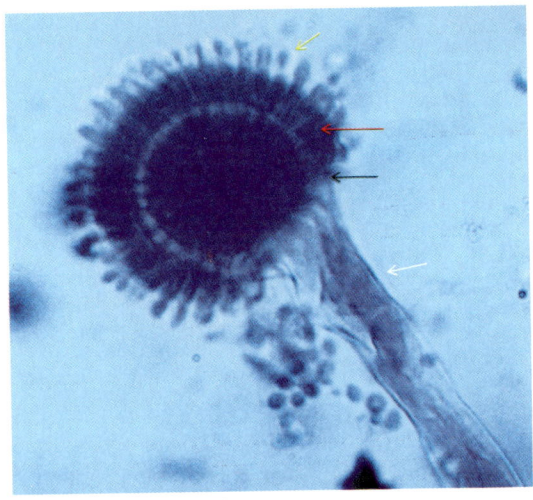

Fig. 5.58: Microscopic morphology of conidial head of an *Aspergillus* species. Identify different structures indicated and the species. This *Aspergillus* species is notorius in causing 'Mycotoxicosis' [LPCB mount ×600].

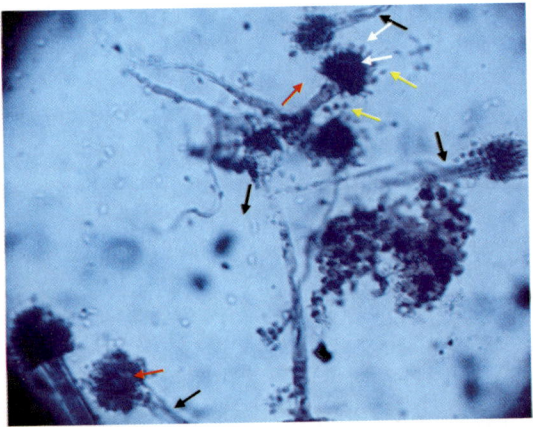

Fig. 5.57: Microscopic morphology of an *Aspergillus* species isolated from a case of otomycosis. Identify the indicated structures and the likely fungus. This species produce abundant yellow cleistothecia [LPCB mount ×400].

ANSWERS

- **Fig. 5.58:** Phialides/Sterigmata (red arrow); *Aspergillus parasiticus*.
- **Fig. 5.57:** Vesicle (red arrow), Conidiophore (black arrow), Conidia (yellow arrow), Phialides/Sterigmata (white arrow); *Aspergillus amstelodami*
- **Fig. 5.56:** *Bipolaris specifera*
- **Fig. 5.55:** *Fusarium solani*
- **Fig. 5.54:** *Curvularia lunata*
- **Fig. 5.53:** *Fusarium solani*
- **Fig. 5.52:** *Fusarium chlamydosporum*

Museum Specimens

In clinical practise one can come across rare and uncommon isolates. It then becomes very necessary to preserve these isolates for future reference and teaching purposes. An isolate can be maintained as a viable source, which will allow the laboratory to continue to subculture and maintain it. Methods to maintain a viable isolate include:

- Periodic transfer on agar slants
- Distilled water method
- Freezing technique
- Freezing and storage in liquid nitrogen
- Oil sealing technique
- Freeze—drying (Lyophilisation)

Sometimes though a less cumbersome, time consuming and labour intensive process may be required. Stock cultures are not usually display worthy in a museum and sometimes students require visual corroboration to appreciate the changing attributes of colony morphology with time. An answer to the entire dilemma is preservation of fungal colonies as "Museum Specimens". These mounted specimens can be preserved for more than five years without any additional effort or intervention.

Method to Preserve Museum Specimens

- Fungi isolated from clinical specimens are grown onto SDCA slants in tubes.
- Colonies appearing are then further subcultured onto SDCA slant poured in a "flat blood culture bottle". (The purpose of this is to get a wider surface for colonies to flourish and reduce the chances of contamination.)
- Colonies which appear in the 'Flat Blood Culture Bottle' are observed regularly. Once the appropriate features intended to be displayed, in terms of colours, textures, etc are obtained—the colonies are ready to be preserved.
- 5–10 drops of 40% Formalin is poured carefully on to the flat surface opposite to the SDCA slant taking care not to spill it on to the colony (as this may corrode the growth).
- The screw cap of the Flat Blood Culture Bottle is kept partially unscrewed to allow ventilation of the contents. The bottle is left in horizontal position with the flat Formalin soaked side down and the SDCA slant with the colony above. The bottle is left undisturbed for 5–6 days.
- The specimen is then ready to be displayed.

The following are some of the museum specimens from our collection.

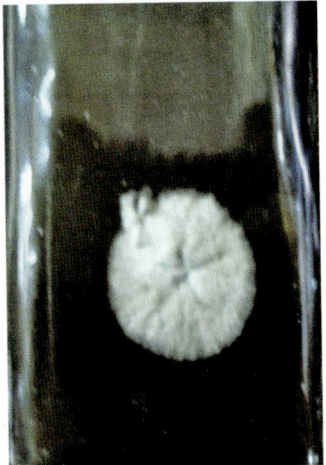

Fig. 6.1: *Trichophyton mentagrophyte*

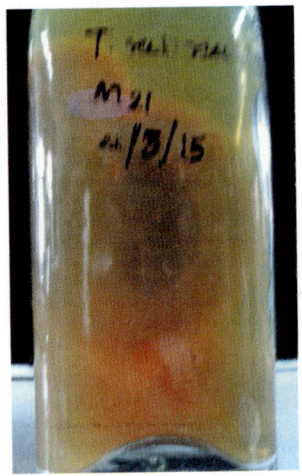

Fig. 6.2a: *T. rubrum* (reverse)

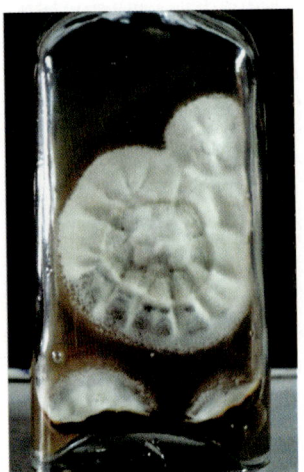

Fig. 6.2: *Trichophyton rubrum*

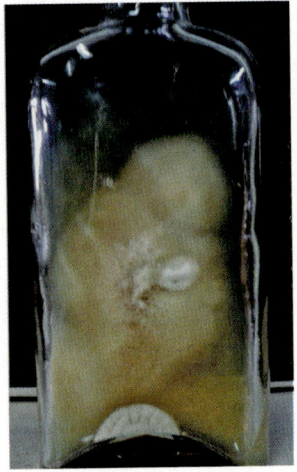

Fig. 6.3: *Trichophyton tonsurans*

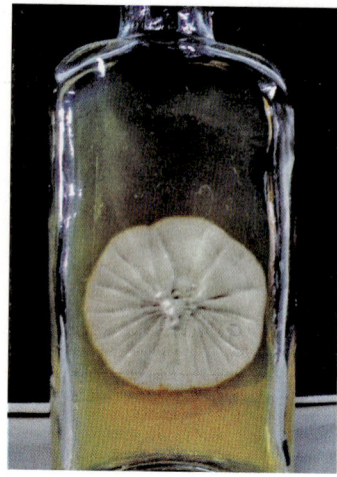

Fig. 6.4: *Trichophyton schoenleinii*

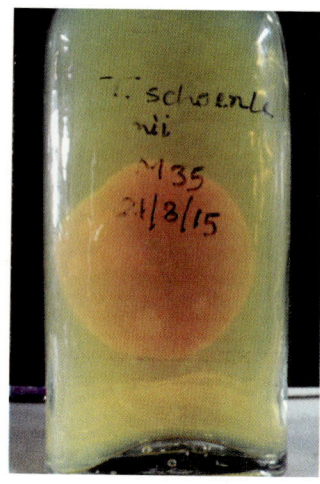

Fig. 6.4b: *Trichophyton schoenleinii* (reverse)

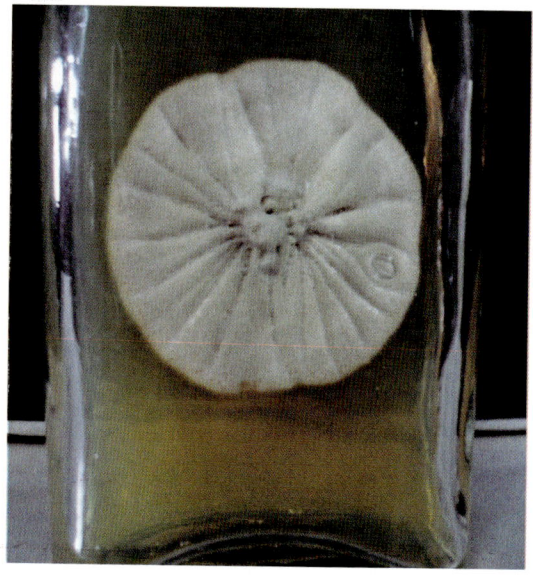

Fig. 6.4a: *Trichophyton schoenleinii* (close view)

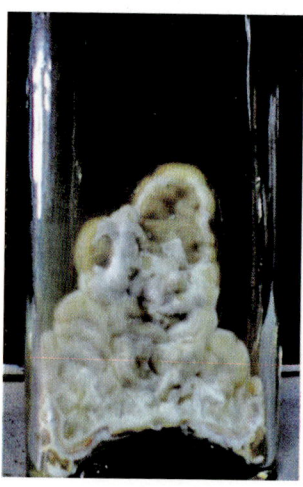

Fig. 6.5: *Trichophyton soudanense* (obverse)

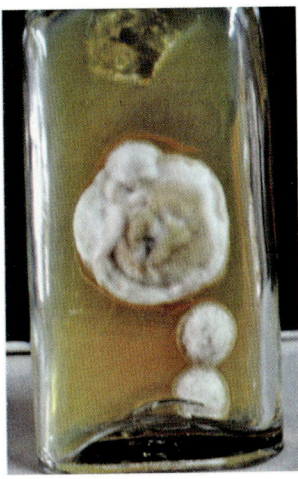

Fig. 6.6: *Trichophyton equinum* (obverse)

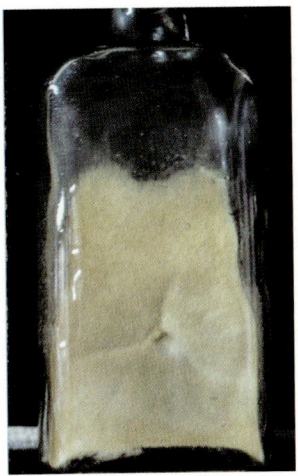

Fig. 6.7: *Microsporum audouinii*

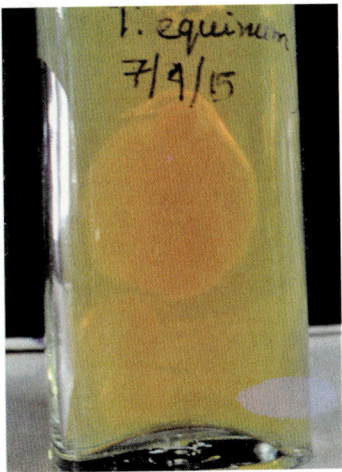

Fig. 6.6a: *Trichophyton equinum* (reverse)

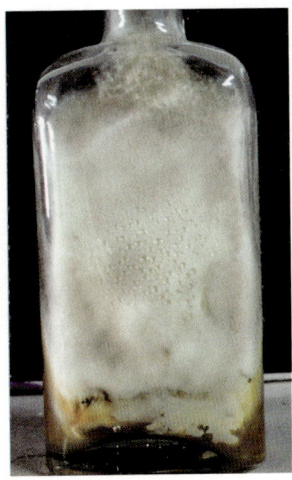

Fig. 6.8: *Microsporum canis* (obverse)

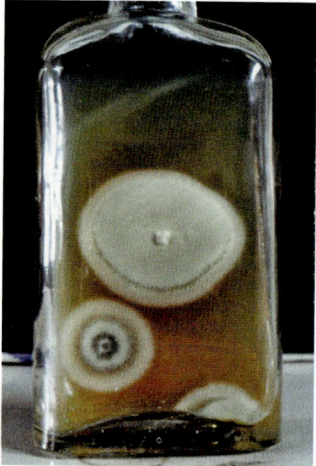

Fig. 6.9: *Microsporum persicolor* (obverse)

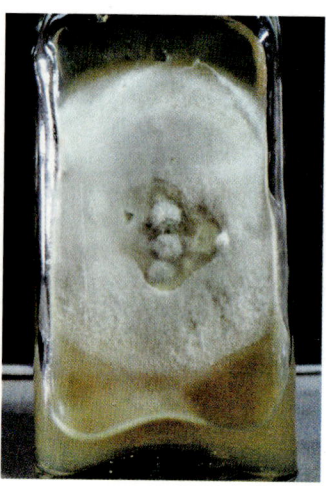

Fig. 6.10: *Microsporum gallinae* (obverse)

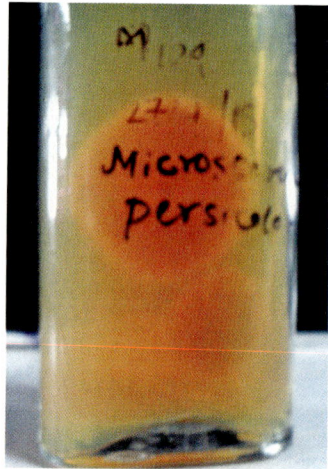

Fig. 6.9a: *Microsporum persicolor* (reverse)

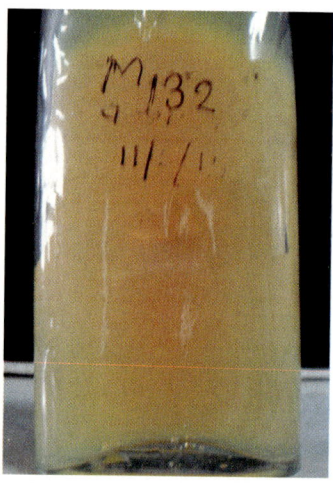

Fig. 6.10a: *Microsporum gallinae* (reverse)

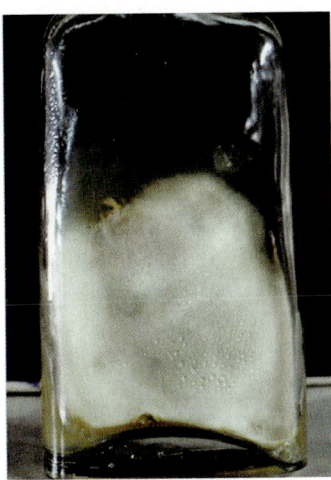

Fig. 6.11: *Epidermophyton floccosum* (obverse)

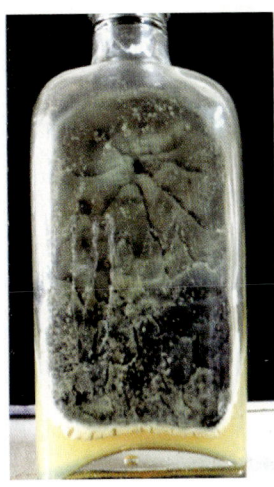

Fig. 6.13: *Aspergillus fumigatus* (obverse; old culture)

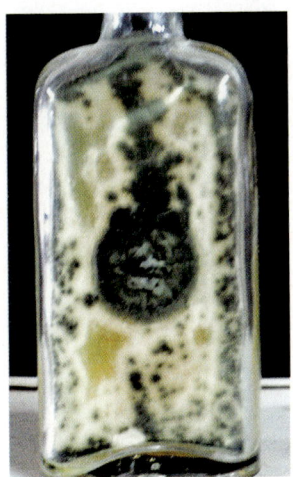

Fig. 6.12: *Aspergillus fumigatus* (obverse)

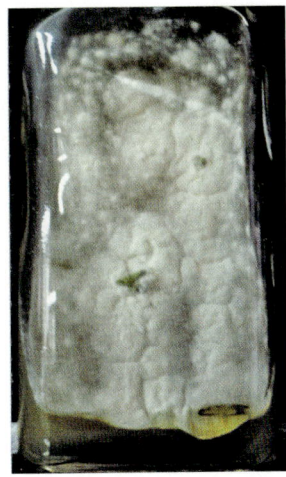

Fig. 6.14: *Aspergillus flavus* (obverse; young culture)

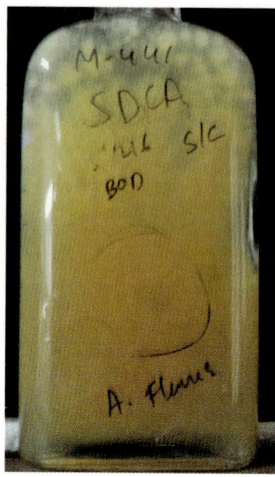

Fig. 6.14a: *Aspergillus flavus* (reverse)

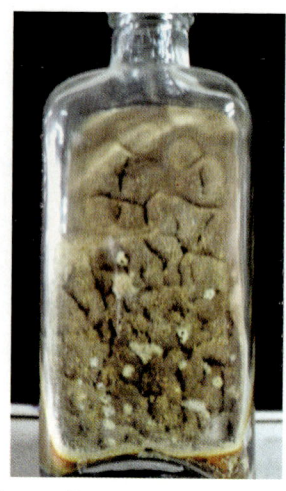

Fig. 6.16: *Aspergillus terreus* (obverse; old culture)

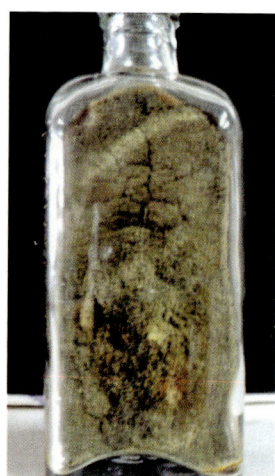

Fig. 6.15: *Aspergillus terreus* (obverse; young culture)

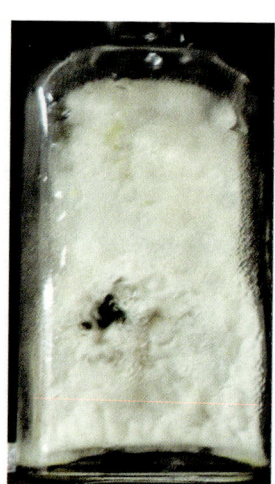

Fig. 6.17: *Aspergillus niger* (obverse)

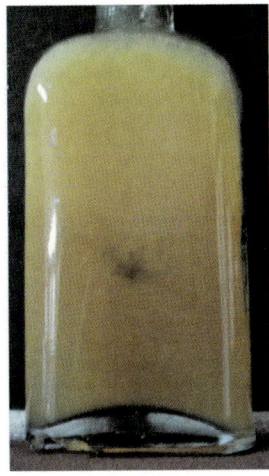

Fig. 6.17a: *Aspergillus niger* (reverse)

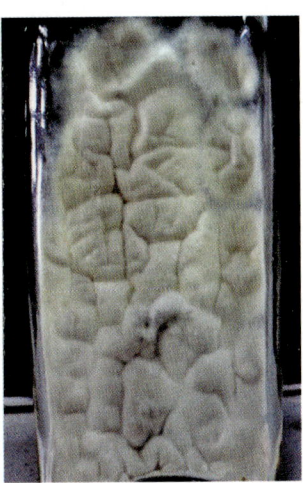

Fig. 6.19: *Fusarium oxysporum* (obverse; aging culture)

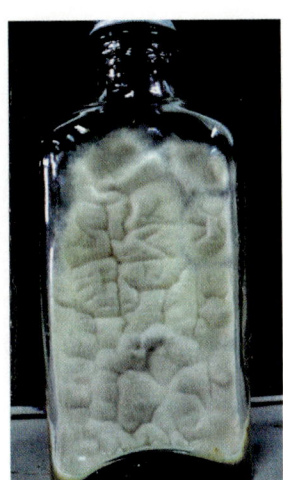

Fig. 6.18: *Fusarium oxysporum* (obverse; young culture)

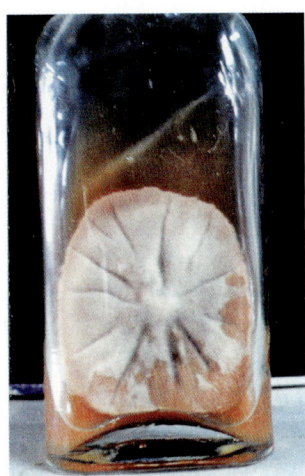

Fig. 6.20: *Fusarium moniliforme* (obverse)

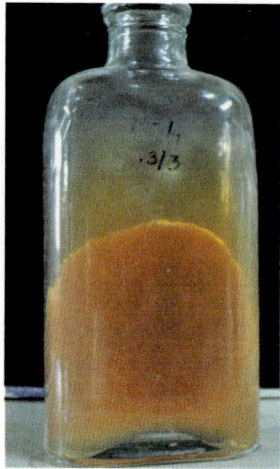

Fig. 6.20a: *Fusarium moniliforme* (reverse)

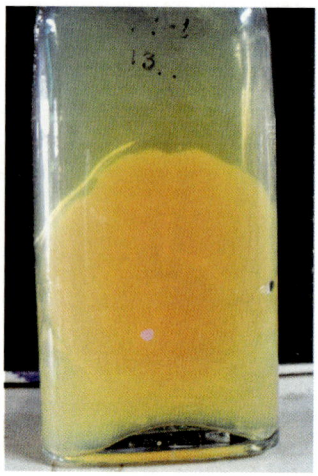

Fig. 6.21a: *Fusarium solani* (reverse)

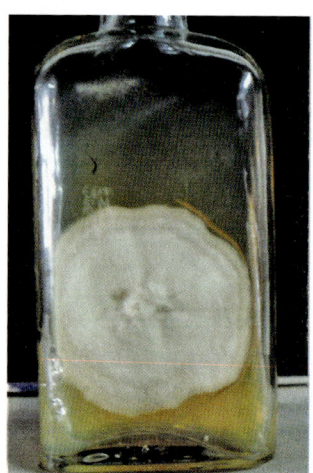

Fig. 6.21: *Fusarium solani* (obverse)

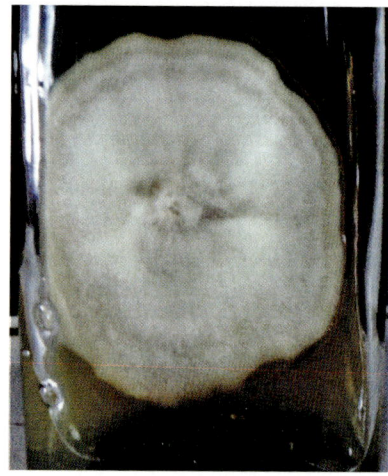

Fig. 6.22: *Fusarium solani* (obverse, close view)

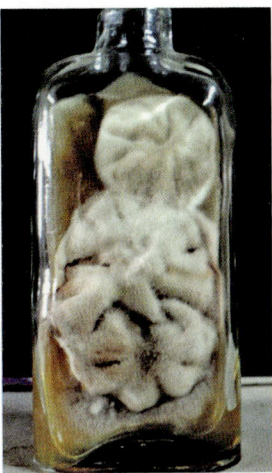

Fig. 6.23: *Fusarium chlamydosporum* (obverse)

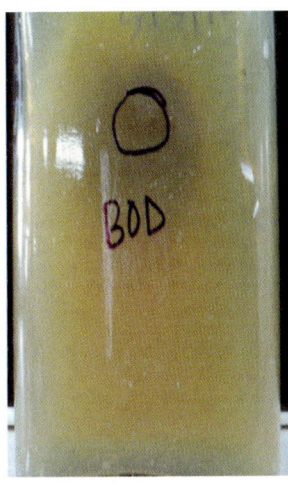

Fig. 6.24a: *Trichophyton violaceum* (reverse)

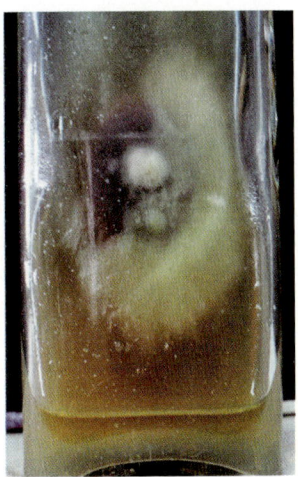

Fig. 6.24: *Trichophyton violaceum*

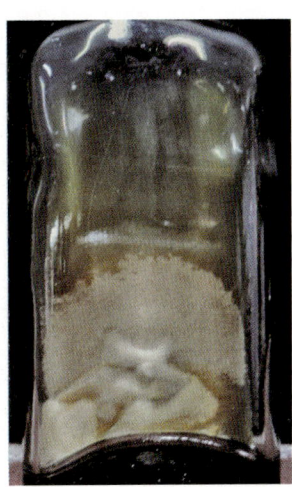

Fig. 6.25: *Madurella species*

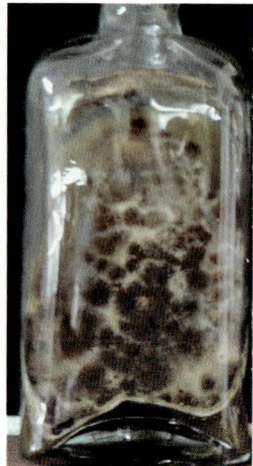

Fig. 6.26: *Sporothrix schenckii*

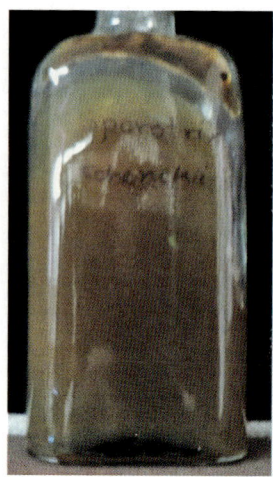

Fig. 6.26b: *Sporothrix schenckii* (reverse)

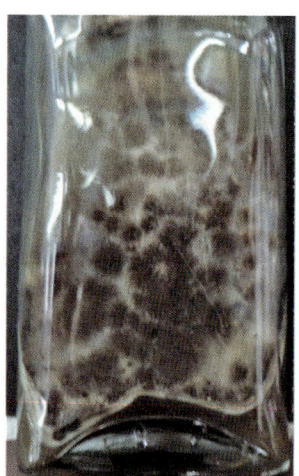

Fig. 6.26a: *Sporothrix schenckii* (close view)

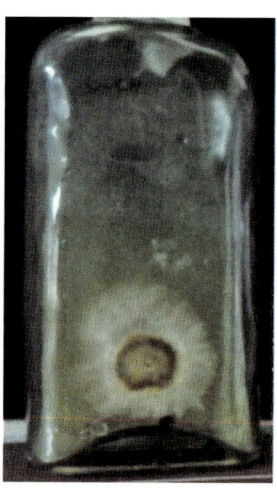

Fig. 6.27: *Microsporum gypseum*

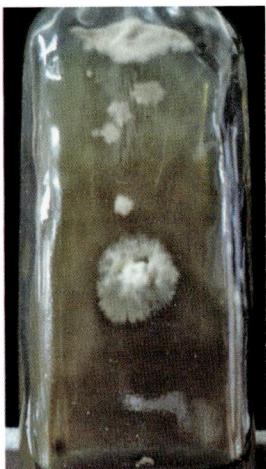

Fig. 6.28: *Microsporum gypseum*

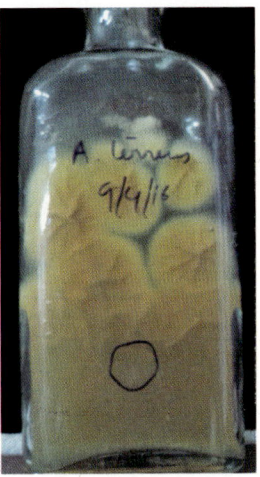

Fig. 6.29a: *Aspergillus terreus* (reverse)

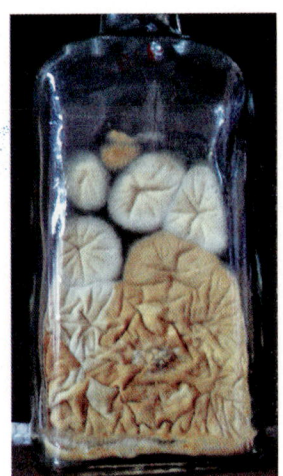

Fig. 6.29: *Aspergillus terreus*

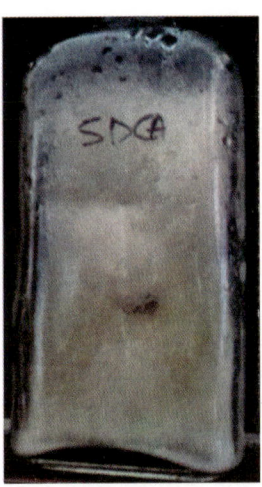

Fig. 6.30: *Lichtheimia corymbifera*

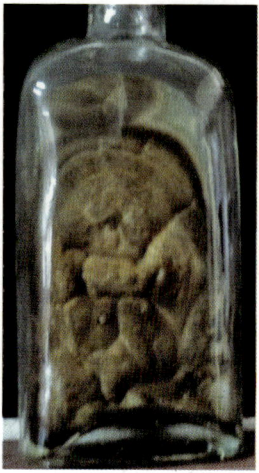

Fig. 6.31: *Curvularia geniculata*

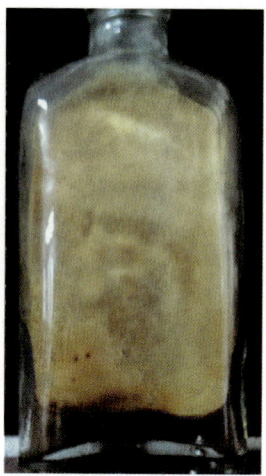

Fig. 6.32: *Paecilomyces lilacinous*

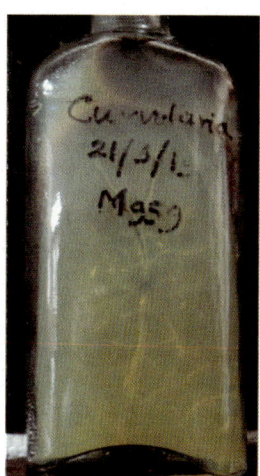

Fig. 6.31a: *Curvularia geniculata* (reverse)

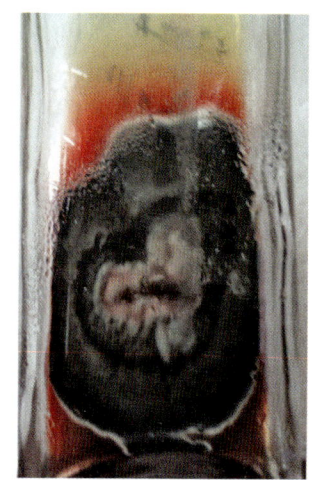

Fig. 6.33: *Penicillium marneffei*

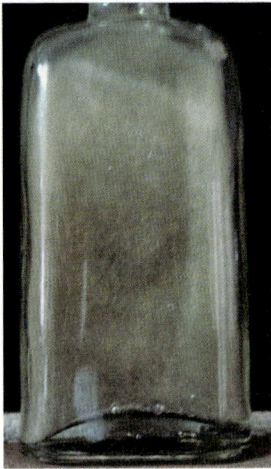

Fig. 6.34: *Rhizopus oryzae* (young culture)

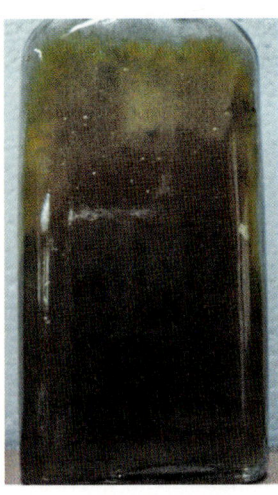

Fig. 6.34b: *Rhizopus oryzae* (reverse)

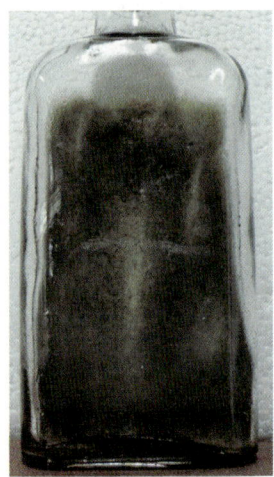

Fig. 6.34a: *Rhizopus oryzae* (old culture; obverse)

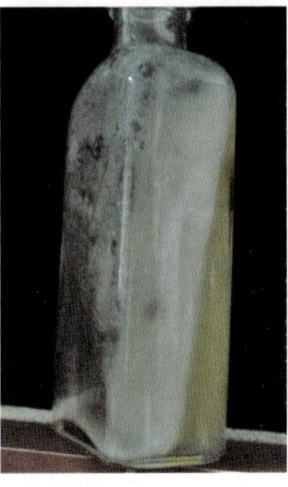

Fig. 6.35: *Mucor species* (side view showing aerial mycelia)

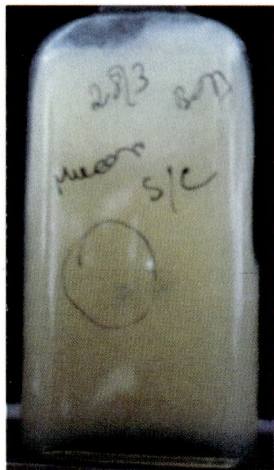

Fig. 6.35a: *Mucor species* (reverse)

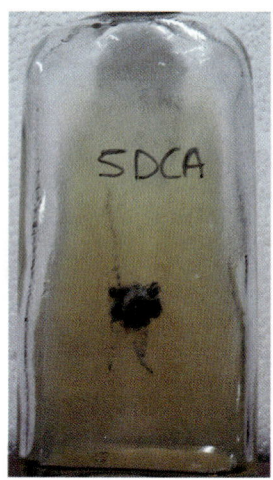

Fig. 6.36: *Cladophialophora carionii* (obverse)

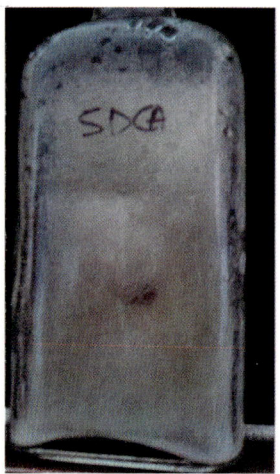

Fig. 6.35b: *Mucor species*

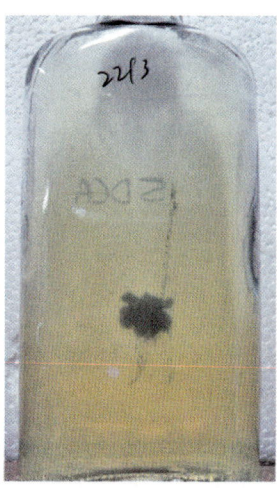

Fig. 6.36a: *Cladophialophora carionii* (reverse)

Index